The Yoga Anatomy Coloring Book

POSE by POSE

Learn the Anatomy and Enhance Your Practice

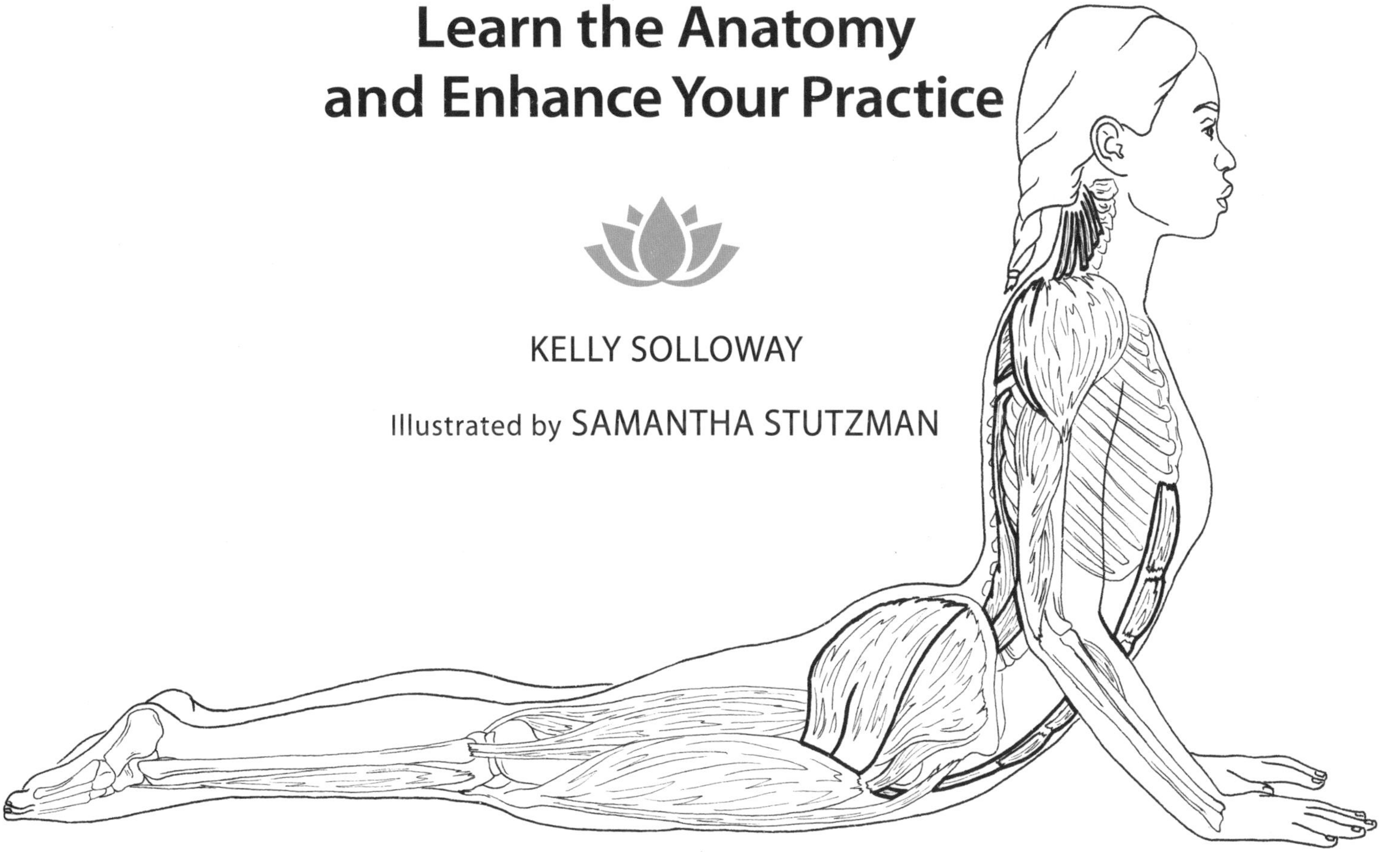

KELLY SOLLOWAY

Illustrated by SAMANTHA STUTZMAN

Get Creative 6

Get Creative 6
An imprint of Mixed Media Resources
19 West 21st Street
Suite 601, New York, NY 10010

Connect with us on Facebook at
facebook.com/getcreative6

Senior Editor
MICHELLE BREDESON

Art Director
IRENE LEDWITH

ISBN: 978-1-68462-013-5

Manufactured in China

3 5 7 9 10 8 6 4

First Edition

This book is dedicated to all you yoga nerds out there who love anatomy, and to those who are just starting to think that it's pretty cool to know what you're made of.—KS

Acknowledgments

This book would not have been possible if not for all the hard work done on my first book, *The Yoga Anatomy Coloring Book*, by all the wonderful people working at Mixed Media Resources. I want to thank Caroline Kilmer for the opportunity to write my first book and this one and her hard work to make them a reality. I also want to thank Michelle Bredeson, whose editing skills are unsurpassed; Irene Ledwith, for her creative genius in putting it all together; along with the rest of the folks I don't even know who made the first book and now this second one possible. Last, but not least, I want to thank Samantha Stutzman for her artistic skill and knowledge of anatomy in creating such beautiful illustrations. And for agreeing to work with me again.

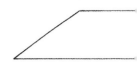

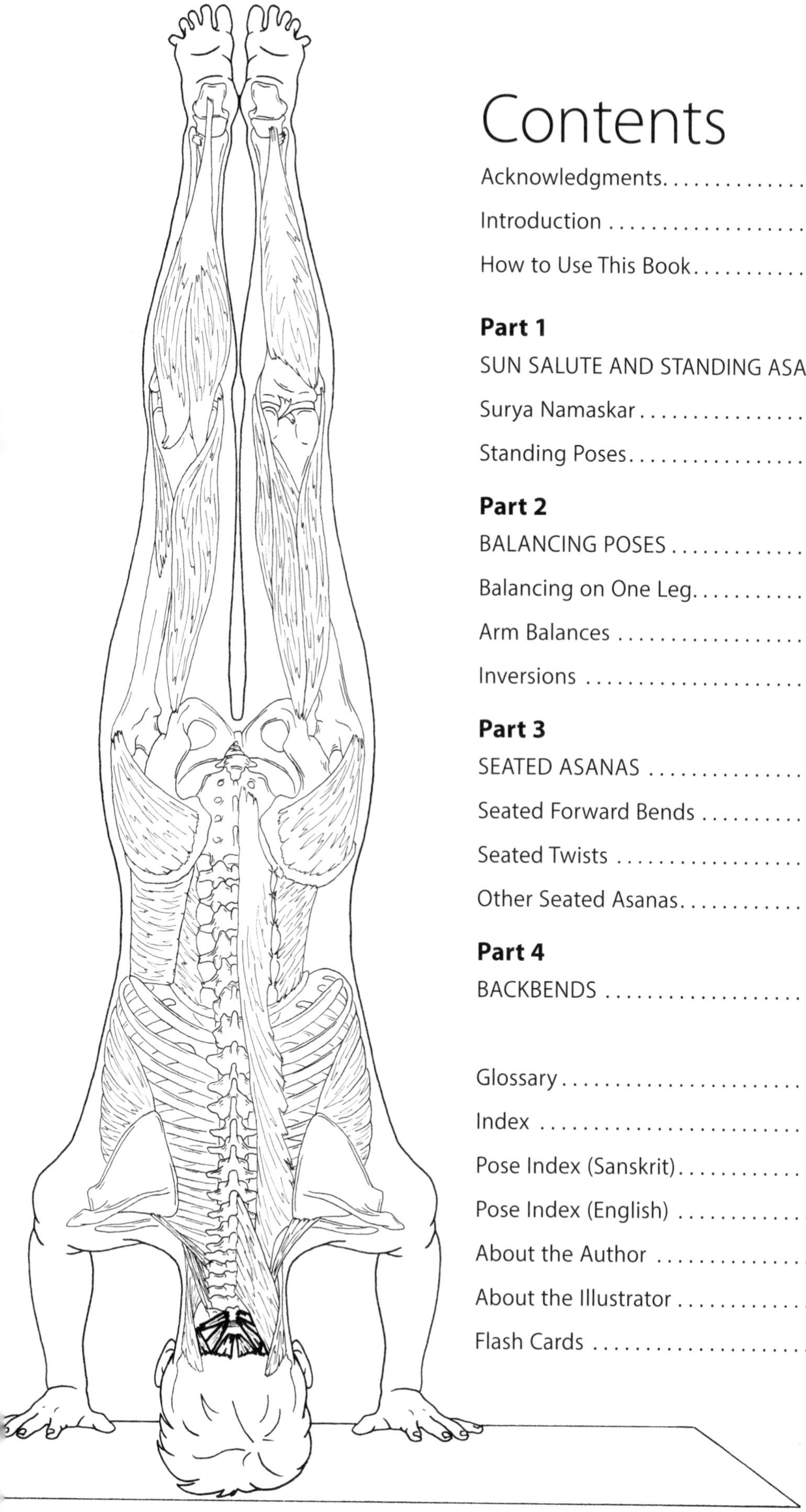

Contents

Acknowledgments. 2

Introduction 4

How to Use This Book. 6

Part 1

SUN SALUTE AND STANDING ASANAS. 8

Surya Namaskar 10

Standing Poses. 22

Part 2

BALANCING POSES 38

Balancing on One Leg. 40

Arm Balances 48

Inversions 60

Part 3

SEATED ASANAS 64

Seated Forward Bends 66

Seated Twists 80

Other Seated Asanas. 88

Part 4

BACKBENDS 102

Glossary 114

Index 117

Pose Index (Sanskrit). 119

Pose Index (English) 119

About the Author 120

About the Illustrator 120

Flash Cards 120

"The study of asana is not about mastering posture. It's about using posture to understand and transform yourself."

—B. K. S. Iyengar

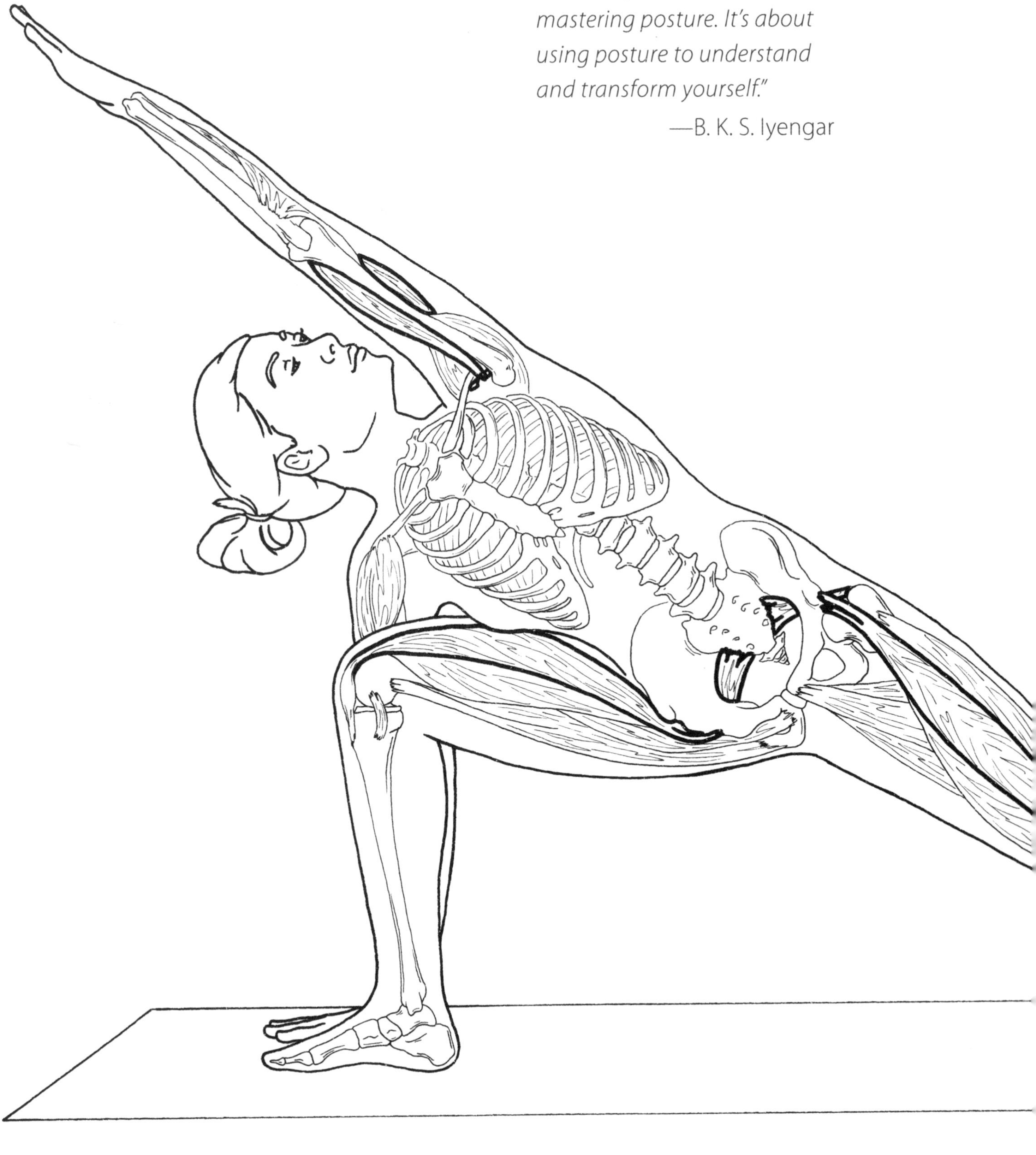

Introduction

I hope this book will provide a greater understanding of what your body is actually doing as you practice the yoga asanas (poses), anatomically speaking. It highlights which muscles need to be working for you and which muscles need to be stretching to achieve proper alignment in each asana. We will take it asana by asana and get more tuned in to what we're actually doing in the posture. We will cover how the big joints are moving and which muscles have to contract and lengthen to make this happen. If you have my first book, *The Yoga Anatomy Coloring Book,* you probably already have a good deal of anatomy under your belt. This book includes a glossary of anatomy terms; if you come across something unfamiliar, be sure to look it up.

Our bodies, though basically the same, are still unique. How we express an asana must take into account the body that is doing it. This explains why there are so many different styles of asana practice: Ashtanga, Iyengar, Kundalini, to name just a few. These teachers found a way of practicing the asanas that worked for the bodies they were in and, in turn, taught this to their students. And we are all very grateful for it. There are certain underlying principles, such as good alignment, keeping joints strong, keeping your ground, not hurting yourself, and paying attention, that should be adhered to, but beyond that, the asana should fit the body, not the other way around. As with all things involving humans, not everyone agrees on everything in yoga. I will give the best information I know on alignment and how to achieve the asana—what I feel the muscles, joints, and other anatomy should be doing, or not doing. But please keep in mind that some may disagree where that foot should be pointed, which muscles should be doing what, or where you should be gazing. You get the idea.

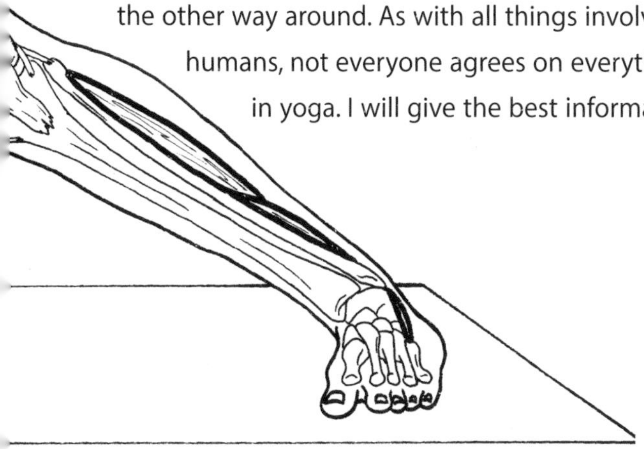

In every asana we do, we do it with our whole body. Some parts have to engage; some parts have to relax. Even if one part is doing nothing, being consciously aware of doing nothing is just as important, maybe more so, as doing something. That being said, it would be a fool's errand to try to "flesh out" what everything is doing in each asana, so we will be focusing more on what's really working and what's really stretching, while peppering in some of the smaller, less "famous" muscles to expand our repertoire of anatomy and add to your anatomy toolbox. Repetition is a good teacher; the bigger, stronger muscles will make many appearances.

Please remember: It is the present body doing the asana, not the ego, not the intellect, not the body you were in 10 or 50 years ago. Honor that. This is a celebration of what your body can do, not an act of frustration for what it can't do (yet). And don't get too hung up on any of the postures. They are just a way to get you to pay more attention.

Om shanti.

—Kelly

I would love to see how you color the poses. Feel free to share your work on Instagram: #yogaanatomycoloring

How to Use This Book

My first book, *The Yoga Anatomy Coloring Book*, is organized by anatomy, and the illustrations of yoga postures highlight the muscles and bones being described. This book takes a different approach and instead focuses on the critical anatomy that is engaged in each pose. The poses are organized by type—standing, balancing, seated, and backbends.

You can work your way through the book, reading about each posture and studying and coloring the anatomy, or you can skip to the asanas that interest you. The text for each pose describes a safe and correct way to practice the pose and the anatomy that makes it happen. Of course, many asanas have variations. I am describing the ones I have found to be most effective through years of practice and teaching.

There are many illustrations to color—please do! This will provide another layer of learning that can really help things stick. I think reading is great, but I believe that by actively "filling it in" you will develop a more intimate knowledge of how this body is put together. Once you have that, you can be more sensitive to what is happening in the body as you (and/or your students) are practicing the yoga asanas. Not only will your knowledge of the body grow, but you will have some great artwork to show for it.

At the back of the book, you'll find a detailed index, a glossary of anatomy terms used throughout, indexes of the yoga asanas in both English and Sanskrit, and perforated flash cards you can use to quiz yourself, study yoga anatomy on the go, and put the postures in sequences to customize your practice!

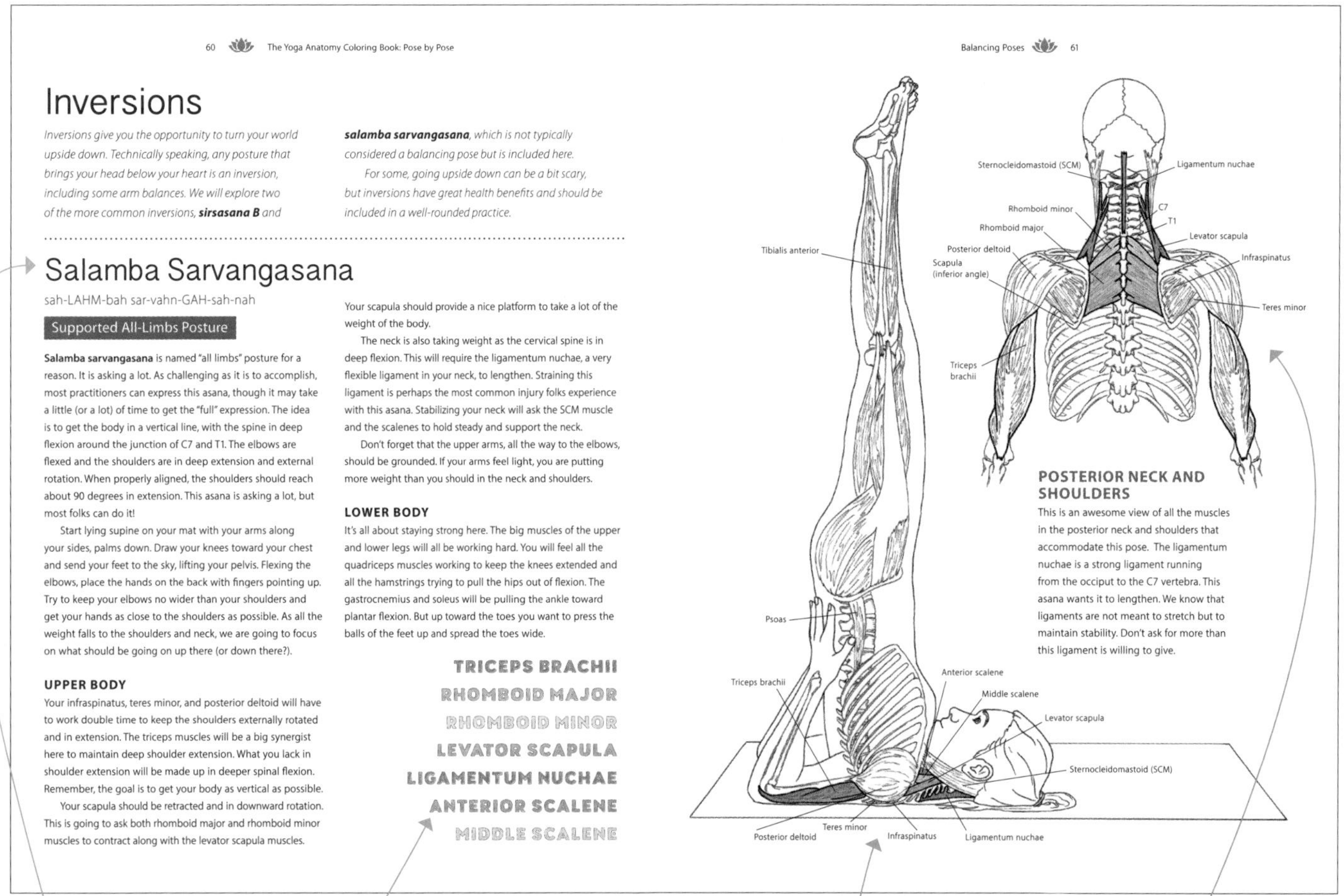
60 The Yoga Anatomy Coloring Book: Pose by Pose

Inversions

Inversions give you the opportunity to turn your world upside down. Technically speaking, any posture that brings your head below your heart is an inversion, including some arm balances. We will explore two of the more common inversions, ***sirsasana B*** *and* ***salamba sarvangasana****, which is not typically considered a balancing pose but is included here.*

For some, going upside down can be a bit scary, but inversions have great health benefits and should be included in a well-rounded practice.

Salamba Sarvangasana

sah-LAHM-bah sar-vahn-GAH-sah-nah

Supported All-Limbs Posture

Salamba sarvangasana is named "all limbs" posture for a reason. It is asking a lot. As challenging as it is to accomplish, most practitioners can express this asana, though it may take a little (or a lot) of time to get the "full" expression. The idea is to get the body in a vertical line, with the spine in deep flexion around the junction of C7 and T1. The elbows are flexed and the shoulders are in deep extension and external rotation. When properly aligned, the shoulders should reach about 90 degrees in extension. This asana is asking a lot, but most folks can do it!

Start lying supine on your mat with your arms along your sides, palms down. Draw your knees toward your chest and send your feet to the sky, lifting your pelvis. Flexing the elbows, place the hands on the back with fingers pointing up. Try to keep your elbows no wider than your shoulders and get your hands as close to the shoulders as possible. As all the weight falls to the shoulders and neck, we are going to focus on what should be going on up there (or down there?).

UPPER BODY

Your infraspinatus, teres minor, and posterior deltoid will have to work double time to keep the shoulders externally rotated and in extension. The triceps muscles will be a big synergist here to maintain deep shoulder extension. What you lack in shoulder extension will be made up in deeper spinal flexion. Remember, the goal is to get your body as vertical as possible.

Your scapula should be retracted and in downward rotation. This is going to ask both rhomboid major and rhomboid minor muscles to contract along with the levator scapula muscles. Your scapula should provide a nice platform to take a lot of the weight of the body.

The neck is also taking weight as the cervical spine is in deep flexion. This will require the ligamentum nuchae, a very flexible ligament in your neck, to lengthen. Straining this ligament is perhaps the most common injury folks experience with this asana. Stabilizing your neck will ask the SCM muscle and the scalenes to hold steady and support the neck.

Don't forget that the upper arms, all the way to the elbows, should be grounded. If your arms feel light, you are putting more weight than you should in the neck and shoulders.

LOWER BODY

It's all about staying strong here. The big muscles of the upper and lower legs will all be working hard. You will feel all the quadriceps muscles working to keep the knees extended and all the hamstrings trying to pull the hips out of flexion. The gastrocnemius and soleus will be pulling the ankle toward plantar flexion. But up toward the toes you want to press the balls of the feet up and spread the toes wide.

TRICEPS BRACHII
RHOMBOID MAJOR
RHOMBOID MINOR
LEVATOR SCAPULA
LIGAMENTUM NUCHAE
ANTERIOR SCALENE
MIDDLE SCALENE

Balancing Poses 61

POSTERIOR NECK AND SHOULDERS

This is an awesome view of all the muscles in the posterior neck and shoulders that accommodate this pose. The ligamentum nuchae is a strong ligament running from the occiput to the C7 vertebra. This asana wants it to lengthen. We know that ligaments are not meant to stretch but to maintain stability. Don't ask for more than this ligament is willing to give.

Pose Names
Sanskrit and English names and pronunciations of the Sanskrit names.

Labels to Color
The main terms that are presented in the text and shown in the pose and can be colored to strengthen the connection between the names and the anatomy.

Poses to Color
Detailed black-and-white drawings of key yoga poses that highlight the major anatomy at work in the posture.

Alternative Views
Additional illustrations provide a detailed look at important areas of the body or another view of the posture.

COLORING TIPS

- Colored pencils are readily available, easy to use, and won't bleed through the paper. If you don't have enough colors to use a different one for every label or anatomical feature, you can vary the pressure or layer colors to create new colors.
- Lighter colors are best because they won't obscure the texture of the muscles or the leaders that connect the labels and anatomy.
- The main muscles and bones featured in each pose are listed in type that can be colored. Color them the same as the anatomy in the illustration. This will help strengthen the connection between the muscle or bone and its name.
- When coloring the muscles, lighten up as you get closer to the bone. This will represent the tendon of the muscle.
- Color individual muscles in a group different shades of the same color. For example, there are four quadriceps muscles; if you color them four different blues, you will easily see and remember that they are separate but related.
- Some illustrations may feature bones and/or muscles that are not specifically mentioned in the text for that pose, and vice versa. You'll already be familiar with some from earlier postures, while you will add others to your repertoire as you read and color through the book. (Extra credit: Further test your knowledge by adding labels to muscles and bones that are shown but not labeled!)
- If you go out of the lines, don't worry; the body is messy like that anyway.
- There are more coloring tips throughout the book!

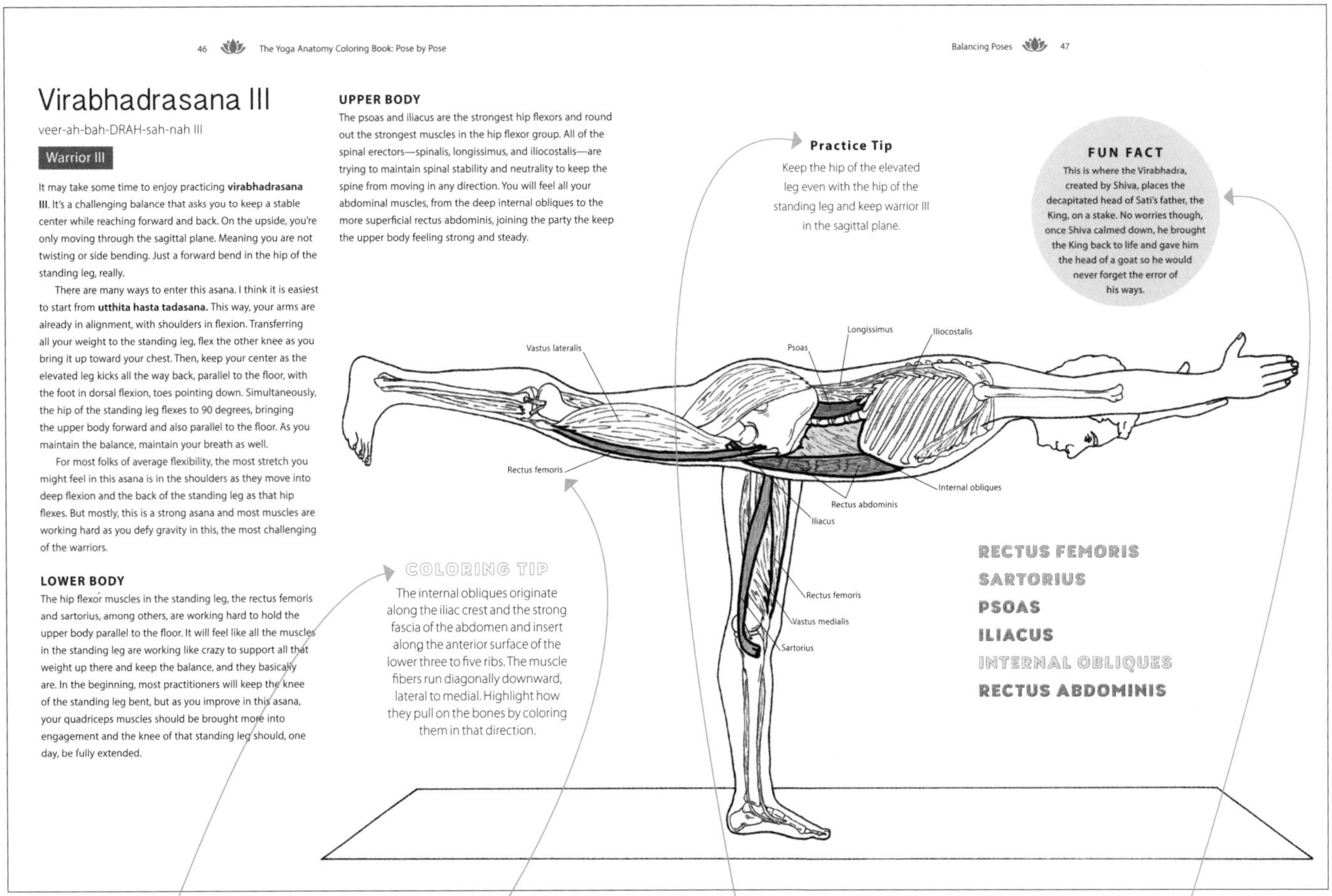
46 The Yoga Anatomy Coloring Book: Pose by Pose

Virabhadrasana III

veer-ah-bah-DRAH-sah-nah III

Warrior III

It may take some time to enjoy practicing **virabhadrasana III**. It's a challenging balance that asks you to keep a stable center while reaching forward and back. On the upside, you're only moving through the sagittal plane. Meaning you are not twisting or side bending. Just a forward bend in the hip of the standing leg, really.

There are many ways to enter this asana. I think it is easiest to start from **utthita hasta tadasana.** This way, your arms are already in alignment, with shoulders in flexion. Transferring all your weight to the standing leg, flex the other knee as you bring it up toward your chest. Then, keep your center as the elevated leg kicks all the way back, parallel to the floor, with the foot in dorsal flexion, toes pointing down. Simultaneously, the hip of the standing leg flexes to 90 degrees, bringing the upper body forward and also parallel to the floor. As you maintain the balance, maintain your breath as well.

For most folks of average flexibility, the most stretch you might feel in this asana is in the shoulders as they move into deep flexion and the back of the standing leg as that hip flexes. But mostly, this is a strong asana and most muscles are working hard as you defy gravity in this, the most challenging of the warriors.

LOWER BODY

The hip flexor muscles in the standing leg, the rectus femoris and sartorius, among others, are working hard to hold the upper body parallel to the floor. It will feel like all the muscles in the standing leg are working like crazy to support all that weight up there and keep the balance, and they basically are. In the beginning, most practitioners will keep the knee of the standing leg bent, but as you improve in this asana, your quadriceps muscles should be brought more into engagement and the knee of that standing leg should, one day, be fully extended.

UPPER BODY

The psoas and iliacus are the strongest hip flexors and round out the strongest muscles in the hip flexor group. All of the spinal erectors—spinalis, longissimus, and iliocostalis—are trying to maintain spinal stability and neutrality to keep the spine from moving in any direction. You will feel all your abdominal muscles, from the deep internal obliques to the more superficial rectus abdominis, joining the party the keep the upper body feeling strong and steady.

COLORING TIP

The internal obliques originate along the iliac crest and the strong fascia of the abdomen and insert along the anterior surface of the lower three to five ribs. The muscle fibers run diagonally downward, lateral to medial. Highlight how they pull on the bones by coloring them in that direction.

Practice Tip

Keep the hip of the elevated leg even with the hip of the standing leg and keep warrior III in the sagittal plane.

Balancing Poses 47

FUN FACT

This is where the Virabhadra, created by Shiva, places the decapitated head of Sati's father, the King, on a stake. No worries though, once Shiva calmed down, he brought the King back to life and gave him the head of a goat so he would never forget the error of his ways.

RECTUS FEMORIS
SARTORIUS
PSOAS
ILIACUS
INTERNAL OBLIQUES
RECTUS ABDOMINIS

Coloring Tips
Specific suggestions for making the most of coloring the anatomy are sprinkled throughout the book.

Identifying Labels
The names of the muscles and bones described in the accompanying text, as well as other key anatomy.

Practice Tips
Helpful hints enhance your yoga practice, help you avoid injury, and deepen the connection between the asana and the anatomy.

Fun Facts
Interesting trivia about anatomy or the stories behind the postures to break the ice in yoga class.

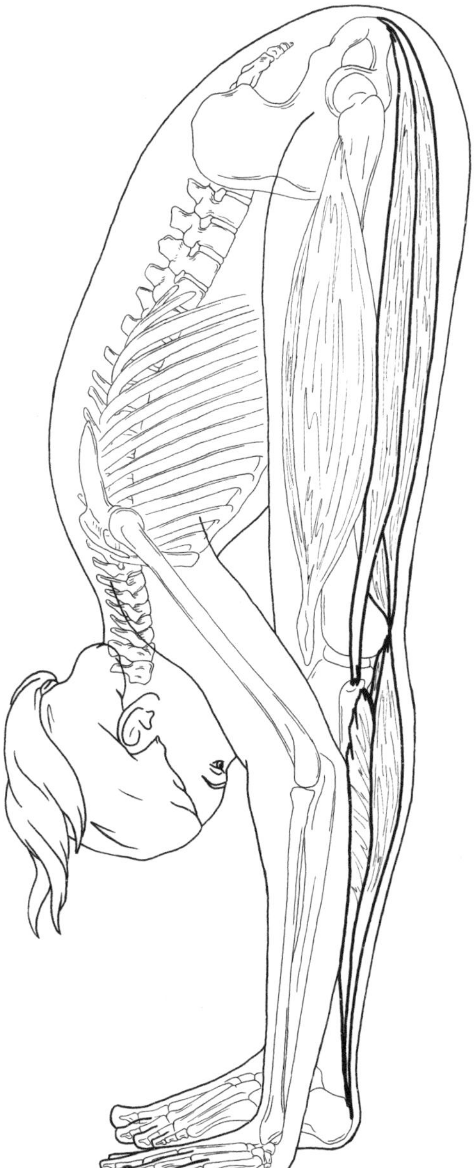

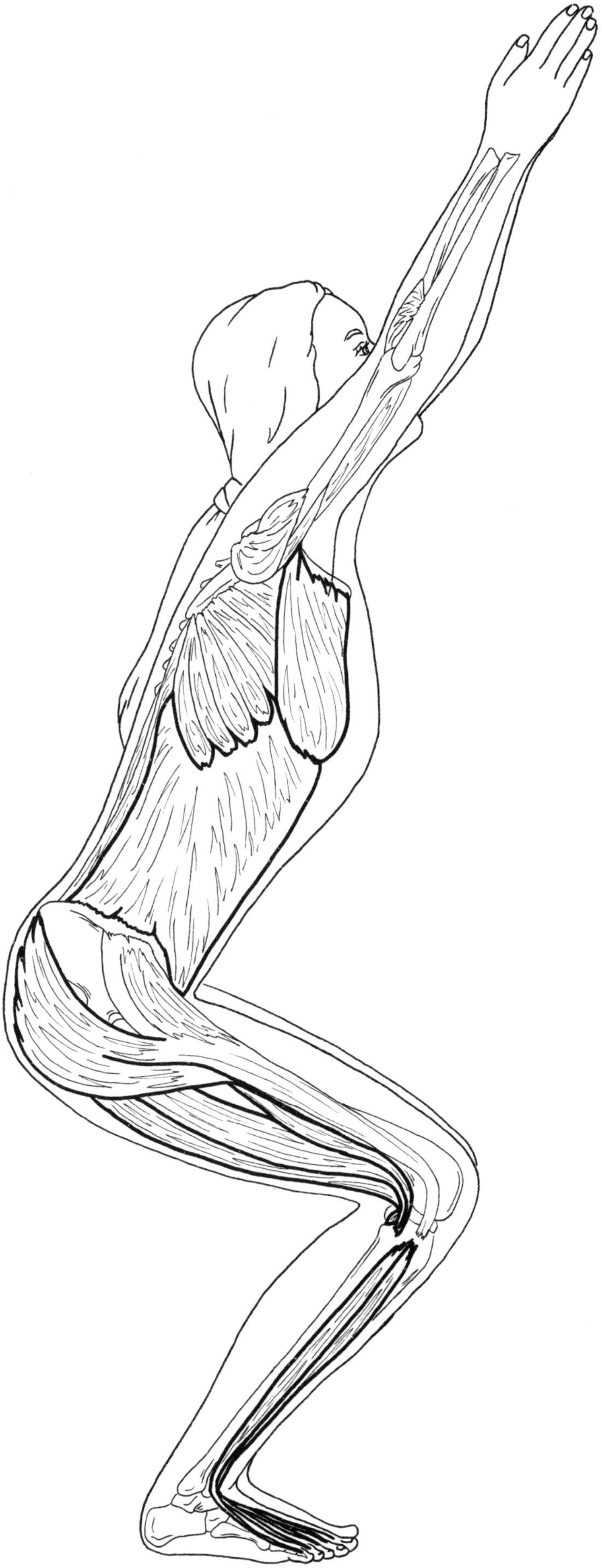

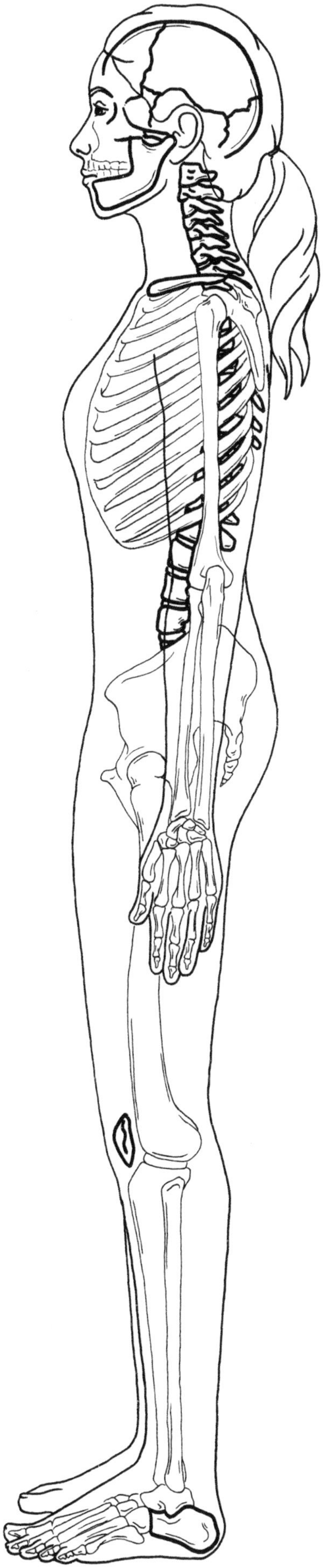

PART 1

Sun Salute and Standing Asanas

The sun salute, or surya namaskar, is the sequence many yogis use to begin their practice. It's a great way to warm up your muscles and joints. There are many variations on the sequence. The sun salute I share in this chapter is very basic and the one I use most often. Once you become familiar with it, feel free to try variations.

The sun salute includes two standing asanas, and a number of standing asanas round out this chapter. These are the poses most people begin with after surya namaskar. They require both feet to be grounded. Holding the asanas, as opposed to flowing through a sun salute, will give you more time to check in on your alignment and make sure everything is where you think it is! And that you are keeping a consistent, full, complete breath. Once you feel all your body parts are where you want them, make sure the breath is there as well.

Surya Namaskar

The sun salute, or surya namaskar, is the warm-up where you start for most traditions of yoga practice. There are many different styles of sun salutes. I have chosen a classical hatha yoga sun salute to explore here. Even within the classical hatha yoga traditions, there are variations on this. This is just my take. As you flow through surya namaskar, do your best to find the full expression of each asana in the time your breath will allow. Let the messages from your body reach your brain with no filter so you can make intelligent choices, not just in the pose, but always.

Tadasana

tah-DAH-sah-nah

Mountain

Tadasana is where the sun salute starts. Standing up straight sounds simple enough, but getting perfect alignment can be complex. Tadasana is asking you to arrange your bones so they line up with the force of gravity. In other words, finding the path of least resistance: neutrality. Tadasana does not mean just standing there waiting for what's next. In tadasana you are constantly making adjustments to find the perfect balance and relationship with gravity. When you first try to get proper alignment, it may not feel natural. That may be a sign that you have not been standing up straight and need to change some bad postural habits.

LOWER BODY

Tadasana starts with the feet getting grounded. Make certain you're evenly distributing the weight in the feet, right and left, front to back. All the phalanges (toes) should be pointing forward and relaxed. Toes are your first line of defense to make adjustments and find a better balance. Don't grip with your toes. Ground with the calcaneus (heel bone) and at the base of the big toe and the base of the pinky toe to create a tripod effect. I know some prefer to ground the inner and outer heel. For tadasana, go with the anatomy and ground the bone!

The patellas (kneecaps) should be pointing forward and the knees should be fully extended. Keep your knees lined up over your ankles.

The pelvis should be neutral. No anterior or posterior tilt. Your center should feel strong with the lower abdominal muscles working evenly with the lower back muscles. Be mindful to line up your acetabulofemoral (hip) joint over the knees. Lining up all the joints in the lower body and keeping the pelvis neutral and balanced will maintain the even distribution of weight in the feet.

UPPER BODY

The spine should be neutral. The five vertebrae (L1–L5) that make up the lumbar spine will naturally form a concave curve and arc toward the anterior body. There are a lot of big strong muscles in the lower back, so it is important not to let them overpower the opposing groups of muscles in the front. Be an equal opportunity employer for a strong, balanced center. The twelve vertebrae that make up the thoracic spine (T1–T12) are smaller than the lumbar vertebrae and naturally form a convex curve that arcs toward the posterior body. The thoracic spine is where all twelve pairs of your ribs attach posteriorly. The five vertebrae that make up your cervical spine (C1–C5) are smaller yet and form a concave curve.

Your shoulders are neutral. This means that the arms are relaxed, hanging along the side body, palms facing in. The distance between the shoulders across the chest and across the upper back should be even. Ideally, the clavicles should form a horizontal line across the upper chest. The shoulders should line up over the hips to keep even distribution of weight.

The skull should be evenly balanced on top of the cervical spine with the ears lining up over the shoulders and the mandible (lower jaw) parallel to the floor.

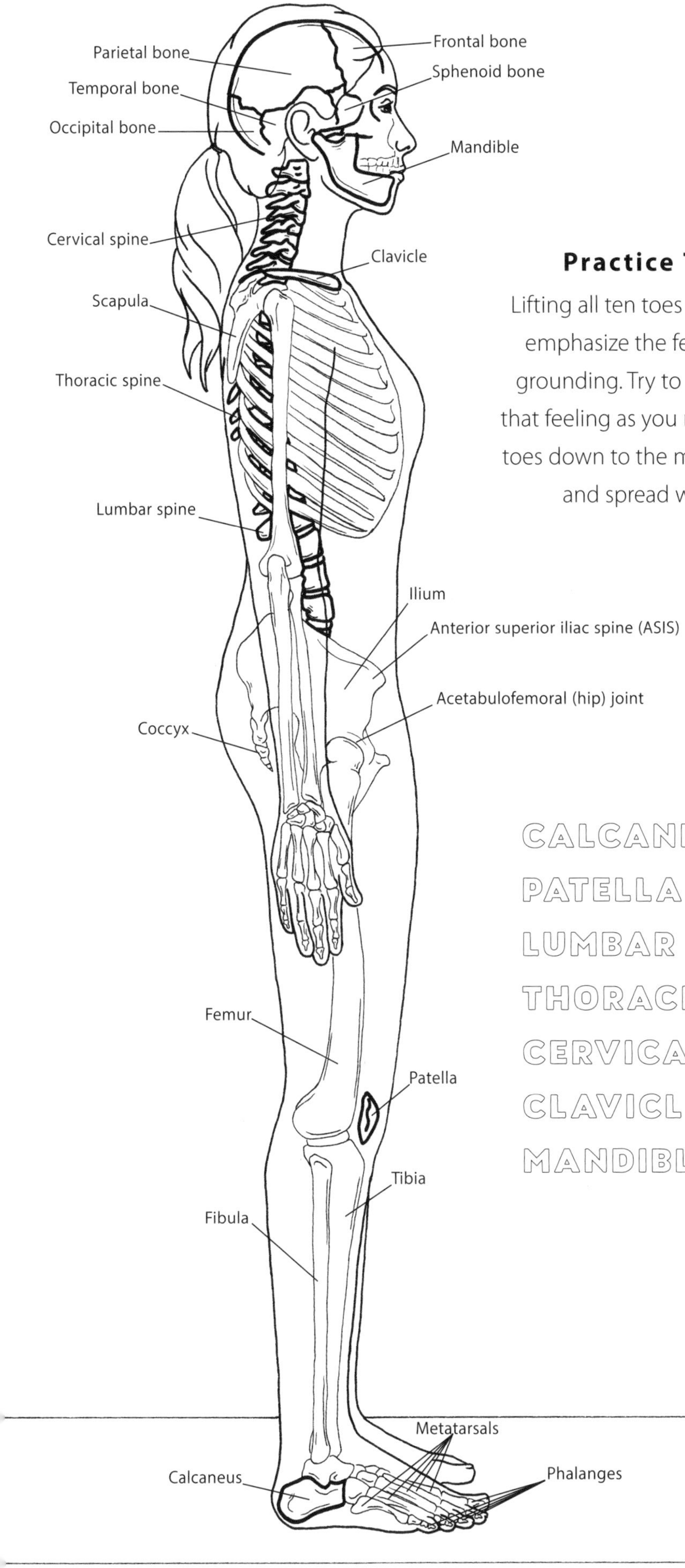

Practice Tip

Lifting all ten toes will really emphasize the feeling of grounding. Try to maintain that feeling as you release the toes down to the mat relaxed and spread wide.

CALCANEUS
PATELLA
LUMBAR SPINE
THORACIC SPINE
CERVICAL SPINE
CLAVICLE
MANDIBLE

THE SPINE

Your spine is an amazing piece of engineering. It protects the spinal cord and moves the body through all the planes of motion. The bones, called vertebrae, are divided into three sections: the cervical spine (labeled C1–C7), the thoracic spine (T1–T12), and the lumbar spine (L1–L5).

With this lateral view, you can see the natural curves and unique qualities of each section.

Lateral View

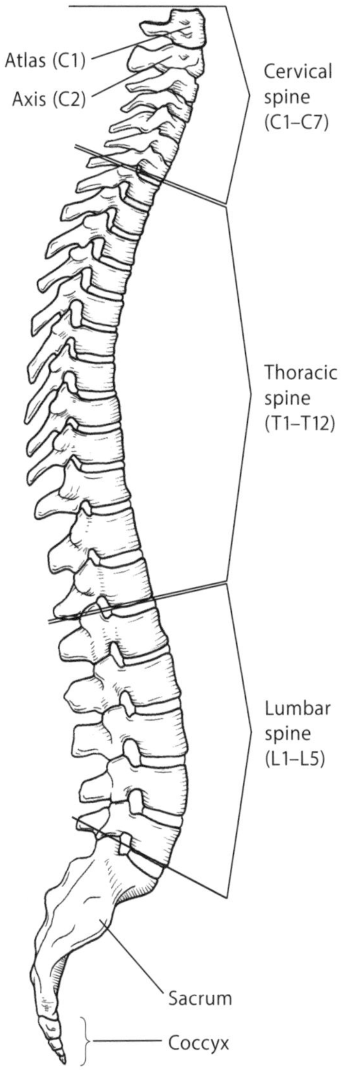

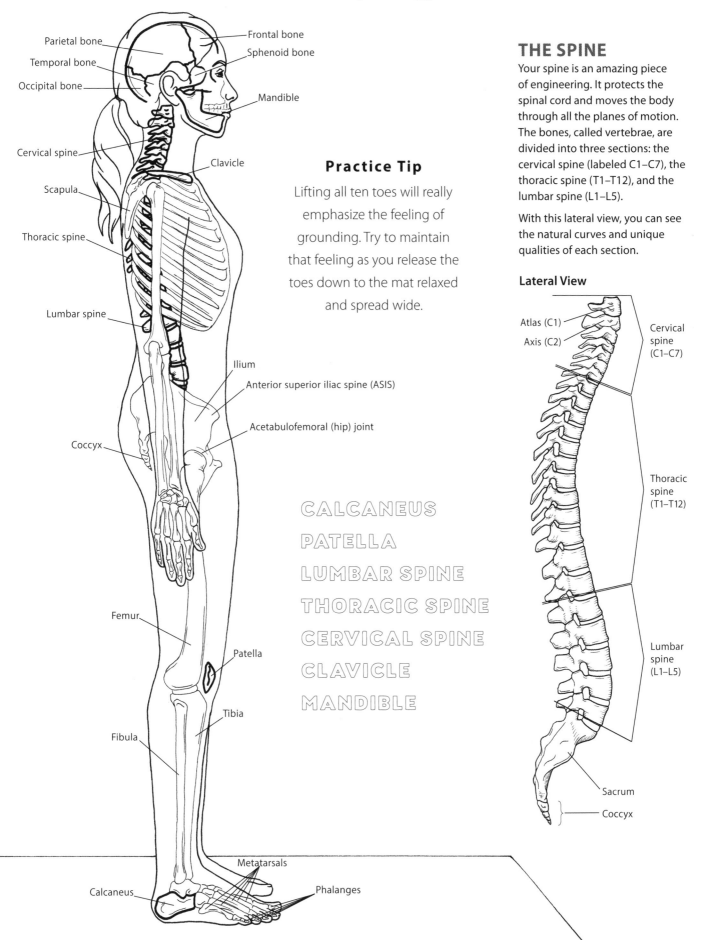

Uttanasana

OOT-tahn-AH-sah-nah

Intense Stretch Posture

Uttanasana is most commonly translated into English as "standing forward bend." Very descriptive for what it looks like, but the literal translation of "intense stretch posture" describes how this asana feels. It is an intense stretch for most all of the muscles along the posterior body.

Starting in **tadasana**, some folks will inhale and bring the arms up and over the head, and some will lean the whole body back toward a backbend; either way, you will exhale into **uttanasana**. Flex at the hips to bring the upper body as close to the legs as possible. Do not flex your spine to "help" with this. It's important to keep the spine as neutral as possible. Only in the full expression of this posture, with the upper body meeting the legs, should you allow for some flexion in the spine. The palms of the hands are down on the mat, along the lateral edges of the feet, fingers pointing forward. Until the hamstrings are long enough, you should modify the hand position and maybe flex the knees a little. Remember, this should feel like a nice deep stretch for the back of the legs; don't torture yourself.

LOWER BODY

It is the deep flexion in the hips and extension in the knees that give the back of the legs that deep stretch. Deep hip flexion requires your hip flexor muscles to pull the upper body toward the legs, taking the hips through their full range of motion through the sagittal plane. Deep hip flexion will lengthen all three of your hamstring muscles: biceps femoris, semimembranosus, and semitendinosus. All three of these muscles originate at the ischial tuberosity. As you flex the hips you are pulling the origin site of these muscles (i.e. the ischial tuberosities) away from the insertion sites at the tibia for the semimembranosus and semitendinosus and the fibula for the biceps femoris muscle. Since your hip flexors are so strong, be careful they don't overpower the asana and cause any of the hamstring tendons to strain, or even worse, tear.

All four of your quadriceps muscles will be working hard here to keep the knees in extension. Whether you can keep the knees in full extension, or require a little flexion to accommodate the length of the hamstrings, the knees should always feel strong and stable.

Some folks may feel the stretch in the lower leg more than in the hamstrings. The biggest muscles you will feel lengthening here are the gastrocnemius and soleus muscles. The smaller, and sometimes overlooked, plantaris muscle will also get a stretch. The plantaris muscle originates on the medial condyle of the femur, and though it is a small muscle, with its belly located in the posterior compartment of the knee, it has one of the longest tendons in the body and inserts all the way down at the calcaneus.

UPPER BODY

I think the most important thing in the upper body is what you're not doing. You are not flexing at the spine; rather the spine should remain neutral until you just run out of room. Too often folks bend at the waist and pull on the lower back; don't do that, it can cause your back to hurt. Also, you are not extending your neck to look forward. The cervical spine should be relaxed, and your gaze should be looking back. If you are flexible enough to get your hands to the floor, your wrists will be in extension, keeping your phalanges (fingers) pointing forward. If your hamstrings are really long and your elbows flex, bend them straight back, no wider than your shoulders.

Practice Tip

Bend your knees if you feel any strain in the back of the legs. Since the biggest muscles in the posterior leg cross over the knee joint, flexing at the knees will give the tendons some slack so you can keep the stretch in the bellies of the muscles, where you want it. Remember: your knees should bend the same direction as the toes, which is straight ahead, and should always feel strong and aligned.

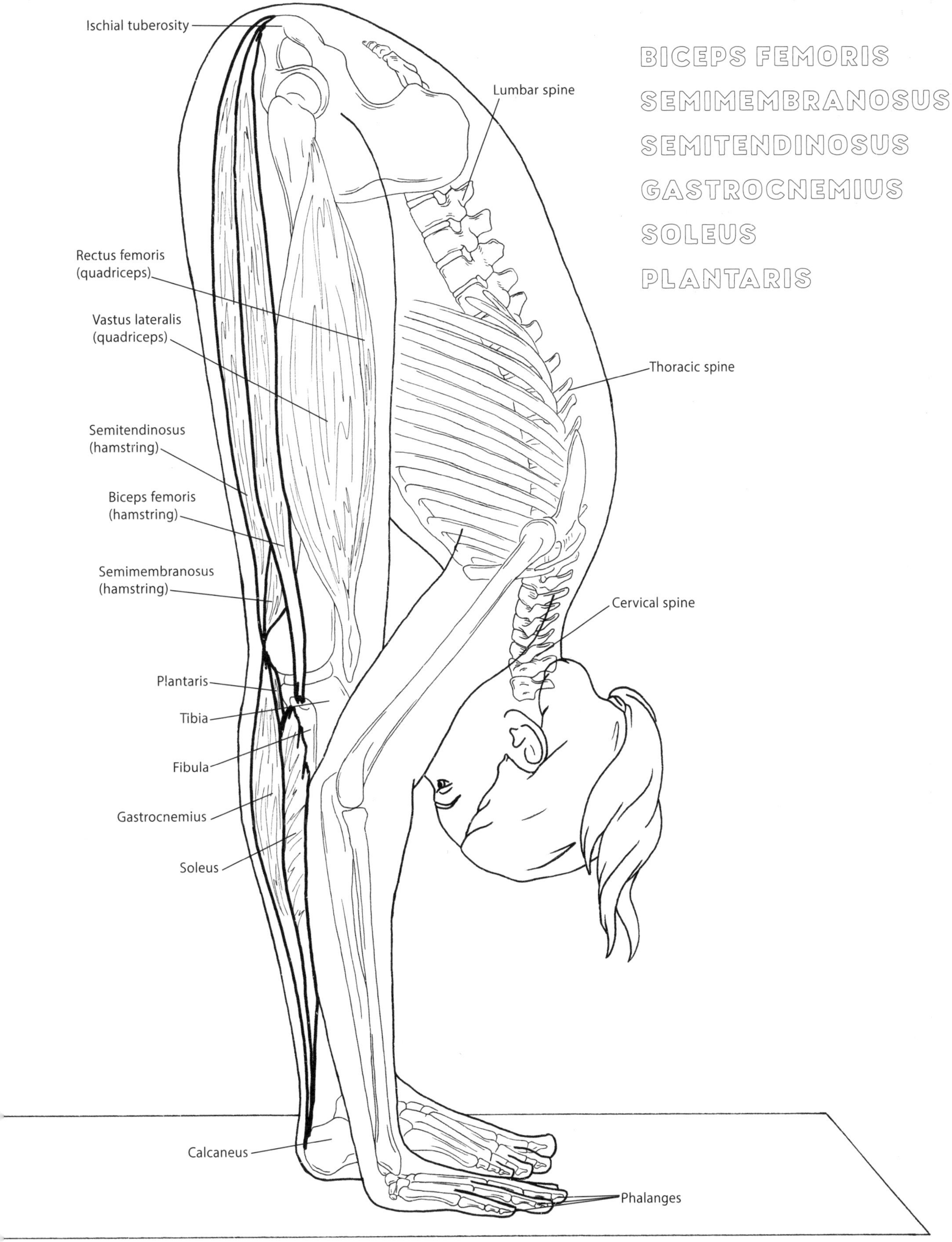
Ischial tuberosity
Lumbar spine
BICEPS FEMORIS
SEMIMEMBRANOSUS
SEMITENDINOSUS
GASTROCNEMIUS
SOLEUS
PLANTARIS
Rectus femoris (quadriceps)
Vastus lateralis (quadriceps)
Thoracic spine
Semitendinosus (hamstring)
Biceps femoris (hamstring)
Semimembranosus (hamstring)
Cervical spine
Plantaris
Tibia
Fibula
Gastrocnemius
Soleus
Calcaneus
Phalanges

Anjaneyasana

ahn-jahn-ay-AH-sah-nah

Low Lunge

Anjaneyasana is a great hip opener that most everyone can do. It can be modified and propped as necessary to relieve weight in the knee of the back leg and/or to keep the heart lifted. And anjaneyasana wants you to raise your heart high. It does have a very devotional quality to it. The strength, balance, and flexibility required for this posture is available to most, and the benefits of this asana should not be missed.

As surya namaskar progresses and you find yourself at the end of your exhale and in the deepest **uttanasana** you can find, inhale and step a foot all the way back. Gently bring that knee down to the mat. It is a personal choice to either tuck the back toes or keep them pointing back. Go where you feel more grounded. The front knee is flexed and parked right over the ankle. Keep the knee pointing forward, the same direction as the toes. The knee and ankle joints of both legs should stay lined up with the hips. The pelvis should move toward posterior tilt as you lift out of your lower back and raise your heart, bringing the spine into extension. Most commonly, the hands will reach for the sky and your gaze will be up, but feel free to play with this.

LOWER BODY

The acetabulofemoral (hip) joint of the front leg is in deep flexion. This is going to ask the gluteus maximus on that side to stretch. The hip joint of the back leg is in deep extension, which needs your hip flexors—primarily the iliacus, psoas, rectus femoris, and sartorius—to stretch. As you are trying to keep your pelvis in a posterior tilt, you should feel the rectus abdominis and external oblique muscles working to pull the anterior pelvis up, while the gluteus maximus and hamstring muscles work posteriorly to pull the pelvis in a downward motion. Some folks describe this as "tucking the hips" or "scooping the hips."

The iliotibial (IT) band will be working here to stabilize the front knee and keep it properly aligned. Try to keep the tibia and fibula, the two bones that make up your lower leg, perpendicular to the ground.

The ankle in the front foot will be in slight dorsal flexion, while the ankle in the back leg will be in deep plantar flexion if you keep the toes pointing back or in deep dorsal flexion if you choose to keep the toes tucked.

UPPER BODY

The spine should be in extension, but not at the expense of the posterior tilt of the pelvis. Lifting the arms high brings the shoulders into flexion, which will ask the anterior deltoid, upper fibers of the pectoralis major, biceps brachii, and coracobrachialis muscles to get working and keep those arms lifted high.

Practice Tip

If there is too much pressure on the back knee, place a soft blanket or towel under it. As you increase the range of motion in your hips, particularly when it comes to extension in the back leg, the pressure on the knee will lessen.

FUN FACT

This asana is named after Anjaneya, who later became the mighty warrior we know today as Hanuman. Legend has it this posture depicts Hanuman's contemplation prior to leaping over the sea to find the kidnapped princess Sita.

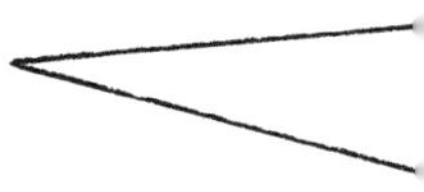

GLUTEUS MAXIMUS
ILIACUS
PSOAS
SARTORIUS
RECTUS ABDOMINIS
EXTERNAL OBLIQUE
ILIOTIBIAL (IT) BAND
ANTERIOR DELTOID
PECTORALIS MAJOR (UPPER FIBERS)
BICEPS BRACHII
CORACOBRACHIALIS

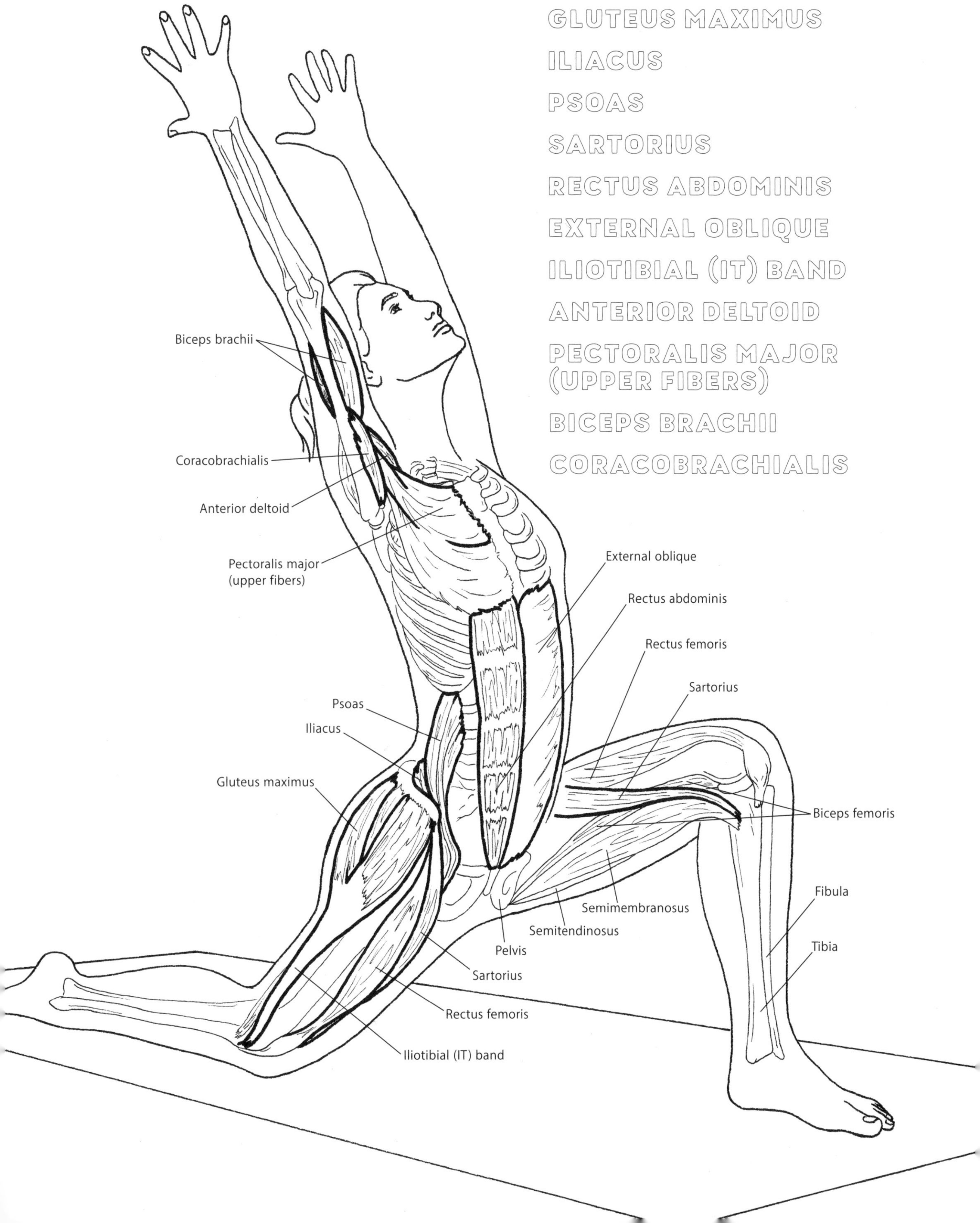

Ashtangasana

ahsh-tahn-GAH-sah-nah

Eight-Limbs Posture

The "eight limbs" or "parts" here refer not to the eight limbs of yoga philosophy, but to actual body parts: the two feet, two knees, two hands, chest, and chin that are grounding as you hold this asana. **Ashtangasana** is most often encountered during a classical hatha yoga sun salute or sometimes in place of a **chaturanga** (yoga "push-up") as part of a vinyasa sequence. But make no mistake, this is very different from chaturanga. **Ashtangasana** is doable for most folks. It is the degree of spinal extension that matters here. Don't ask for too much too soon.

After you complete your inhale in **anjaneyasana** (low lunge), exhale and step your front foot back toward a plank. Keeping the heels lifted, bend the knees down to the mat, then bring your chest and chin down to rest on the mat as well. The pelvis, more specifically the sit bones, or the ischial tuberosities, should be as high as possible. The elbows should be flexed and hugging the side body. The closer the chest is to your knees is what determines how deep you take this posture. So if you can control that, which you can, this asana is doable. As your spinal extension deepens and shoulder extension improves, you will be able to take this posture deeper. If you can't get your chest and chin down at first, keep coming forward with your chest until you touch down.

LOWER BODY

The lower body is held in place by gravity in **ashtangasana** and none of the joints are taken to such a deep range of motion so you may not feel that deep a stretch. The hips and knees are in flexion, but not so much. The feet are in deep dorsal flexion, but since the knees are also flexed, there may still be lengthening of the muscles in the lower leg. And, even though gravity is working for you, there is still strong engagement required in the muscles of the lower body to maintain this asana. The attention here is to keep proper alignment with the ankles and knees hip-distance apart.

UPPER BODY

It is here that you will feel most of the work being done. The spine is in deep extension. The strongest extensors of the spine are a group of muscles called the spinal erectors, or erector spinae. This group consists of three smaller groups of muscles. The spinalis muscle lies closest to the spine and is the smallest of the erector spinae. It is divided into the spinalis thoracis, which runs along the thoracic spine, and the spinalis cervicis, which runs along the cervical spine. Just lateral to the spinalis is the longissimus muscle. As the name implies, it is a long muscle that runs the entire length of the spine. The iliocostalis muscles is the most lateral of the group with origin and insertion sites along all twelve pairs of ribs. Acting together, these are the strongest backbending muscles you have, and you will be using them.

The deeper the spinal extension, the deeper the shoulder extension, so you will need to negotiate this. As your shoulders go into deeper and deeper extension, it will ask for more and more length from your anterior deltoid, biceps brachii, and coracobrachialis muscles along with the upper fibers of the pectoralis major muscle. You're working with a lot of strong muscles here, so be careful that the strong muscles of the back don't overpower the shoulders.

ANTERIOR DELTOID
SPINALIS
LONGISSIMUS
ILIOCOSTALIS
BICEPS BRACHII
PECTORALIS MAJOR

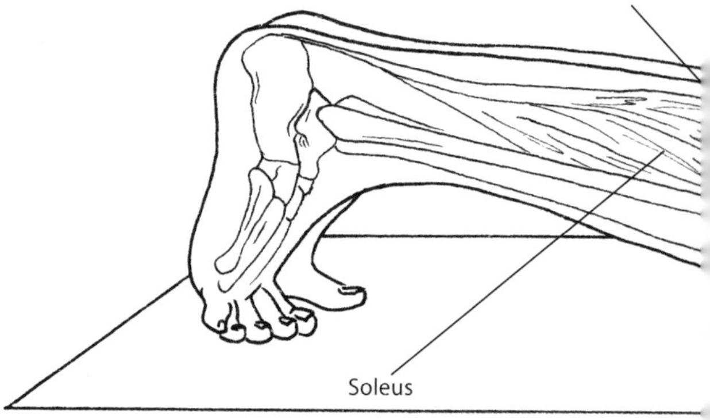

THE SPINAL ERECTORS

Here is a beautiful view of the spinal erectors—the spinalis thoracis, spinalis cervicis, longissimus, and iliocostalis—in their individual glory. Bring them together and you have a heck of a lot of power running from your sacrum all the way up to your occiput. Use all that strength wisely.

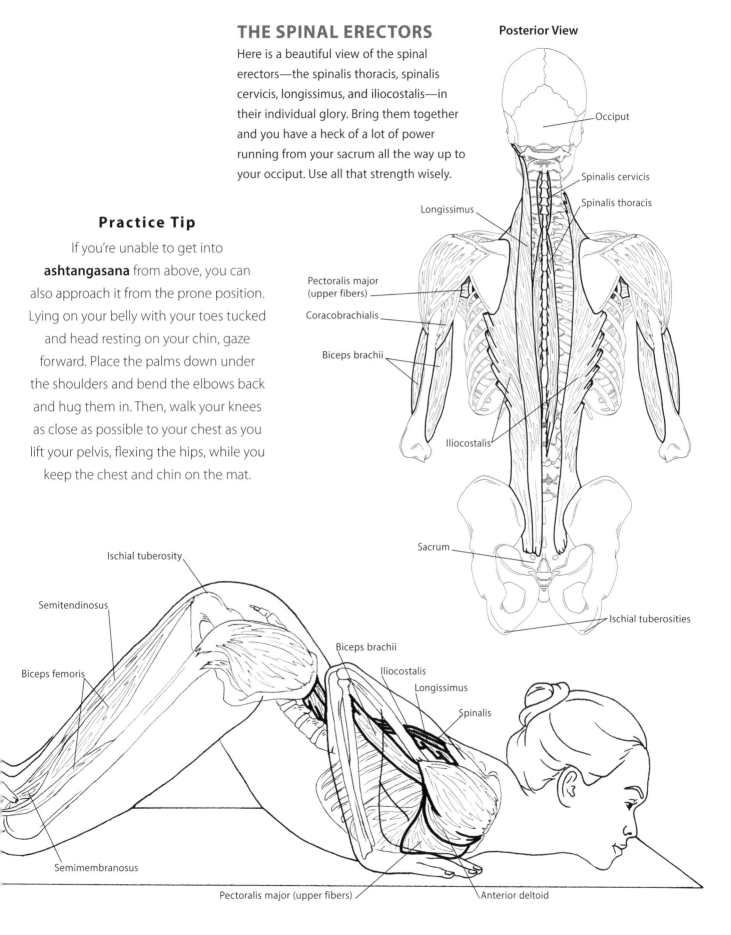

Posterior View

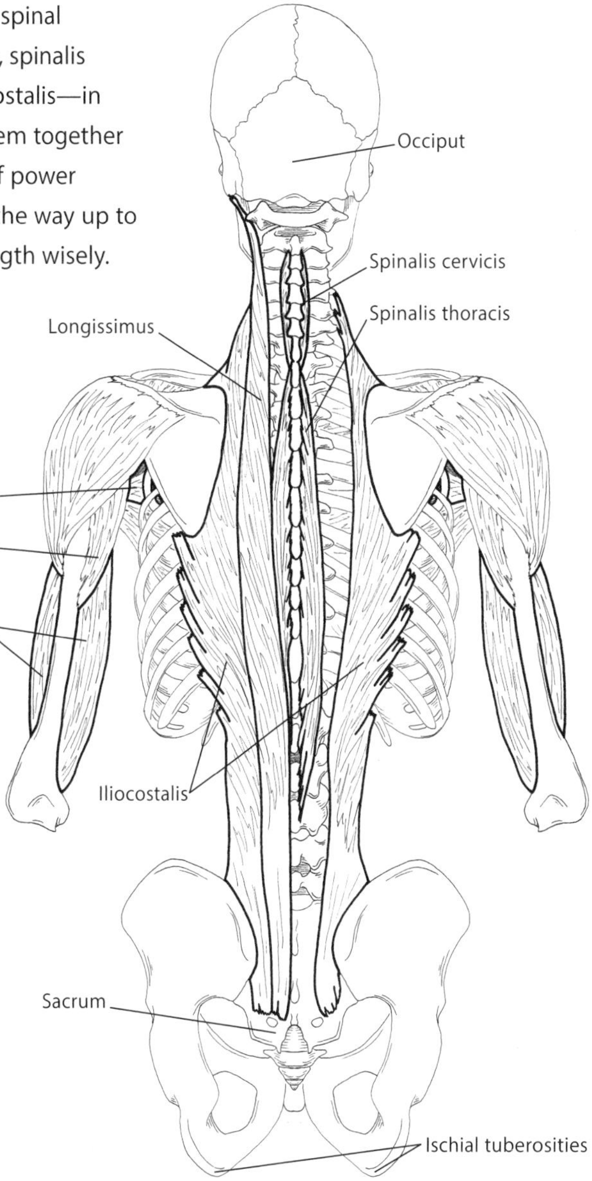

Practice Tip

If you're unable to get into **ashtangasana** from above, you can also approach it from the prone position. Lying on your belly with your toes tucked and head resting on your chin, gaze forward. Place the palms down under the shoulders and bend the elbows back and hug them in. Then, walk your knees as close as possible to your chest as you lift your pelvis, flexing the hips, while you keep the chest and chin on the mat.

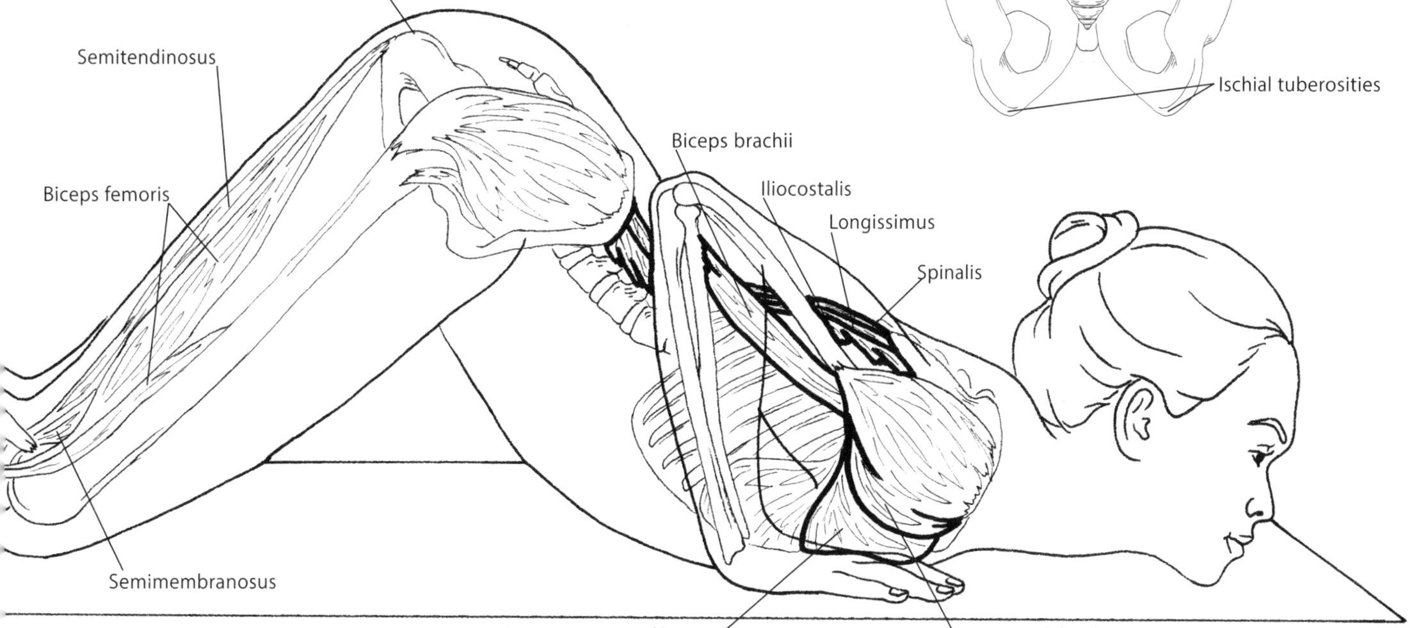

Bhujangasana

boo-jun-GAH-sah-nah

Cobra

Bhujangasana is a basic and foundational backbending posture. It will help to start working just about all of the muscles along the posterior body. And, since you have a lot of surface area to ground in this posture, that means you have just as much opportunity to lift. Take advantage of it!

Following the classical hatha yoga tradition of surya namaskar, you would enter **bhujangasana** from **ashtangasana**. Inhale as you transition the ankles to plantar flexion and extend the knees. As the pelvis moves forward, establish a deep posterior tilt and bring the pelvis to the mat. You should be grounding from the pelvis to the toes. The scapula moves toward upward rotation (that's the feeling of your scapula coming up and under the heart and lungs, drawing the shoulders down and lifting the heart center) and the shoulder (glenohumeral joint) moves toward external rotation as the spine goes into deep extension. The elbows should move toward extension and kept shoulder-distance apart. Don't let the elbows move away from the body; this can put your shoulders in a more vulnerable position.

LOWER BODY

The pelvis should be in the full range of motion of posterior tilt. This is the feeling of the spine of the ilium, the most anterior of the pelvic bones, being pulled back as the coccyx, or tailbone, pulls anteriorly. The hips will be in extension and internal rotation. The gluteus maximus is the strongest muscle in the body and the strongest to perform both posterior pelvic tilt and hip extension. The hamstrings will all be working hard here for both of these actions as well. The external obliques and lower portion of the rectus abdominis muscles will be engaged to maintain the posterior pelvic tilt. The gluteus medius and minimus will also be working pretty hard here to maintain internal rotation in the hips. So all your glutes will have the opportunity to strengthen here.

All four quadriceps muscles will be engaged to keep the knees fully extended; however, rectus femoris, along with the rest of the hip flexors, will get a stretch as the hips move toward deep extension. The strongest of the hip flexor group is the psoas muscle and its partner, iliacus; they are so close, some just refer to them as the iliopsoas.

The ankles will be in deep plantar flexion. This will give the tibialis anterior muscles, the strongest muscles of the anterior lower leg, a deep stretch.

UPPER BODY

Primarily, **bhujangasana** is a backbend, or in technical terms, a deep spinal extension. The strongest spinal extensors, the spinal erectors, will all be working hard here. They will get a lot of help from a deeper group of muscles known as the transversospinalis group. Like the spinal erectors, they consist of three groups of muscles; the multifidi muscles are the biggest and most superficial of the group. They originate at the sacrum and transverse processes of the spine and run superiorly, inserting at the spinous processes a few vertebrae above the origin site all the way up to the cervical spine. The rotatores muscles are deep to the multifidi and originate a little higher at the transverse processes of the lumbar spine. They insert directly at the next superior spinous process. The smallest of the group, the semispinalis capitis, originates even higher, at the transverse processes of the thoracic spine, and inserts at the occipital bone.

Keeping your heart lifted will require the scapula to be in upward rotation and the glenohumeral joint in external rotation. Pulling the scapula inferiorly and then tilting the inferior angle of the scapula anteriorly and superiorly (forward and up) will work both the upper and lower fibers of the trapezius muscle. It is the posterior deltoid, infraspinatus, and teres minor muscles that will hold the shoulders in external rotation.

The triceps muscles will be in eccentric contraction as you try to fully extend the elbows and resist gravity, while the pronator teres muscles helps to keep the forearm in pronation. Keep your elbows feeling strong here and hugged with muscle.

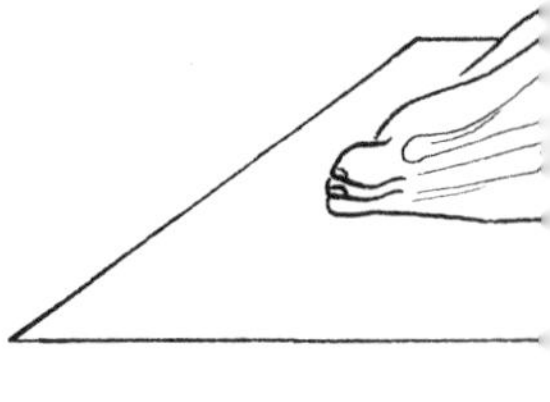

THE TRANSVERSOSPINALIS MUSCLES

These muscles, which include the multifidi, rotatores, and semispinalis capitis muscles, act directly on the vertebrae. Keeping these muscles strong helps maintain the spaces between the vertebrae, which gives the discs between the vertebrae all the space they need to function properly.

GLUTEUS MAXIMUS
EXTERNAL OBLIQUE
RECTUS ABDOMINIS
PSOAS
ILIACUS
MULTIFIDI
ROTATORES
SEMISPINALIS CAPITIS
POSTERIOR DELTOID
INFRASPINATUS
TERES MINOR

Posterior View

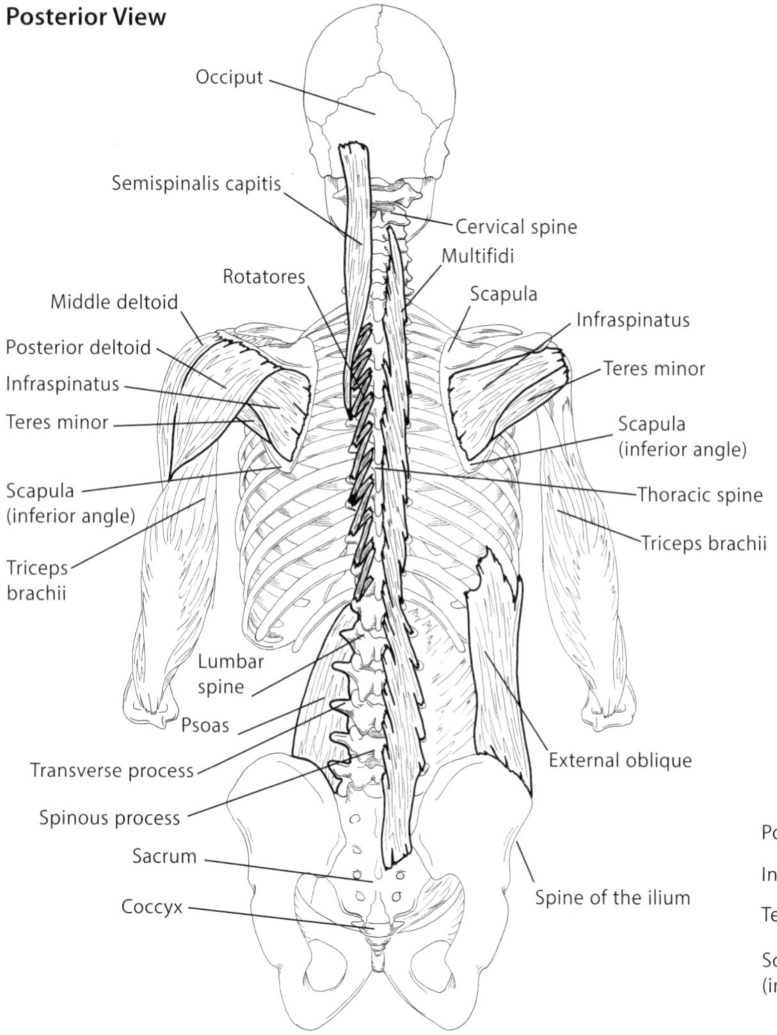

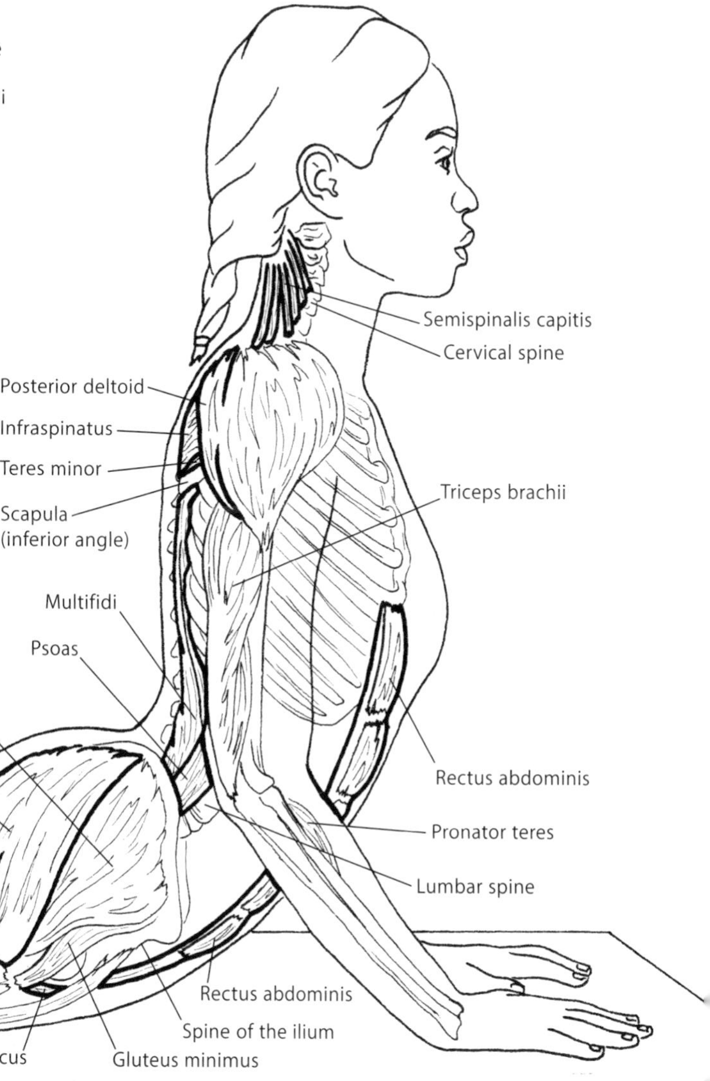
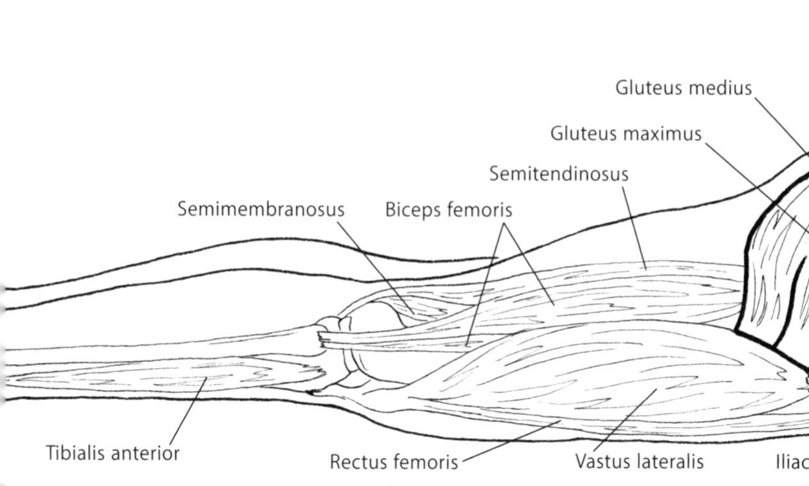

Adho Mukha Svanasana

AH-doh MOO-kah shvah-NAH-sah-nah

Downward-Facing Dog

Adho mukha svanasana today is ubiquitous with hatha yoga practice. Most people who have never practiced yoga are probably aware that downward-facing dog is something that yogis do. And they're right. This is a posture not to be missed. It will strengthen and lengthen the biggest, strongest muscles in the body. You should include this in your practice, a lot.

As you move through the sun salute, **bhujangasana** will lead you to **adho mukha svanasana**. If possible, roll over your toes to move from plantar flexion to dorsal flexion; otherwise, just flip your feet. Lifting the pelvis up, the hips will move into flexion and the spine should move to neutral. The arms and legs are fully extended and the knees and elbows should feel strong. The feet should be about hip-distance apart and the hands about shoulder-distance apart. All the phalanges should be spread wide and the weight as evenly distributed as possible between the hands and the feet. Remember, you always ground with what is on the ground!

LOWER BODY

With your hips in flexion, the knees fully extended, and the ankles in dorsal flexion, all the muscles along the posterior leg are going to get a deep stretch. Perhaps the deepest stretch is felt in the hamstring muscles. All three hamstring muscles—biceps femoris, semimembranosus, and semitendinosus—originate at the ischial tuberosities. (The biceps femoris, as the name suggests, has a second, shorter head that originates along the posterior femur.) You do not want to feel the stretch of any muscle at the origin site. As the hamstrings make their way down the posterior upper leg, you get to the bellies of the muscles, and that's where you want to feel the stretch. Too often I hear of strains, and worse, tears, at the origin site of the hamstring muscles. Don't let your ego hurt your body.

As your heels reach for the earth, the gastrocnemius and soleus muscles will feel the biggest stretch in the posterior lower leg. The Achilles tendon attaches your gastrocnemius muscle to your calcaneus, or heel bone. Don't overtax it as the tibialis anterior muscle tries to deepen the dorsal flexion in the ankle.

UPPER BODY

Most of the work here is in the shoulders and arms. With a lot of your body weight eventually ending up in your hands, you want to make sure you're creating a strong structure. The shoulders will be in deep flexion and external rotation. This will put your deltoid muscles in quite a dilemma. While the anterior deltoid will have to work to maintain shoulder flexion, it will have to lengthen to accommodate the external rotation. Similarly, the posterior deltoid will have to lengthen to accommodate the shoulder flexion, in addition to having to work to maintain external rotation. There is a lot to negotiate there as the deltoid muscle is a strong actor on the shoulder. Keep your shoulders and upper back feeling strong.

The forearms should be in pronation, working the pronator teres, with some help from the pronator quadratus and brachioradialis muscles.

*From **adho mukha svanasana,** to complete the sun salute, inhale as you step up with the same foot you stepped back with to find **anjaneyasana** on the other side. Then exhale as you step the back foot up to the front and find **uttanasana** again. Finally, inhale as you stand tall with arms reaching up and then exhale back to **tadasana**.*

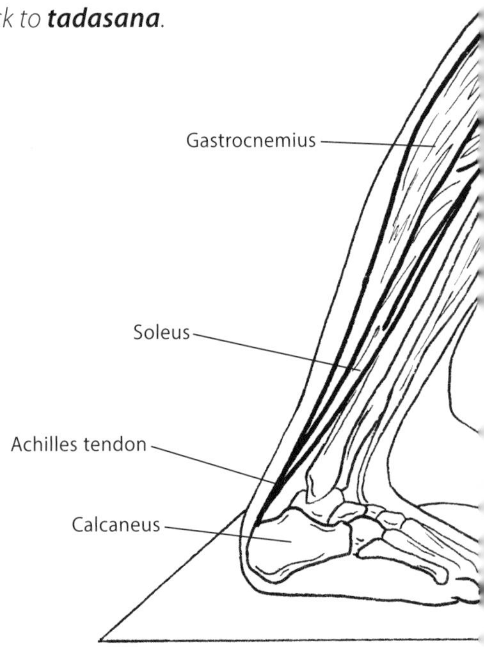

Practice Tip

Slightly flex the knees if you feel the stretch more in the tendinous attachments than the bellies of muscles, whether in the upper or lower leg. If your wrists get tired really fast, make sure you are distributing the weight equally throughout the palmar surface of the hand.

FUN FACT

Downward-facing dog is actually named after the posture dogs take when they give themselves a good stretch. We can learn a lot from our four-legged friends!

BICEPS FEMORIS
SEMIMEMBRANOSUS
SEMITENDINOSUS
GASTROCNEMIUS
SOLEUS
POSTERIOR DELTOID

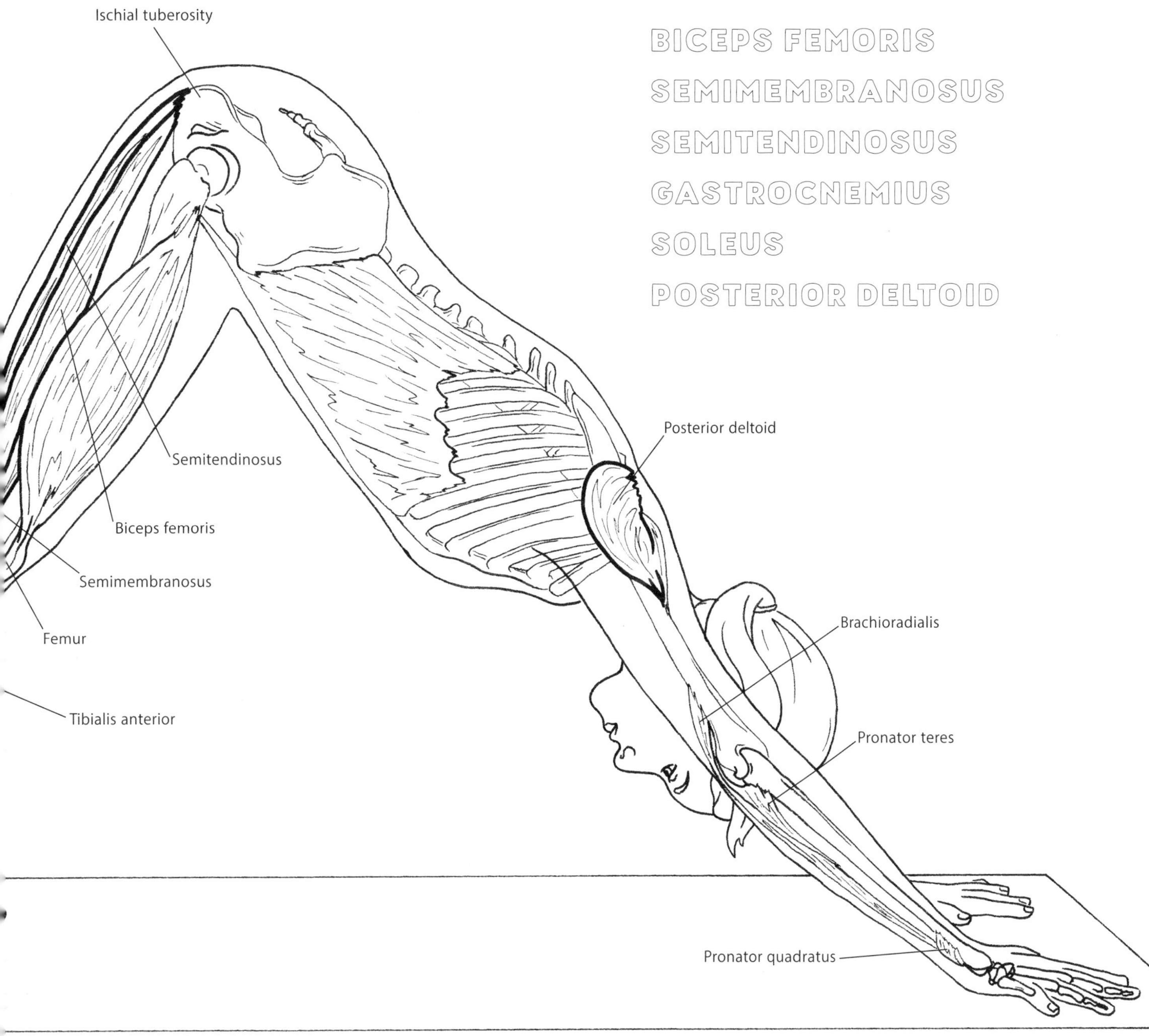

Standing Poses

For most folks first encountering the yoga postures, after warming up, you start with the standing asanas. These are meant to condition the biggest and strongest muscles of the body. The standing postures in this section require both feet on the mat. All standing asanas require the feet to be evenly grounded to provide a strong foundation as you move through your hips and shoulders, arms and legs. Focus on excellence, not perfection.

Padahastasana

pah-dah-hahs-TAH-sah-nah

Foot-Hand Posture

This is essentially **uttanasana** with a different hand position. Beyond getting a good stretch in the back of the legs inherent in most forward bends, **padahastasana** will also give all those extensor muscles in the forearms and wrists a nice stretch. Some folks may have to bend the knees to get the hands under the feet. It all depends on the body practicing the asana.

Start standing with your feet hip-distance apart, toes pointing forward. Flex at the hips as you keep your spine as neutral as possible. Slip your hands under your feet with palms up, getting your toes right up to the crease in your wrist. Extend the knees as much as possible while you keep the head and neck relaxed.

LOWER BODY

The hips are in deep flexion. The muscles of the posterior leg, primarily the gluteus maximus, hamstrings, gastrocnemius, and soleus muscles, will all lengthen and feel a deep stretch. The quadriceps muscles in front should all contract to keep the knees in extension, with the rectus femoris muscle (the biggest of the quadriceps muscle group) working double time as it is also helping to deepen the hip flexion. The strongest muscle in hip flexion is the psoas muscle, and you should be using it here.

UPPER BODY

Whether you flex your elbows or not will depend on how deep you can flex your hips and how flexible the muscles in the posterior leg are. If the elbows do bend, you should flex them out to the sides. The wrists will be in deep flexion no matter what. The major extensor muscles of the wrists and hands include the extensor carpi radialis longus, extensor carpi radialis brevis, extensor digitorum, and extensor carpi ulnaris. The extensor pollicis brevis, extensor pollicis longus, and extensor digiti minimi muscles are smaller, deeper extensors of the wrist. All of these muscles that run along your posterior forearm will lengthen. This should feel pretty good. You have probably figured out by the names that the extensor carpi radialis longus and brevis are on the radial, or thumb, side of the arm and that extensor carpi ulnaris is on the ulnar, or pinky, side of the arm because you know the bones of the forearm.

Ideally the spine maintains neutrality, the chest stays broad, and the head and neck can just relax.

GLUTEUS MAXIMUS

SEMITENDINOSUS

BICEPS FEMORIS

GASTROCNEMIUS

SOLEUS

EXTENSOR CARPI RADIALIS LONGUS

EXTENSOR CARPI RADIALIS BREVIS

EXTENSOR DIGITORUM

EXTENSOR CARPI ULNARIS

EXTENSOR MUSCLES

These muscles run along the posterior side of the forearm and are responsible for a lot of the strength in your hands. You will feel these muscles working hard anytime you put weight in your hands. Enjoy the stretch here.

Posterior View

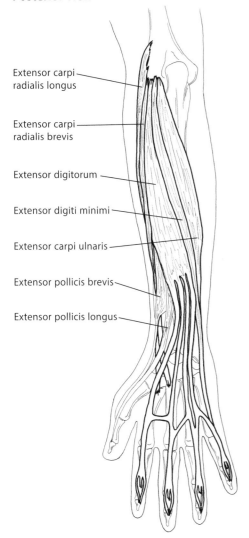

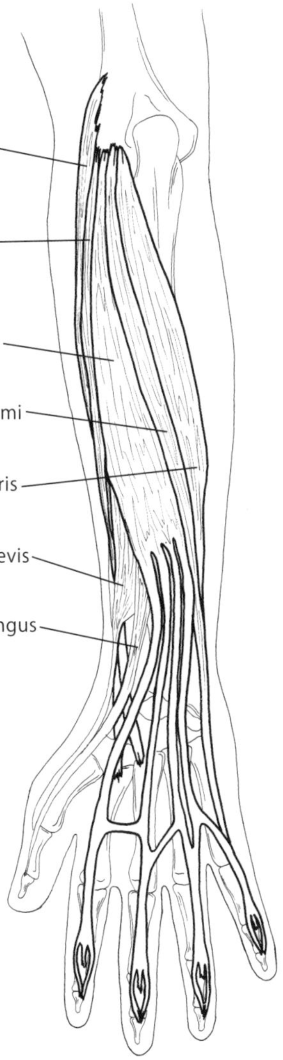

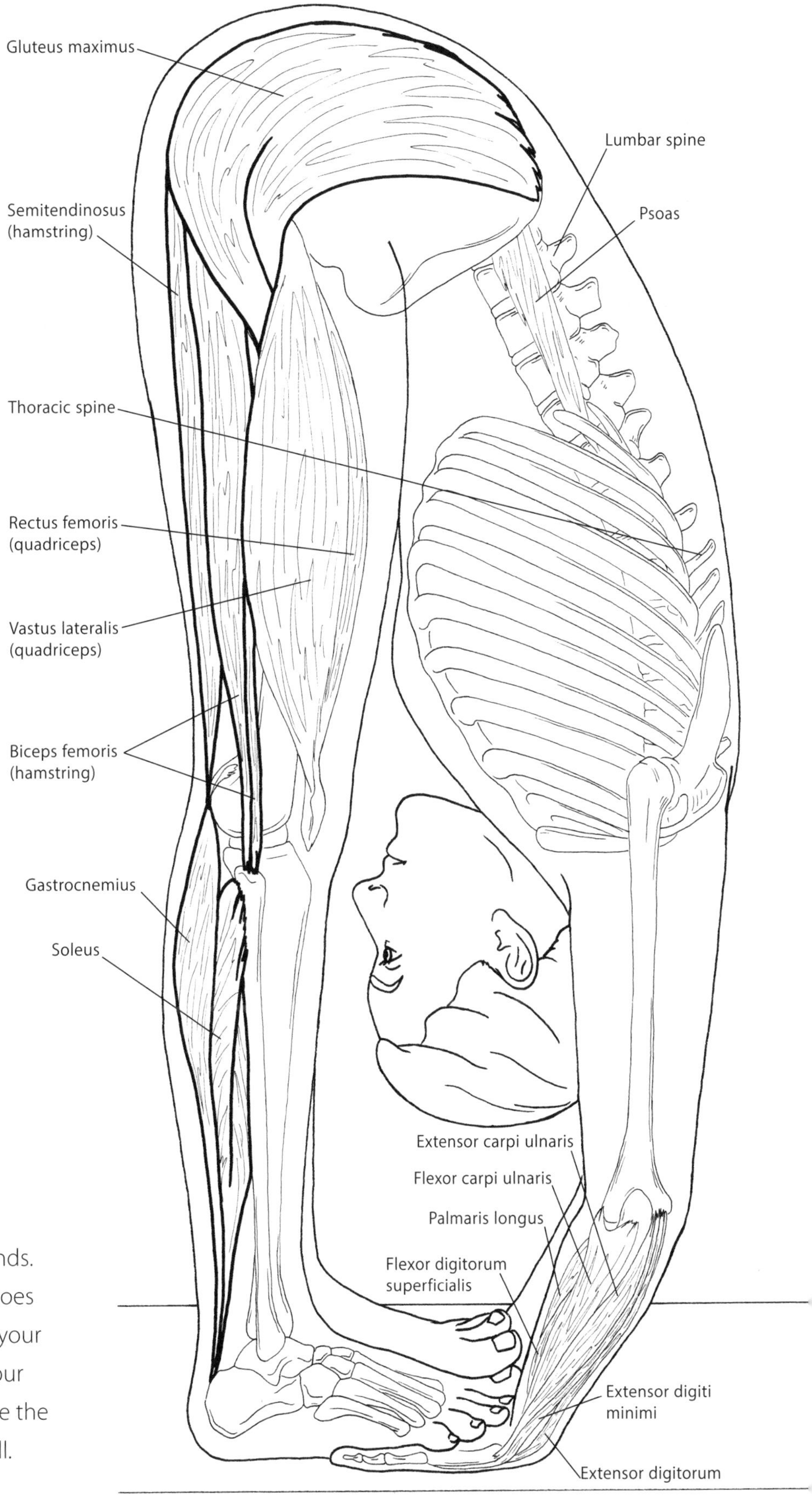

Practice Tip

The feet should be pressing into the hands. To make this feel even better, curl your toes and give the big muscles in the heels of your hands a nice massage. Trying to pull your hands from under your feet can extenuate the stretchy feeling in the forearms as well.

Utthita Trikonasana

oo-TEE-tah trik-oh-NAH-sah-nah

Extended Triangle

Utthita trikonasana is an essential yoga asana and an amazing hip opener. Finding and constantly improving correct alignment in this asana will keep you feeling open and strong. Too many folks don't use available props or feel they have to get the bottom hand to the floor before it's ready and end up collapsing the pose and losing all the benefit. Don't be that person.

Start standing on your mat in a wide straddle with your feet about a leg-distance apart. Turn the front foot so the toes are pointing straight ahead. Rotate the back foot slightly toward the front, lining up the heels front to back. If you are unsteady, take the front foot a little wider so you feel grounded. Externally rotate the front hip to line up the patella with the phalanges (kneecap with toes). Flex at the front hip to bring the upper body toward the front leg and the spine as close to being parallel to the floor as you can get. Once the hips have given all they have to give, the shoulders should be in abduction to bring the bottom hand toward the floor on the lateral side of the leg and the top hand toward the sky. Both arms are fully extended with shoulders externally rotating so the palms of the hands are facing anteriorly. The arms should form a vertical line perpendicular to the floor. The only movement in your spine is the rotation in the cervical spine, primarily at the atlantoaxial joint, as you gaze upward and try to line up the nose with the thumb of the top hand.

LOWER BODY

There is a lot going on in this asana, but above all, it is a big hip opener, and that is where we will mostly focus. Both hips are abducted to set up this asana requiring some length from the adductor muscles.

The front hip is externally rotating, asking the piriformis muscle, the strongest lateral rotator of the hip, to work hard to maintain the alignment of the knee with the toes. In the front leg, you will feel all of the adductor muscles, particularly the gracilis, and all of the hamstring muscles, notably the medial hamstrings—the semimembranosus and semitendinosus muscles—all getting a good stretch.

The hip of the back leg is in slight internal rotation to keep the back foot turned at about a 45-degree angle. This will keep the semitendinosus and the semimembranosus working as well as lengthening. Also working to maintain internal rotation in the back hip are the anterior fibers of the gluteus medius and the gluteus minimus and the adductor muscles as well. Because this asana started with the hips abducted, you can see that these muscles still have to work as they stretch. So don't get confused when you feel the lengthening in these muscles, along with a little bit of work.

UPPER BODY

The glenohumeral joint of both arms are in abduction, trying to form a vertical line with your arms. The upper arm will work to maintain abduction, asking the deltoid muscles and supraspinatus muscle to do most of that work. The lower arm has gravity doing most of the work!

The forearms are pronated to keep the palm facing anteriorly. The pronator teres muscles are the strongest muscles you have to pronate the forearms, and you will be using them here.

Practice Tip

As you move into the asana, try to move solely through the frontal plane to avoid misaligning the posture. Your spine should maintain neutrality and your heart center should feel lifted to the sky rather than being dragged down toward your mat.

MIDDLE DELTOID

POSTERIOR DELTOID

SUPRASPINATUS

SEMIMEMBRANOSUS

SEMITENDINOSUS

PIRIFORMIS

PSOAS

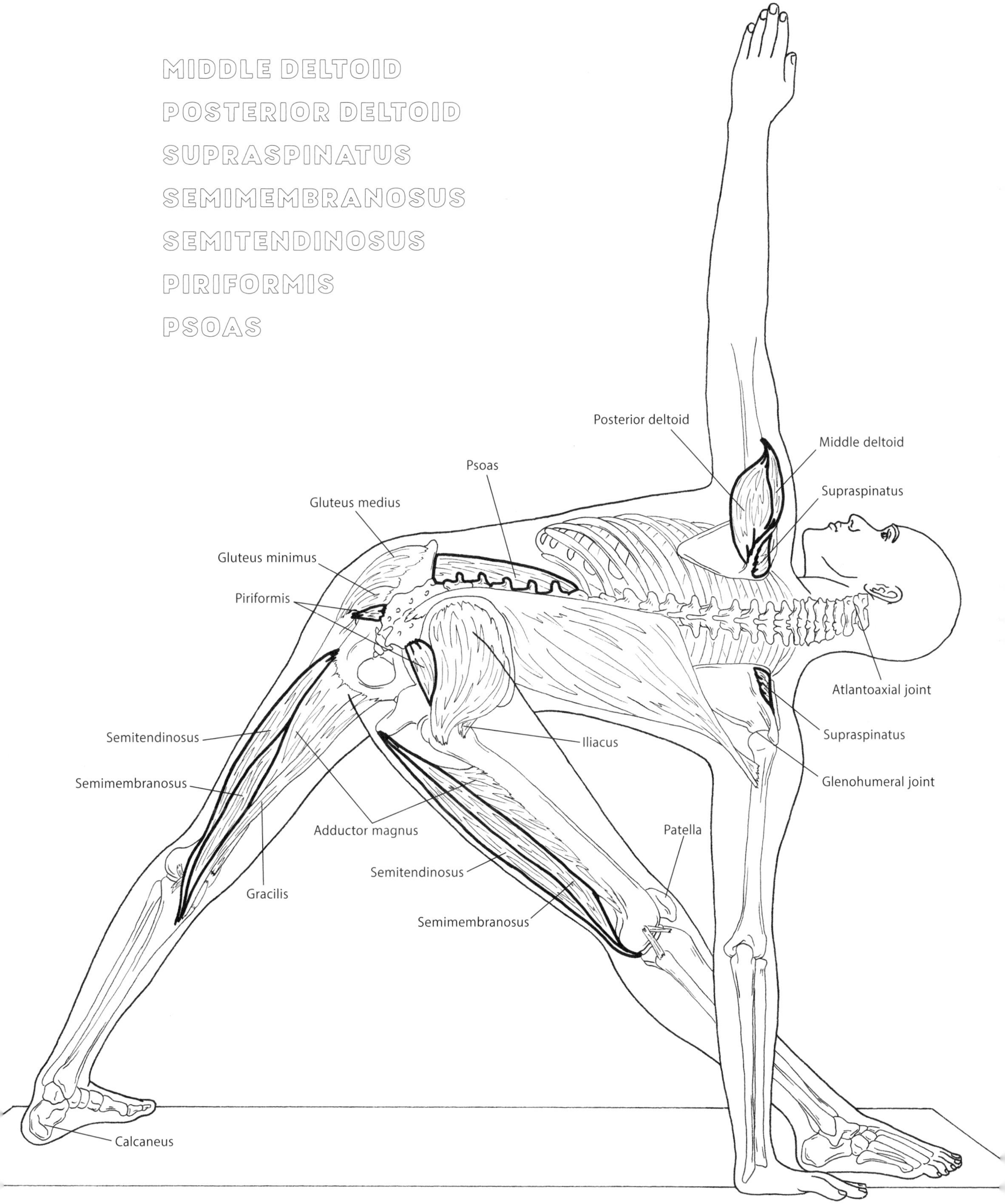

Utthita Parsvakonasana

oo-TEE-tah parsh-vah-coh-NAH-sah-nah

Extended Side Angle

Utthita parsvakonasana is an essential, not to mention classic, yoga asana. It is primarily meant to give the side body a big stretch from the lateral side of the back foot all the way up to the top arm. It's a chance to lengthen along the whole lateral body. Too often practitioners will cheat this posture in an effort to get the bottom hand all the way to the mat before it is ready (much like in **utthita trikonasana**). This will take you out of alignment and you will miss all the benefit this asana has to offer.

Start standing on your mat with feet about a leg's length apart. Point the toes of the front foot forward and flex the knee, bending it in the same direction as the toes and parking it right over the ankle. Slightly angle the back foot forward and keep the back leg fully extended and the back foot firmly grounding as you flex the front hip to bring the front hand down to the mat along the lateral lower leg, trying to move solely through the coronal plane. Form a straight line from the lateral edge of the back foot all the way up to the top hand, careful to not let the top hip and/or shoulder tilt forward. Rotate the neck to bring your gaze up.

LOWER BODY

Both sides of the hips are in abduction. All of the adductor muscles in the back leg will get a nice stretch as you try to bring the pelvis closer toward the earth. Because there is some slight internal rotation in the hip of the back leg (to keep the toes pointing toward the front of the mat), the piriformis, along with the deeper external rotators of the hip, will also have an opportunity for some lengthening.

The hip of the front leg is mostly working. In addition to adducting, the front hip is also flexing, a lot, and in slight external rotation to keep the knee lined up with the toes. The rectus femoris muscle will have to work hard in eccentric contraction up in the hip to defy the force of gravity and maintain flexion, while it lengthens down below, along with the rest of the quadriceps, to accommodate the knee flexion.

The knee of the back leg is fully extended, keeping the back leg straight and keeping your quadriceps muscles on the job to maintain extension. The knee of the front leg is flexed to as close to 90 degrees as you can get. This will depend on how low you can sink your pelvis.

The ankle of the back foot is supinated, which will give the peroneal longus and peroneal brevis muscles that run along the lateral side of the lower leg a deep, delicious stretch. It is important that the back foot stay grounded, particularly the lateral edge, and evenly weighted with the front foot. If you let the lateral edge of the back foot peel away from the mat, you will miss out on the stretch of the peroneal muscles; don't do that, it feels too good!

UPPER BODY

You should do your very best to maintain spinal neutrality. Do not compensate for what you lack in hip flexibility by laterally flexing the spine to get your hand to the floor.

Both shoulders are in abduction, however, the top shoulder much more so. All of the deltoid muscles (anterior, middle, and posterior) in the top shoulder along with the supraspinatus muscle will be fully engaged to reach the arm up and over the head. The forearm up top will be supinated to keep the palm facing down. The biceps brachii and the supinator muscle are your strongest supinators in the forearm with brachioradialis acting as a synergist.

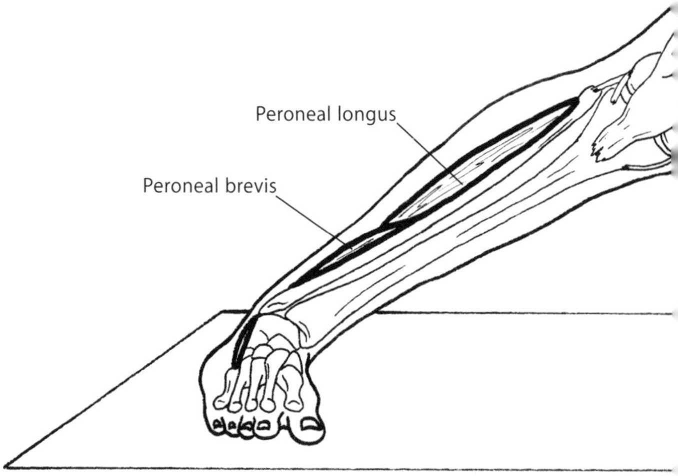

Practice Tip

You will know that your front knee is properly aligned if you can see your big toe on the medial side of your knee and the knee is blocking the other toes. This goes for lunges, and basically any other standing posture asking you to flex the front knee.

PIRIFORMIS
RECTUS FEMORIS
PERONEAL LONGUS
PERONEAL BREVIS
SUPRASPINATUS
BICEPS BRACHII

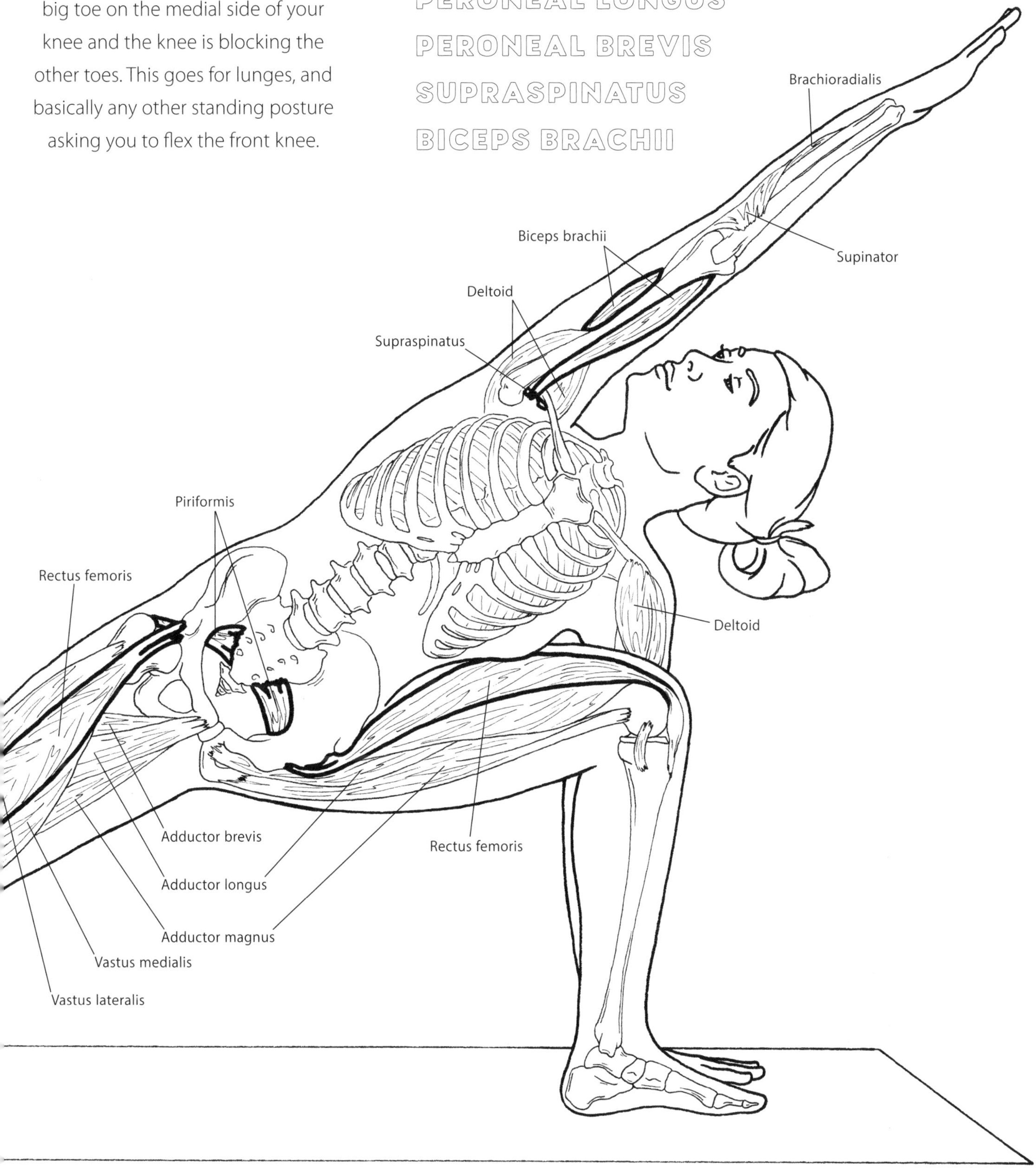

Parsvottanasana

parsh-VOH-tan-AH-sah-nah

Pyramid

The literal English translation, "intense side stretch," for this asana is misleading. The other English name often heard, "pyramid," just describes the shape of the posture. If I were to name this asana it would be the "Oh my God, now I really know where my hamstring muscles are!" asana. **Parsvottanasana** is an easy enough posture to find for most, while it might take a while to fully express it. Arm positions can vary, but, eventually, as you progress in the posture and your overall shoulder flexibility improves, the hands will be brought behind the back in a "reverse" prayer position.

Start standing and either take a step forward or a step back. Keep the front foot pointing forward and the back foot angled toward the front with the heels lined up, front to back. Face the front of the mat with both sides of the pelvis evenly facing forward. Internally rotate your shoulders and pronate your forearms like crazy as you bring your arms behind the back and press the palms together, fingers pointing up. Flexing at the hips, bring the upper body as close to the front leg as possible. While the back leg should remain straight, if the hamstrings in the front leg are not fully on board for this stretch, bend the front knee as much as you need.

LOWER BODY

Both sides of the hips are in flexion, but the hip of the front leg will be in much deeper flexion than that of the back. And it is in the front leg that you will feel the biceps femoris, semitendinosus, and semimembranosus muscles, also known as your hamstring muscles, getting a big stretch. The hip in the back leg will also be internally rotating to keep that back foot pointing toward front and firmly grounded. You may feel a stretch in the hamstrings of the back leg, but the semimembranosus and semitendinosus will have to do some work in the back leg to maintain internal rotation.

The quadriceps in both legs will be working here to keep the knees extended. Consciously engaging your quadriceps muscles (as if you were going to kick the leg forward) can help to keep the message clear to the hamstring muscles to keep stretching through a process known as "reciprocal inhibition." This is another clue to the genius of the body. The body knows that if one group of muscles is contracting, in this case the quadriceps, then the opposite group of muscles, in this case the hamstrings, must stay relaxed, and, in turn, stay in stretching mode. Imagine what would happen if opposing groups of muscles contracted at the same time; your body is too smart for that.

The ankle of the back foot will be in deep dorsal flexion, causing the gastrocnemius and soleus muscles to lengthen.

UPPER BODY

Bringing your arms and hands into a "reverse namaste" position is challenging. Because of the deep internal rotation required in the glenohumeral joint (where the humerus meets the scapula) the posterior deltoid, infraspinatus, and teres minor muscles have to be able to provide the length. Because of the deep pronation, the biceps brachii muscles must also lengthen. Do not force this. Remember: nothing should hurt.

Practice Tip

If you are unable to bring your arms to a "reverse namaste," try reaching behind your back for the opposite elbow. If that doesn't work, bring your hands behind your back and interlace your fingers with arms fully extended, palms together. Have patience.

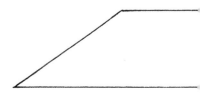

COLORING TIP

The hamstrings are three distinct muscles. Coloring each hamstring a different shade of the same color will symbolize that they are members of the same group.

BICEPS FEMORIS
SEMITENDINOSUS
SEMIMEMBRANOSUS
POSTERIOR DELTOID
INFRASPINATUS
TERES MINOR

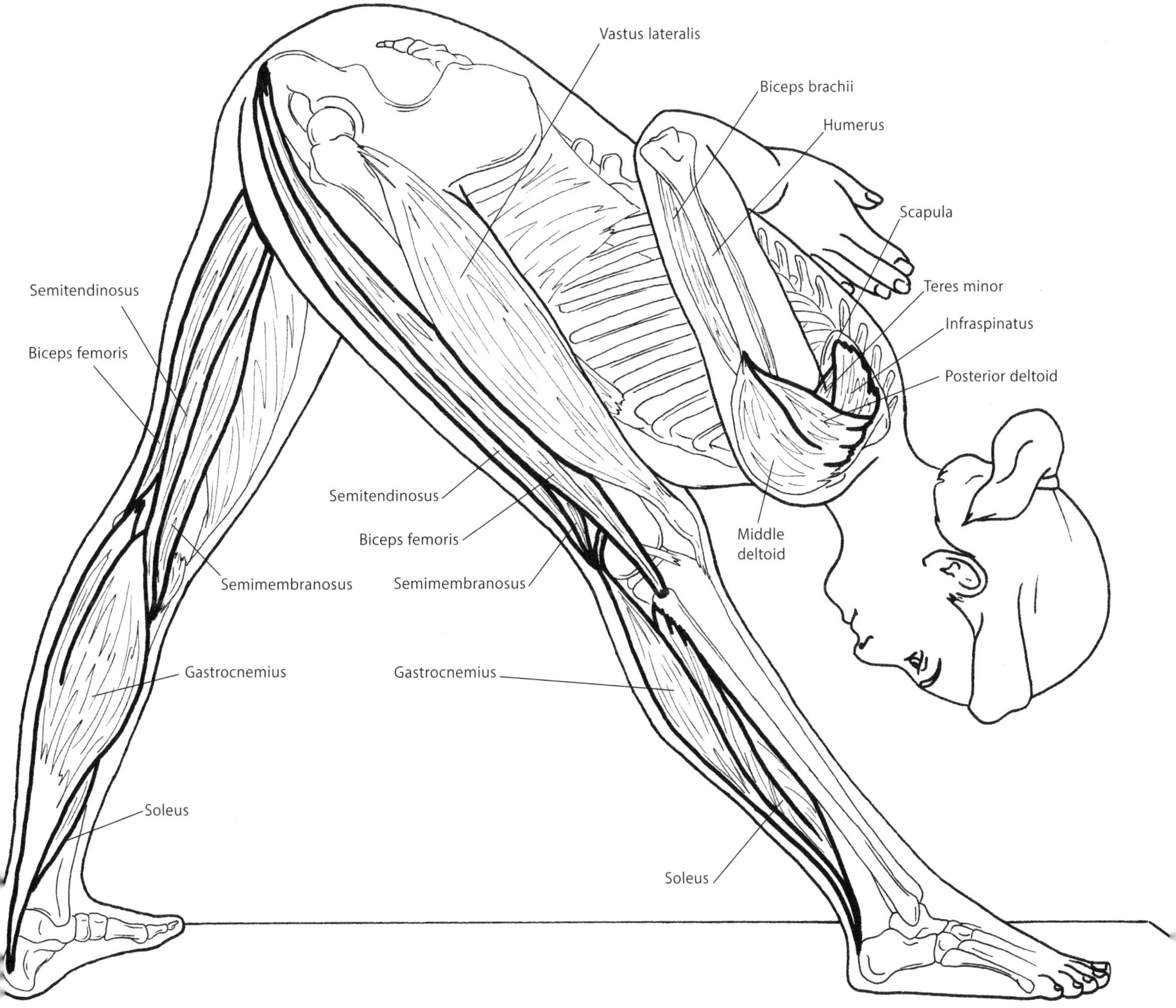

Utkatasana

OOT-kah-TAH-sah-nah

Chair

I don't think anyone finds **utkatasana** easy, but it's an asana that everyone can and should practice. I think the reason most find it so difficult is that utkatasana is asking your lumbar and thoracic spine to bend the opposite way of their natural curves. Utkatasana wants your hips in posterior tilt, bringing your lumbar spine, which is naturally a concave curve, toward flexion. It also wants your thoracic spine, which is naturally a convex curve, to move toward extension. This posture is particularly beneficial for those prone to either lordosis (an exaggeration of the curve of the lumbar spine) or kyphosis (an exaggeration of the curve of the thoracic spine).

Start standing in **tadasana**. Keeping your weight evenly distributed in your feet, flex your knees as much as possible. Then bring your pelvis into full range of motion of posterior tilt. Keep the posterior tilt established as you bring the rest of your spine into extension. Finally, raise your arms as high as you can, flexing at the shoulders.

LOWER BODY

Your pelvis will be in deep posterior tilt and your hips will be in slight flexion. The posterior tilt in the pelvis will employ the external oblique, gluteus maximus, hamstrings, and rectus abdominis. You want full range of motion here so you should feel these muscles really working for you. In addition, the psoas and iliacus muscles, along with the rest of your hip flexors will be eccentrically contracting to maintain hip flexion and resist gravity.

Your knees will also be in flexion, asking all of the hamstring muscles to work double-time here to keep the knees stable and maintain the bend in the knees. It will get help from other knee flexors, including the popliteus. The popliteus is not the strongest knee flexor, but in the posterior knee, it is the deepest muscle and the only muscle that acts solely on the knee.

Most will feel the majority of the effort to hold the posture down in the ankles. The ankles are in deep dorsal flexion, requiring the tibialis anterior, extensor digitorum longus, and extensor hallucis longus muscles to work really hard.

UPPER BODY

While the lumbar spine is being pulled toward flexion because of the posterior tilt of the pelvis, the thoracic spine, along with the cervical spine, is being pulled toward extension. The spinalis thoracis, longissimus thoracis, and iliocostalis muscles, part of the group of muscles known as the erector spinae muscles, will be working to their fullest to bring the backbend to the thoracic vertebrae. Serratus posterior superior will help by contracting to lift the upper ribs. Serratus posterior superior is primarily a respiratory muscle that lifts the upper ribs during inhalation. Try not to let this affect your breath, particularly if you tend to be a chest breather.

The glenohumeral (shoulder) joint is in deep flexion and external rotation. The pectoralis major muscle is your strongest shoulder flexor and you will feel it, primarily in the upper fibers of the muscle. It will get a fair amount of help from the anterior deltoid and biceps brachii. Coracobrachialis, a smaller but still powerful muscle, will be employed as well. The posterior deltoid is your strongest external rotator of the shoulder. The anterior and posterior fibers of the deltoid muscles perform opposing actions. **Utkatasana** is asking both sides of the deltoid to work here, which adds to the challenge of the asana.

The forearms are in supination, which will work the biceps brachii even more. The supinator muscle, as the name implies, will be engaged here as well.

FUN FACT

The literal English translation for this pose is "fierce" or "powerful" pose. It is said to represent Hanuman, the monkey god, as he continually grew his tail longer to intimidate Ravana, the King of the Rakshasas (demons). Performing **utkatasana** teaches us that when things turn out to be harder than they look, we need to fiercely persevere.

EXTERNAL OBLIQUE

GLUTEUS MAXIMUS

HAMSTRINGS

POPLITEUS

TIBIALIS ANTERIOR

EXTENSOR DIGITORUM LONGUS

EXTENSOR HALLUCIS LONGUS

PECTORALIS MAJOR

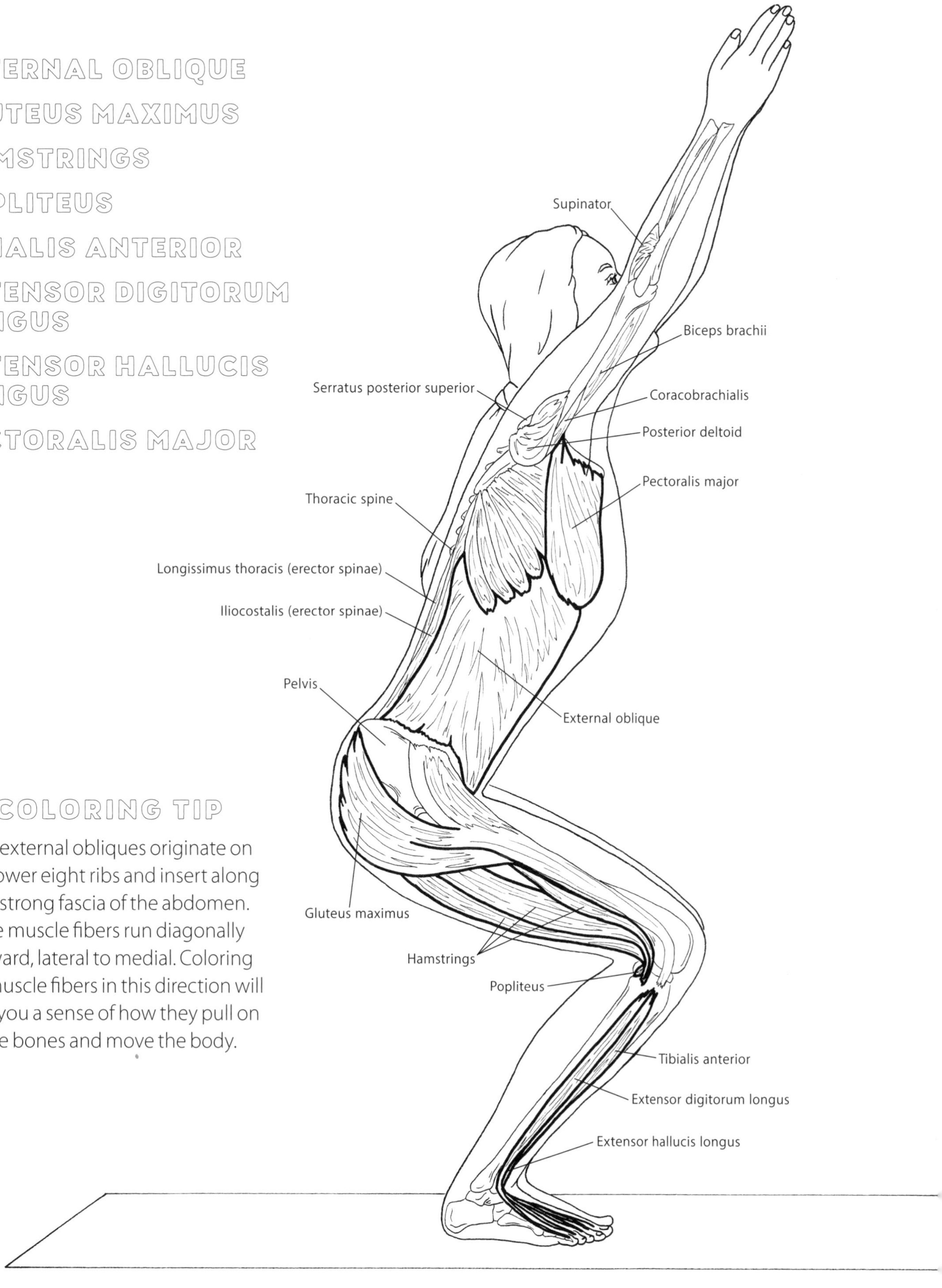

COLORING TIP

The external obliques originate on the lower eight ribs and insert along the strong fascia of the abdomen. The muscle fibers run diagonally upward, lateral to medial. Coloring the muscle fibers in this direction will give you a sense of how they pull on the bones and move the body.

Virabhadrasana I

veer-ah-bah-DRAH-sah-nah I

Warrior I

Virabhadrasana I is a strong standing posture. It is right there in the name: warrior. This asana is primary and foundational in yoga and is practiced from beginner level all the way up to the most challenging yoga asana classes.

Standing with your feet about a leg's length apart, the toes of the front foot should point forward with the knee flexed and right over the ankle. The back foot is angled toward the front of the mat, and the back leg is fully extended. The pelvis faces the front of the mat, or at least as close to that as you can get as you keep your feet evenly grounded. The pelvis is in posterior tilt as you lift your heart and your gaze turn upward with your arms strong and reaching straight up.

LOWER BODY

The pelvis is in posterior tilt. The hip of the front leg is in flexion, as close to 90 degrees as you can get. This will ask the psoas, iliacus, and rectus femoris, some of the strongest flexors of the hip, to work—hard. The hamstrings will also be working hard in that front leg to keep the knee flexed, also as close to 90 degrees as you can get. The front foot is in dorsal flexion and has about half your body weight to support. The tibialis anterior, the strongest dorsal flexor of the ankle will be strengthened as you hold this posture.

You have almost the opposite happening in the back leg. The hip is in extension and also internal rotation. All those muscles that work to flex the hip in the front leg will get a deep stretch here. You may particularly feel rectus femoris having to lengthen to accommodate the posterior tilt in addition to be working in the lower fibers of the muscle along with the other three quadriceps muscles—vastus lateralis, vastus intermedius, and vastus medialis—to keep the back knee fully extended. The back ankle is in dorsal flexion and also supinated, which will give peroneal longus and peroneal brevis some length, especially as you keep the outer edge of the back foot grounded.

UPPER BODY

The spine is in extension, meaning you are going toward a backbend here, all the way up to the cervicals, but not at the expense of losing the posterior tilt in the hips. The lower fibers of the rectus abdominis work hard to maintain the hips in posterior tilt, while the upper fibers will get a nice stretch from the spinal extension.

The glenohumeral joint is in deep flexion to reach the hands up high. This will strengthen your anterior deltoids, biceps brachii, and coracobrachialis, along with the upper fibers of the pectoralis major.

Practice Tip

Emphasize the internal rotation of the back leg to help square the hips to face forward, but be mindful that you keep evenly grounding your feet. If you let the lateral edge of the back foot start to lift, you are just doing a sloppy lunge. Remember, a warrior never wants to lose ground.

FUN FACT

Virabhadra, the Warriors, were created from a dreadlock Shiva yanked from his head in a fit of rage upon learning of the death of his consort, Sati. He created the Warriors to get his revenge on King Daksha, Sati's father, whom he blamed for her death.

TIBIALIS ANTERIOR
RECTUS FEMORIS
VASTUS LATERALIS
VASTUS INTERMEDIUS
VASTUS MEDIALIS
RECTUS ABDOMINIS (LOWER FIBERS)
CORACOBRACHIALIS

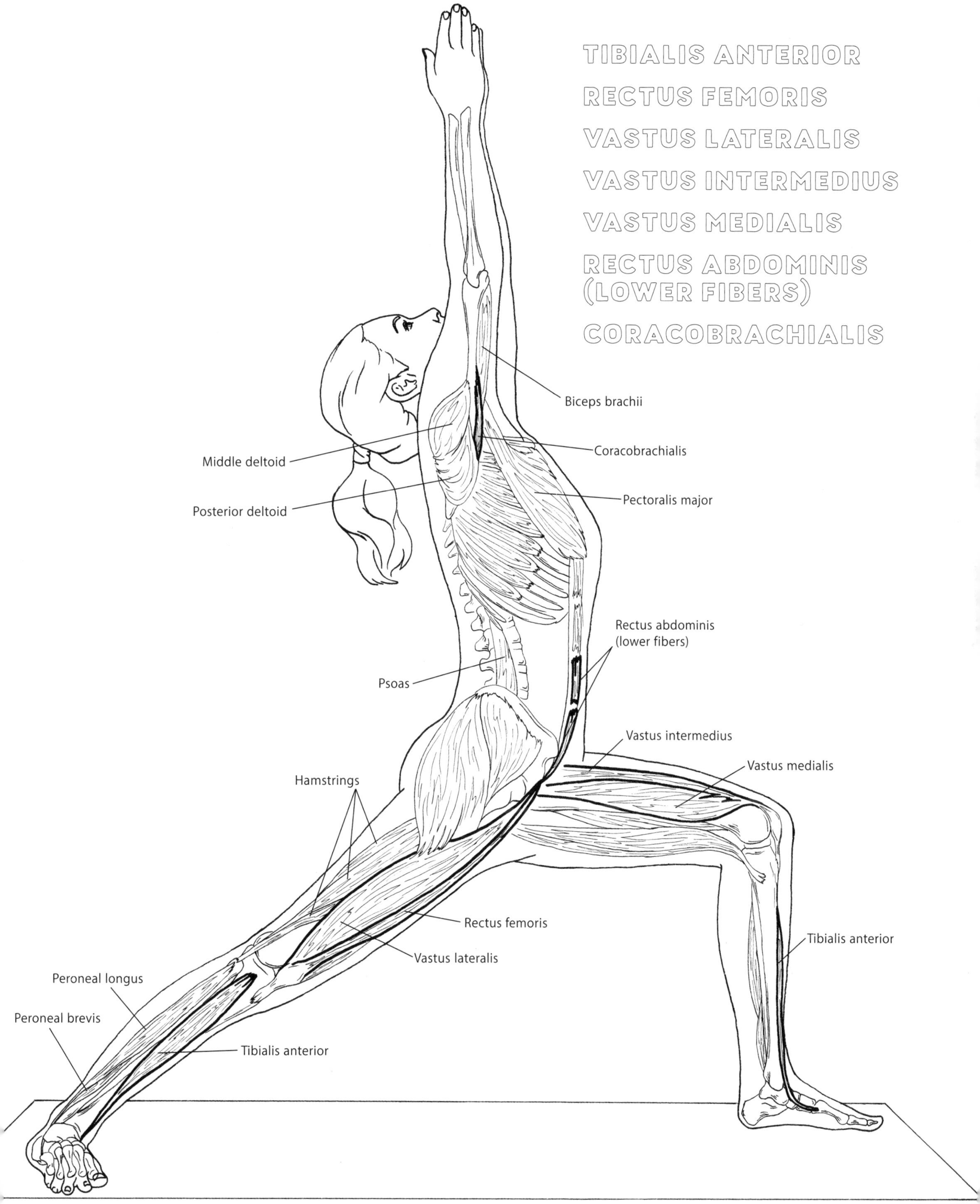

Virabhadrasana II

veer-ah-bah-DRAH-sah-nah II

Warrior II

Most find **virabhadrasana II** easier than **virabhadrasana I**. I believe it's because of the positioning of the pelvis. Warrior I and warrior II feet and knees are the same, but the hips are now in abduction with the front hip also in external rotation. It is a strong solid standing posture that will increase strength and flexibility and can be practiced by just about anyone. It is just a matter of how deep you take it. Alignment is more important than appearing to be deeper in the posture.

Set your feet, legs, and pelvis (just posterior tilt aspect) as described in virabhadrasana I. But, this is where the similarity ends. The pelvis and the upper body are facing the long side of the mat. Your arms should be fully extended and held strong in abduction parallel to the floor. The forearms are pronated to keep the palms facing down. Rotating the cervical spine, gaze softly toward your front fingertips.

LOWER BODY

Holding the pelvis in posterior tilt will work the gluteus maximus and hamstring muscles most of all. Most delicious though is giving almost all the adductor muscles a deep stretch here; "almost" because the gracilis is the only one of the adductor muscle group that crosses the knee, so you won't feel it in the front leg. The adductor muscle group is composed of the pectineus, adductor brevis, adductor longus, adductor magnus, and, as mentioned before, gracilis.

Maybe most important here, because it is the most common misalignment, is keeping the front knee facing forward and lined up with the toes. You will need to engage the external rotators of the hip (the acetabulofemoral joint that's sometimes called the coxal) joint. The strongest external rotator in the hip is your piriformis muscle.

UPPER BODY

Your shoulders are held in abduction, keeping your arms parallel to the floor. All fibers of the deltoid muscle, anterior, middle, and posterior will be working hard to keep the arms elevated, strong, and steady. The supraspinatus muscle, the only one of your rotator cuff muscles that is not involved in rotation, is very involved in abduction at the glenohumeral joint. It is debatable how much the supraspinatus muscle is working here. Some say a whole lot, some say not so much, but all agree, it is working.

The spine should remain neutral, except for the cervical spine, which will be in deep rotation to bring the gaze forward.

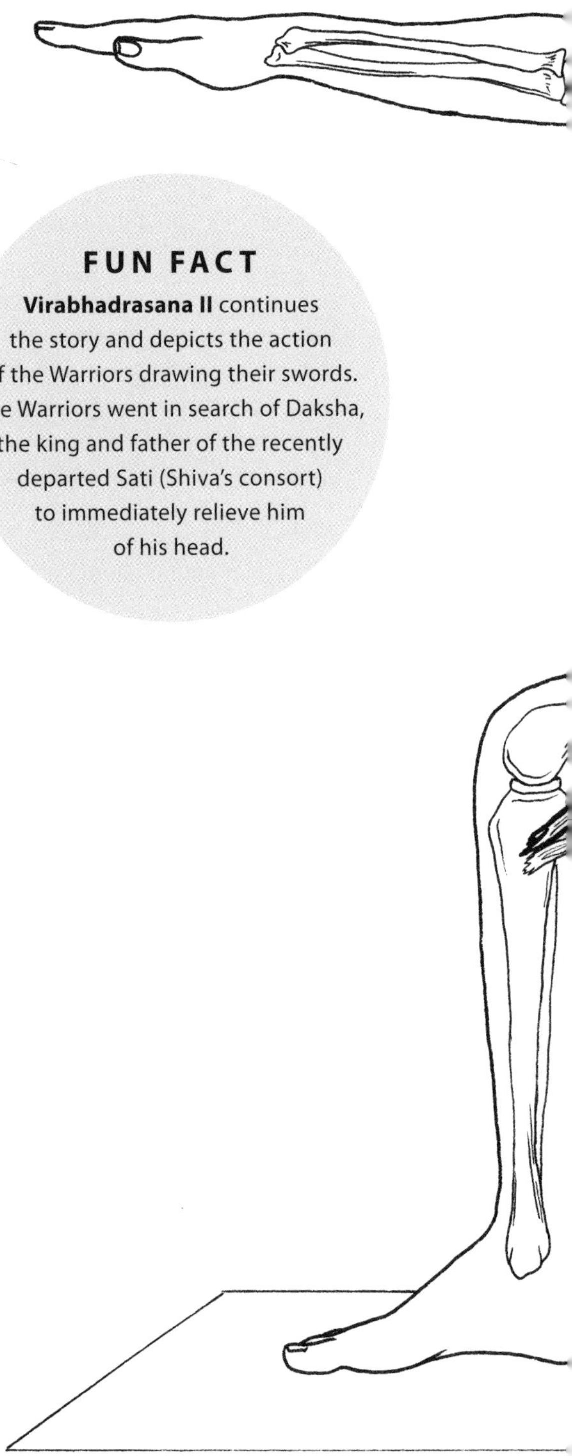

FUN FACT

Virabhadrasana II continues the story and depicts the action of the Warriors drawing their swords. The Warriors went in search of Daksha, the king and father of the recently departed Sati (Shiva's consort) to immediately relieve him of his head.

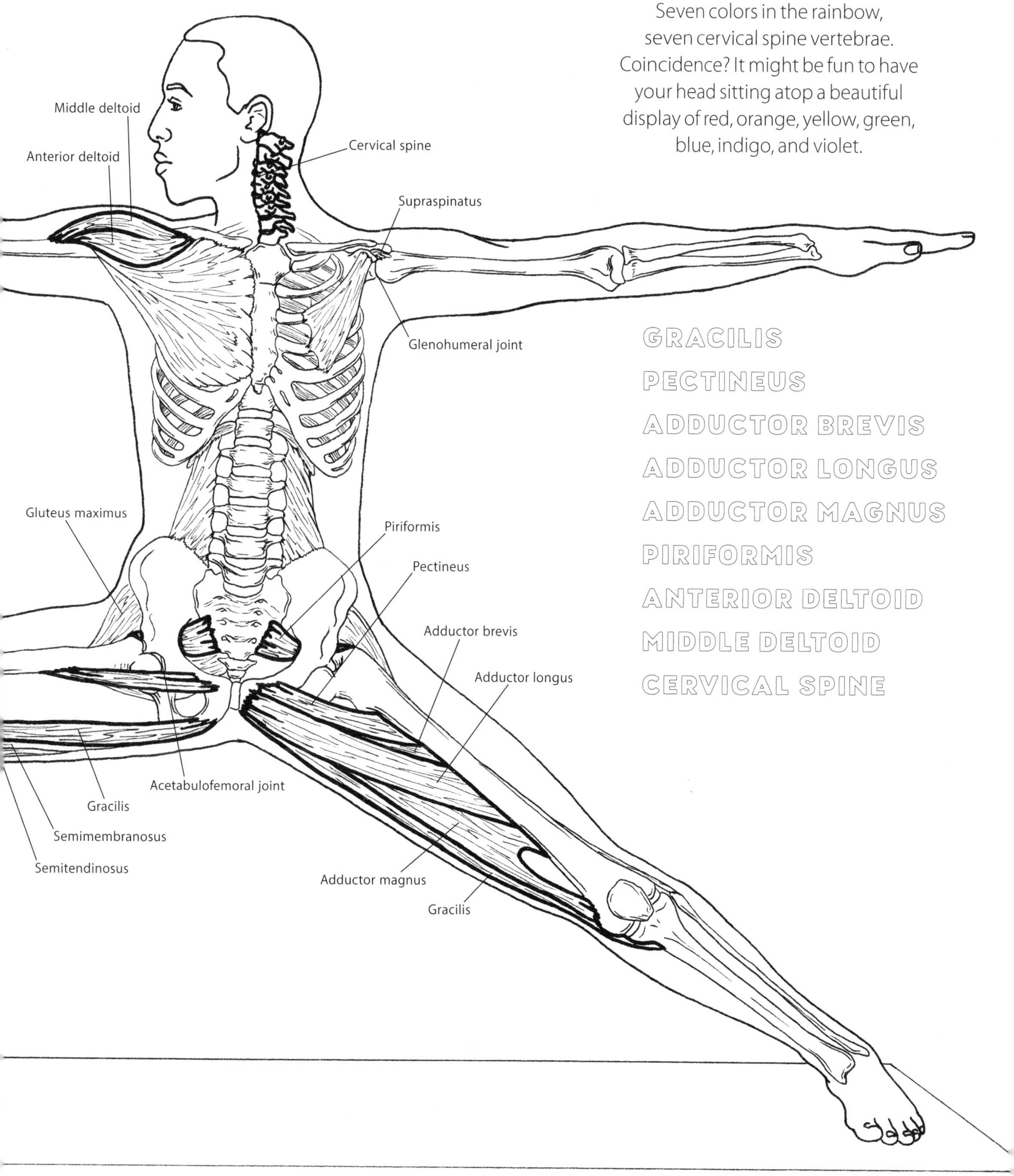

COLORING TIP

Seven colors in the rainbow, seven cervical spine vertebrae. Coincidence? It might be fun to have your head sitting atop a beautiful display of red, orange, yellow, green, blue, indigo, and violet.

GRACILIS
PECTINEUS
ADDUCTOR BREVIS
ADDUCTOR LONGUS
ADDUCTOR MAGNUS
PIRIFORMIS
ANTERIOR DELTOID
MIDDLE DELTOID
CERVICAL SPINE

Parivrtta Trikonasana

par-ee-VRIT-tah trik-oh-NAH-sah-nah

Revolved Triangle

Parivrtta trikonasana takes your triangle for a twist. To bring this posture to its full expression, you will need a fair amount of rotation in the spine, not to mention strength and flexibility in the hips and legs. Most likely, when first approaching this asana, you will need to at least prop the bottom hand. Don't make the mistake of bringing the rotation into the pelvis and misaligning the posture just to get that bottom hand lower. Ideally, your spine is parallel to the floor.

Get started with your feet about a leg's length apart. Point the toes of the front leg forward with the back foot slightly angled toward the front. Keeping the legs straight, turn the pelvis to face forward. As you flex at the hips, rotate the spine to the same side as the front leg as you bring the palm of the opposite hand down outside of the front foot. The other hand is reaching straight up. Your gaze is toward the top hand as the entire spine comes into deep rotation.

LOWER BODY

Both hips will be in flexion, but the hip of the front leg much more so. This will give the gluteus maximus muscle of the front leg a deep stretch. The hamstrings in the front leg will also feel some lengthening; if it feels like too much, you should slightly flex the knee until the hamstrings are ready for full knee extension.

With the hip of the back leg only in slight flexion, you should keep full extension in the knee. The hip of the back leg should be more focused on maintaining internal rotation. This will keep the gluteus medius and gluteus minimus muscles working really hard for you, while your piriformis muscle can enjoy some lengthening. They will get a lot of help from all five muscles that compose the adductor group along with the two hamstring muscles that run medially along the posterior thigh: semimembranosus and semitendinosus. This will help keep the pelvis evenly facing forward. You will feel the quadriceps muscles in both legs working hard to keep the knees extended and the legs feeling strong.

UPPER BODY

The glenohumeral (shoulder) joints of both arms are in abduction with the top shoulder also externally rotating so the palm of the top hand is facing the same as the anterior, or front, of the upper body.

The real work in the upper body in **parivrtta trikonasana** is getting and maintaining deep spinal rotation. The multifidi, rotatores, and external obliques are some of the strongest muscles that rotate the spine. They all work unilaterally to rotate the spine to the opposite side. They get a lot of help from the internal obliques, which work unilaterally to rotate the spine to the same side. As you move up to the cervical spine, there are many more muscles that act on the neck to keep your gaze up. One of the strongest is the levator scapula muscle. Since this muscle works unilaterally to rotate the cervical spine, if it's tight, its paired muscle will not have enough length to accommodate deeper rotation. This is also the muscle that pulls your shoulders up to your ears, so you can bet that there are a lot of tight levator scapula muscles out there.

FUN FACT

Revolved or "twisting" asanas are of great benefit to digestion. You are literally giving your internal organs a nice massage and helping to keep things moving. And when it comes to digestion, the last thing you want is to be stuck.

GLUTEUS MAXIMUS
GLUTEUS MEDIUS
GLUTEUS MINIMUS
SEMIMEMBRANOSUS
SEMITENDINOSUS
MULTIFIDI
ROTATORES
LEVATOR SCAPULA

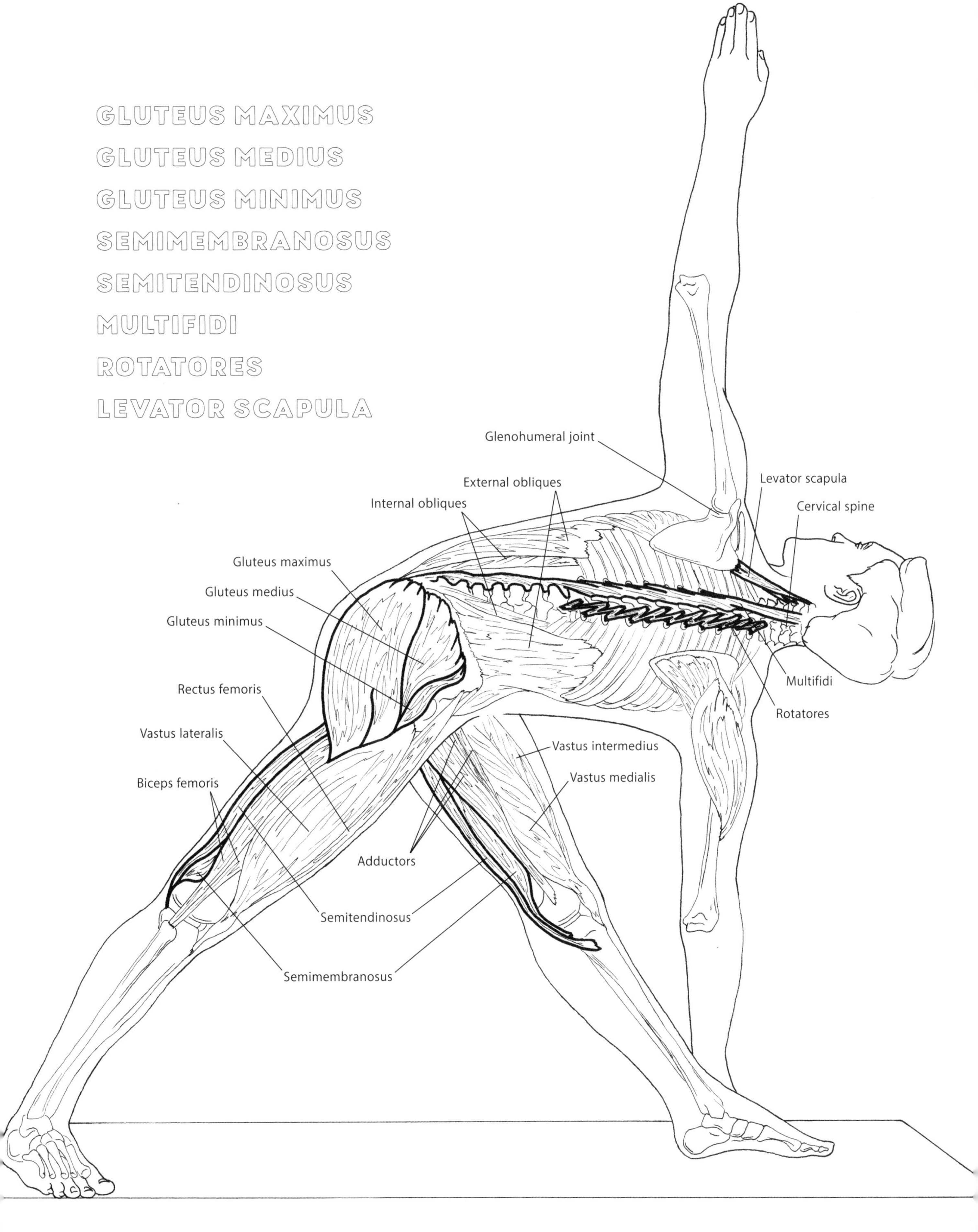

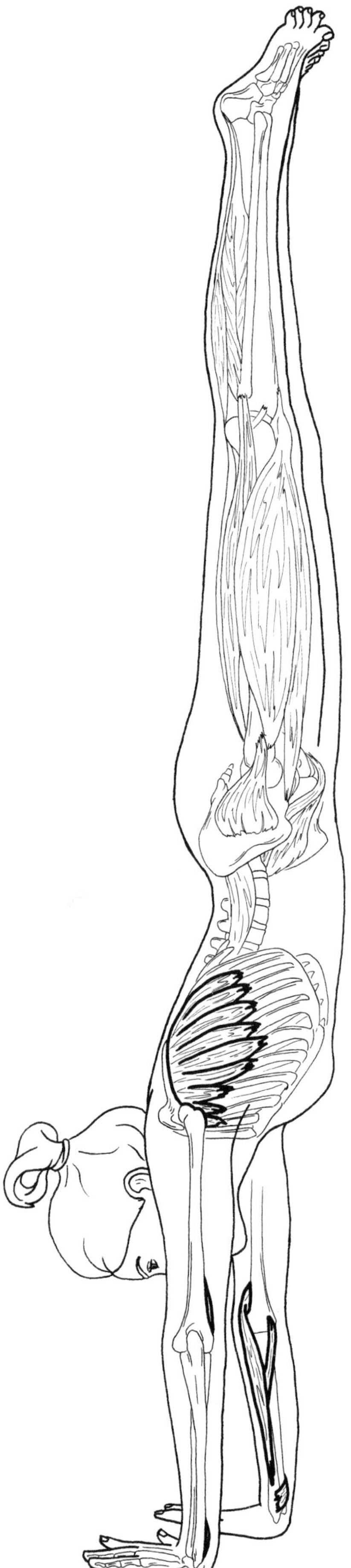
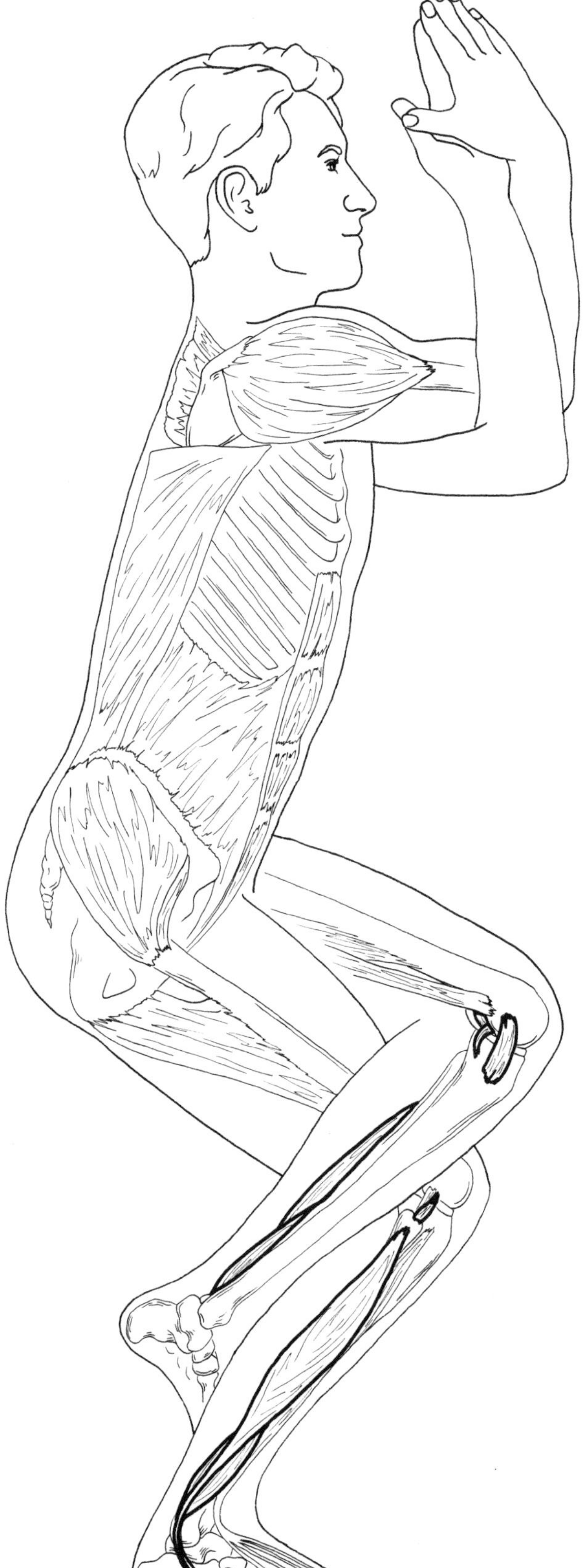

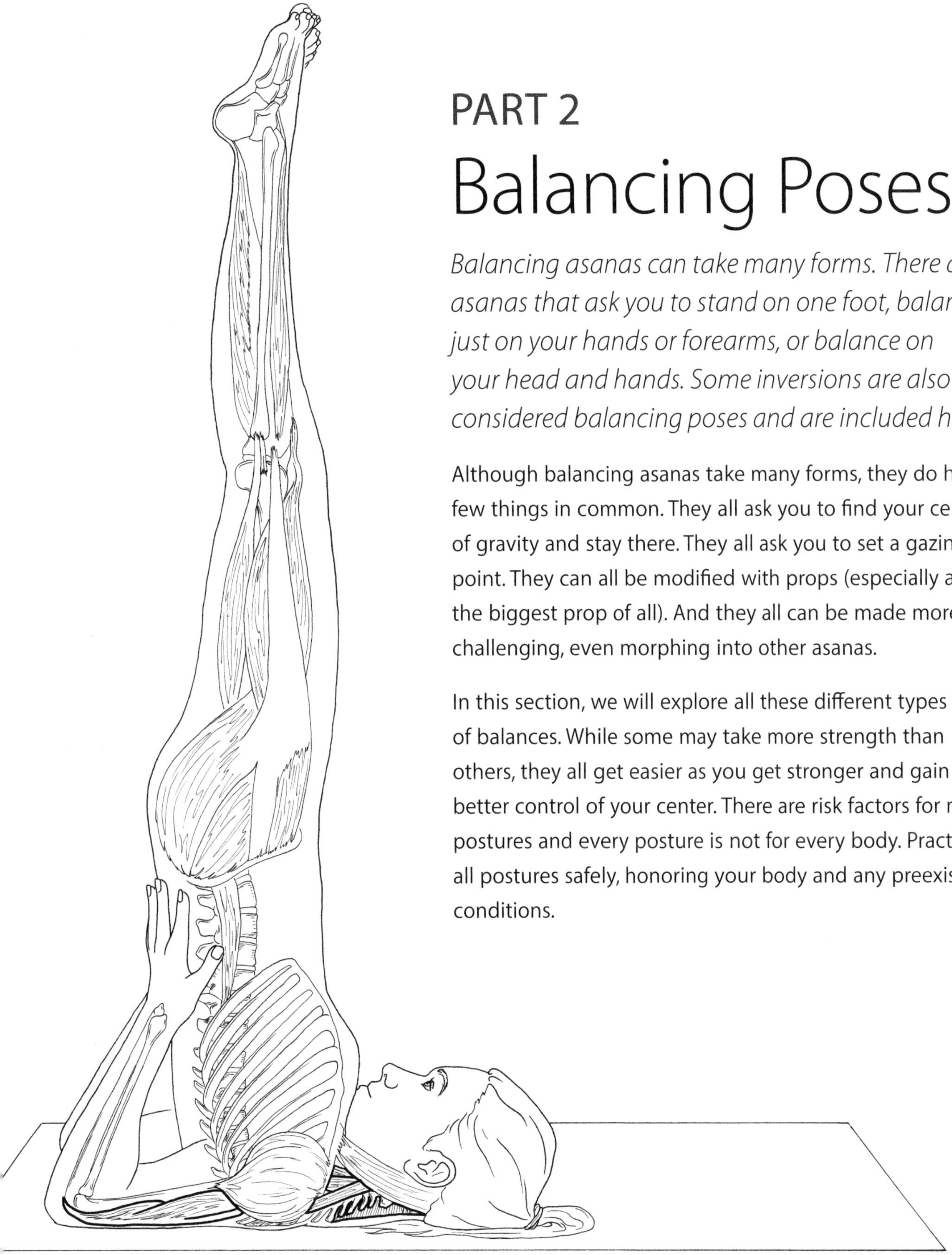

PART 2

Balancing Poses

Balancing asanas can take many forms. There are asanas that ask you to stand on one foot, balance just on your hands or forearms, or balance on your head and hands. Some inversions are also considered balancing poses and are included here.

Although balancing asanas take many forms, they do have a few things in common. They all ask you to find your center of gravity and stay there. They all ask you to set a gazing point. They can all be modified with props (especially a wall, the biggest prop of all). And they all can be made more challenging, even morphing into other asanas.

In this section, we will explore all these different types of balances. While some may take more strength than others, they all get easier as you get stronger and gain better control of your center. There are risk factors for most postures and every posture is not for every body. Practice all postures safely, honoring your body and any preexisting conditions.

Balancing on One Leg

Balancing on one foot is perhaps the easiest way to get your mind to settle down and focus. It is hard to think of anything else. Balancing is a skill that, like everything else, improves with practice. Try not to get frustrated; some days will be better than others. Most important is to get your center of gravity over the balancing leg and leave it there. All balance corrections should be done with what's on the mat. Use your toes and try not to move your center. Setting a gazing point, or drishti, will make balancing easier. Moving your gaze will make a balancing posture more challenging. These postures are a great way to bring control and calm the mind. Remember: Sutra 1.2 of Patanjali's Yoga Sutras define yoga as "the calming of the disturbances of the mind."

Vrksasana

vrik-SHAH-sah-nah

Tree

Vrksasana is the first balancing asana most will encounter. It is a strong asana that strengthens the knee joint and all the surrounding muscles in addition to conditioning the core. Keeping the image of a tree in your mind can be helpful. Root yourself to the earth, grow tall and straight and strong, and extend your limbs. There are many arm and hand variations to explore, even some different leg variations.

Vrksasana will not just improve your balance and strengthen your knee, it will also tone your core and improve your ability to remain calm in the face of challenges as you root your tree and let it breathe.

Start standing in **tadasana**. Set your drishti. Shift all your weight to one leg, moving your center of gravity over that leg. Flex, externally rotate, and abduct the hip of the other leg and flex the knee to place the plantar surface of that foot on the medial side of the standing leg, toes pointing down. The foot must be above or below the knee as you do not want lateral pressure on the knee; it's not supposed to bend that way. As you stand tall, place the hands in anjali mudra (prayer position) in front of your heart center. This is a very traditional gesture for the hands in **vrksasana**.

As always, use what is on the earth to evenly ground your body in the asana. In **vrksasana** and some of the postures to follow, all you will have is one foot. Use it wisely and try to make any balance adjustments (and you will be constantly making balance adjustments, even at the minutest level) with your toes and foot. Making adjustments by moving your hips or shoulders can get you caught up in a compensation pattern you may not be able to find your way out of.

LOWER BODY

You have twenty-six bones in each foot, with fourteen of them making up your toes. These are your phalanges. You should keep them relaxed and allow for movement in the bottom, balancing foot. They are very helpful for making balance corrections on a smaller level, before things get out of hand, and keeping you standing tall. Press the plantar surface of the foot down while lifting the arches.

There are three arches in the foot. The longitudinal medial arch is formed by nine bones, starting at the calcaneus and talus and traveling distally to the navicular, the three cuneiforms, and the first three metatarsals. The longitudinal lateral arch does not lift like the medial one when standing. It is also formed starting at the calcaneus, but then travels distally to the cuboid and the 4th and 5th metatarsals. The transverse arch spans the width of the foot and therefore is in the frontal plane. It is formed starting medially at the cuboid bone, and then spans the three cuneiform bones and the base of the metatarsals. The ligaments of the foot and the thick plantar fascia create the strongest structure known, the arch. They basically form a tripod that will keep you strong and stable. Ground where your arches meet, lift in between, and grow your limbs to the sun.

The knee of the standing leg should be fully extended and hugged with muscle. This means that all of your quadriceps muscles along with the tensor fasciae latae (TFL) will be working to keep that knee feeling strong as it maintains extension.

UPPER BODY

You will feel the abdominal muscles drawing in and working here to keep the torso balanced, stable, and strong. The deep transverse abdominis muscles, the more superficial internal obliques, the even more superficial external obliques, and the most superficial layer, the rectus abdominis muscles, are the biggest and most powerful muscles you will be feeling here.

CALCANEUS

TALUS

CUNEIFORM

METATARSALS

EXTERNAL OBLIQUE

RECTUS ABDOMINIS

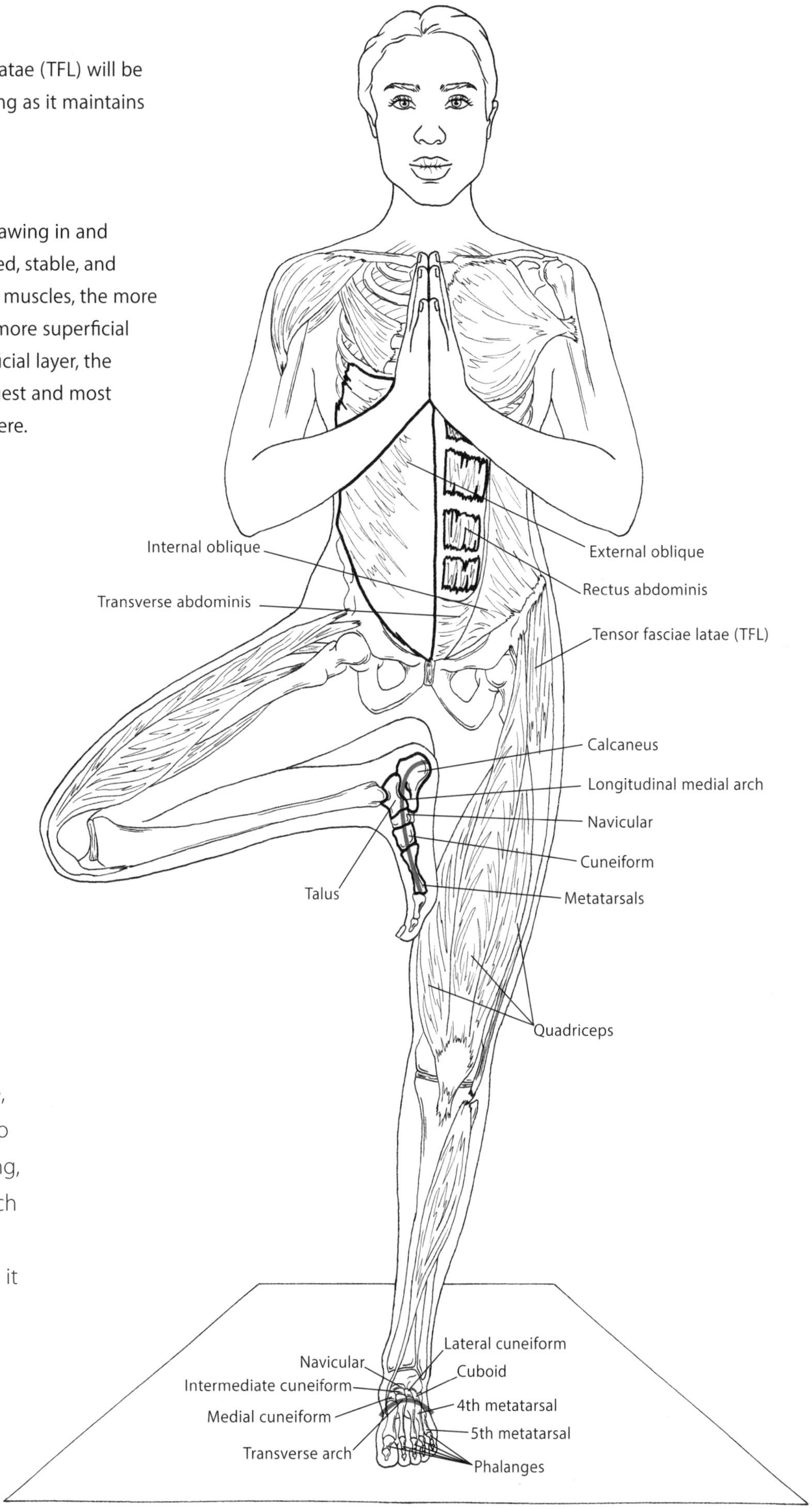

Practice Tip

Once you feel strong and stable, try to shift your drishti upward to make **vrksasana** more challenging, or try different arm variations, such as raising the arms high. If you really want a challenge, try doing it standing on a block!

Garudasana

gah-roo-DAH-sah-nah

Eagle

Garudasana is an inspiring posture. Garuda, the eagle, has a long and storied history and is very revered. Before your eagle takes flight, you first have to get it all together. **Garudasana** asks you to balance on one leg while both arms and legs wrap around each other. Once you get it all together, the trick is to keep it together.

Start balancing on both feet first and set your drishti. Bend the knees a lot, making sure your feet stay evenly weighted. Bring the arms into horizontal abduction (out to the sides and parallel to the floor) to help with balance, then transfer all the weight to one leg. Flexing both knees, bring the other leg around the front of the standing leg. Reach the elevated foot around the back of the calf of the standing leg, bringing the dorsal surface of the foot just above the lateral malleolus of the ankle of the standing leg. The ankle of the elevated foot will be in eversion, meaning the ankle is turning the foot laterally to hold on to that calf. Keeping your center centered, bring the arm on the side of the elevated leg under the other arm, horizontally adducting like crazy, and wrap your forearms around each other, pressing palms together. It's like a prayer with a twist. The hips and knees should be flexed as much as possible as you try to bring the shoulders into flexion as well.

LOWER BODY

Your core muscles will keep your hips in flexion as the adductor muscles, particularly the adductor magnus, work to keep those legs wrapped. The peroneal longus and peroneal brevis along with the extensor digitorum longus will also be working hard at the ankle to keep the foot wrapped around the standing leg. **Garudasana** may cause some medial rotation in the knees, and your knees will afford you some, but any strain felt in the knees must be avoided. You have four big strong ligaments in your knee that are there to keep the knee joint stable; the anterior cruciate ligament (ACL), the posterior cruciate ligament (PCL), the lateral collateral ligament (LCL), and the medial collateral ligament (MCL). Don't test them; knees should always feel strong, never vulnerable.

UPPER BODY

Up above in the shoulders the scapula will protract as the shoulders horizontally adduct, giving both the rhomboid minor and rhomboid major muscles a nice stretch. Flexing at the shoulders to lift the arms will work your shoulder muscles. Lift as high as you can, sending the prayer to heaven while you keep yourself firmly rooted to the earth.

FUN FACT

The story goes that Garuda incubated in his egg for one thousand years before hatching into the beautiful King of All Birds. It is because of Garuda's determination and strength that Vishnu is often seen with Garuda as his mount and mode of transport. Garuda reminds us to be patient and take the time you need to grow and stay strong.

Practice Tip

Keep flexing the knees a lot. This will not only help deepen the wrap in your legs, but it will bring your center of gravity lower, making the balance easier to manage.

PERONEAL LONGUS

PERONEAL BREVIS

ANTERIOR CRUCIATE LIGAMENT (ACL)

POSTERIOR CRUCIATE LIGAMENT (PCL)

LATERAL COLLATERAL LIGAMENT (LCL)

MEDIAL COLLATERAL LIGAMENT (MCL)

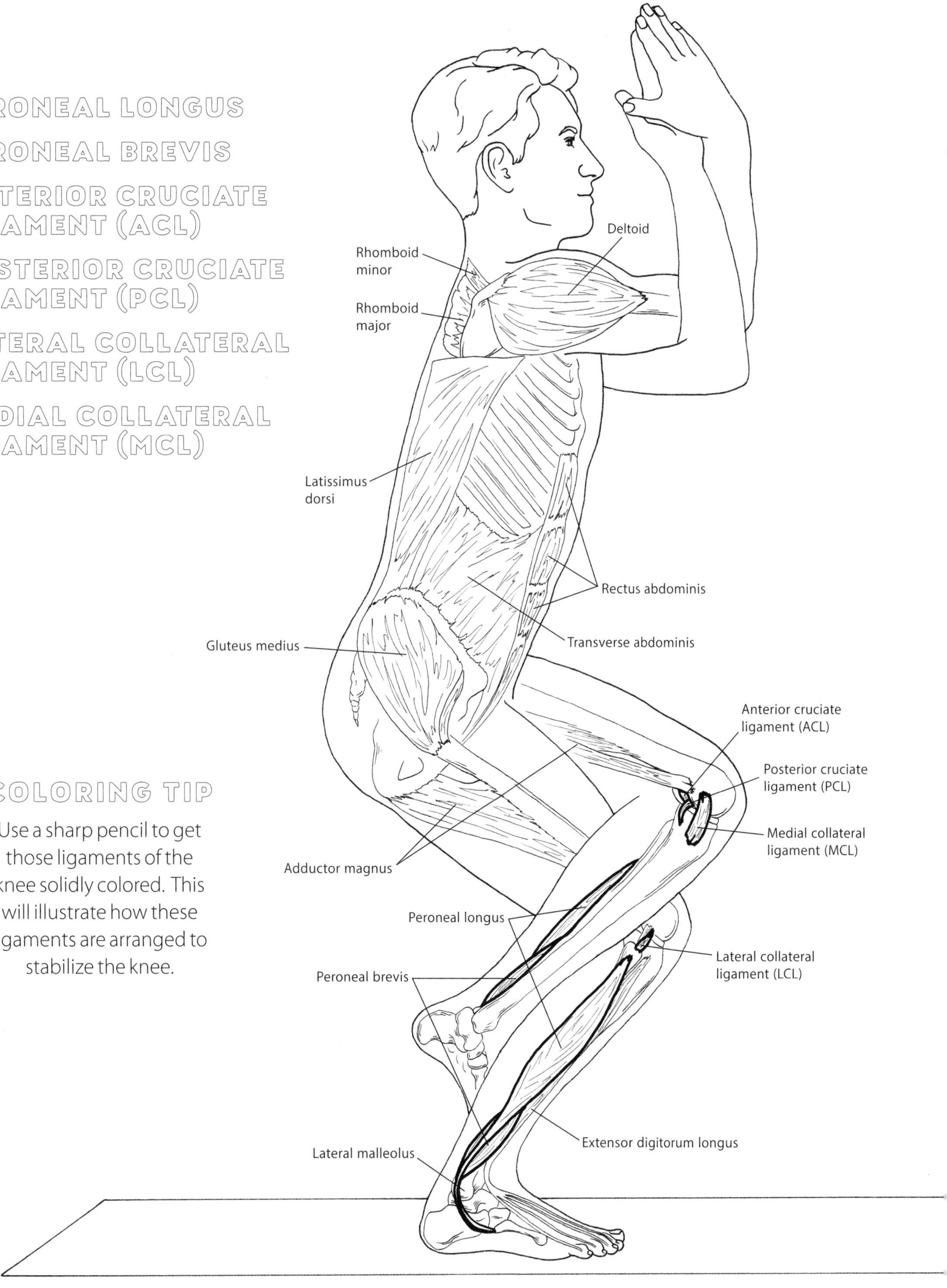

COLORING TIP

Use a sharp pencil to get those ligaments of the knee solidly colored. This will illustrate how these ligaments are arranged to stabilize the knee.

Natarajasana

not-ah-rah-JAH-sah-nah

King Dancer

Natarajasana is a challenging balancing posture that can take many variations. The form shown here is how most will first practice it. Getting proper alignment and becoming more proficient in this asana is a lifelong journey as the body constantly tries to figure out how to get and then maintain balance and stability while lifting that back leg higher and higher.

Start by standing on your mat in **tadasana.** Set your drishti (gazing point) and shift all the weight to one leg, moving your center of gravity over that leg. Reach the hand on the other side for the other foot and send that leg back and up. Simultaneously, flex the hip of the standing leg to bring the upper body forward, reaching the other arm in front of you. Keep the hips even and try to move solely through the sagittal plane as you enter the posture. Work with the counterbalance of weight moving forward and back, and keep your center over that standing leg. Natarajasana will both strengthen and lengthen those big muscles in your legs and give you an opportunity to open up the backbend as well.

LOWER BODY

Your hips will be in opposite ranges of motion. The hip of the standing leg has to maintain some degree of flexion, while the hip of the back leg is in deep extension. The spine is also in deep extension, asking the psoas muscle on the side you are balancing on to work very hard along with the iliacus to maintain flexion while lengthening bilaterally to accommodate the spinal extension.

You will feel the standing leg working hard. Your hamstring muscles will have to give a little to flex the hip, but you mostly feel the quadriceps muscles engaging to maintain knee extension, particularly rectus femoris, the strongest of the quadriceps, as it is also helping to keep the hip in flexion.

It is in the hip of the elevated leg where you will get a deep stretch (provided you can keep your balance!). The entire length of the psoas and iliacus muscles will lengthen along with the other big flexors of the hip, including the rectus femoris, the sartorius, and the tensor fasciae latae (TFL). It is primarily the gluteus maximus that is working here to keep the hip moving toward extension.

UPPER BODY

Like the hips, the shoulders are also working in opposing ranges of motion. The shoulder of the arm holding the foot is in deep extension. This is going to require the latissimus dorsi and teres major muscles along with the posterior deltoid to be fully engaged as you try to pull that foot up toward the sky while you negotiate with the lengthening of the hip flexors to get the fullest expression of this asana. The long head of the triceps muscle along with the lower fibers of the pectoralis major will act as synergists helping with shoulder extension.

In the arm reaching forward, the anterior deltoid and upper fibers of the pectoralis major will be engaged to keep the shoulder flexed. The biceps brachii and coracobrachialis are also strong flexors of the shoulder that will be engaged.

Practice Tip

Keep the hip of the elevated leg even with the hip of the standing leg and be careful not to bring the spine toward rotation by letting the hip of the elevated leg lift up. Remember, you only want to move into this asana through the sagittal plane.

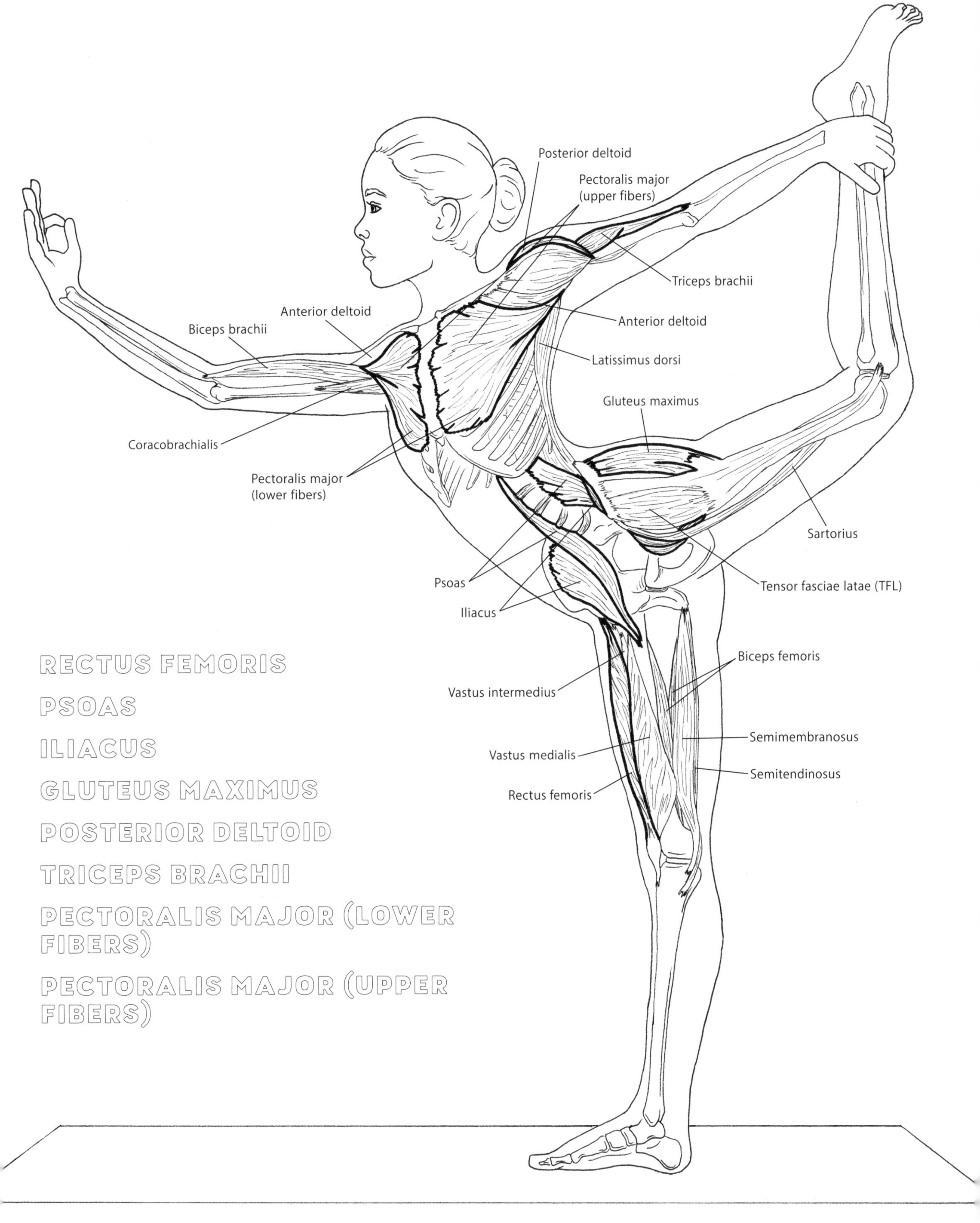

RECTUS FEMORIS

PSOAS

ILIACUS

GLUTEUS MAXIMUS

POSTERIOR DELTOID

TRICEPS BRACHII

PECTORALIS MAJOR (LOWER FIBERS)

PECTORALIS MAJOR (UPPER FIBERS)

Virabhadrasana III

veer-ah-bah-DRAH-sah-nah III

Warrior III

It may take some time to enjoy practicing **virabhadrasana III**. It's a challenging balance that asks you to keep a stable center while reaching forward and back. On the upside, you're only moving through the sagittal plane. Meaning you are not twisting or side bending. Just a forward bend in the hip of the standing leg, really.

There are many ways to enter this asana. I think it is easiest to start from **utthita hasta tadasana** (like **tadasana**, but with arms reaching above the head). This way, your arms are already in alignment, with shoulders in flexion. Transferring all your weight to the standing leg, flex the other knee as you bring it up toward your chest. Then, keep your center as the elevated leg kicks all the way back, parallel to the floor, with the foot in dorsal flexion, toes pointing down. Simultaneously, the hip of the standing leg flexes to 90 degrees, bringing the upper body forward and also parallel to the floor. As you maintain the balance, maintain your breath as well.

For most folks of average flexibility, the most stretch you might feel in this asana is in the shoulders as they move into deep flexion and the back of the standing leg as that hip flexes. But mostly, this is a strong asana and most muscles are working hard as you defy gravity in this, the most challenging of the warriors.

LOWER BODY

The hip flexor muscles in the standing leg, the rectus femoris and sartorius, among others, are working hard to hold the upper body parallel to the floor. It will feel like all the muscles in the standing leg are working like crazy to support all that weight up there and keep the balance, and they basically are. In the beginning, most practitioners will keep the knee of the standing leg bent, but as you improve in this asana, your quadriceps muscles should be brought more into engagement, and the knee of that standing leg should, one day, be fully extended.

UPPER BODY

The psoas and iliacus are the strongest hip flexors and round out the strongest muscles in the hip flexor group. All of the spinal erectors—spinalis, longissimus, and iliocostalis—are trying to maintain spinal stability and neutrality to keep the spine from moving in any direction. You will feel all your abdominal muscles, from the deep internal obliques to the more superficial rectus abdominis, joining the party the keep the upper body feeling strong and steady.

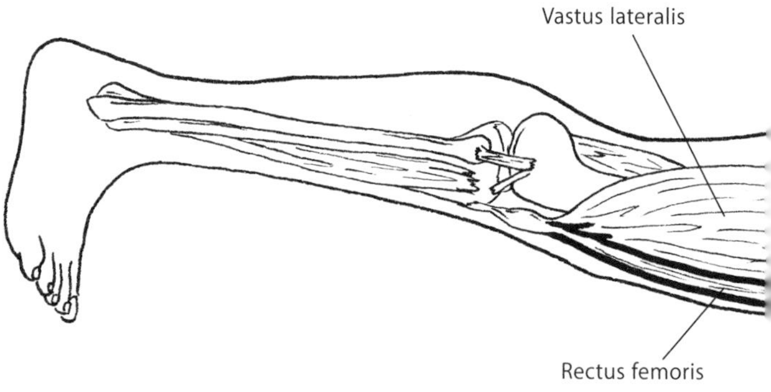

COLORING TIP

The internal obliques originate along the iliac crest and the strong fascia of the abdomen and insert along the anterior surface of the lower three to five ribs. The muscle fibers run diagonally downward, lateral to medial. Highlight how they pull on the bones by coloring them in that direction.

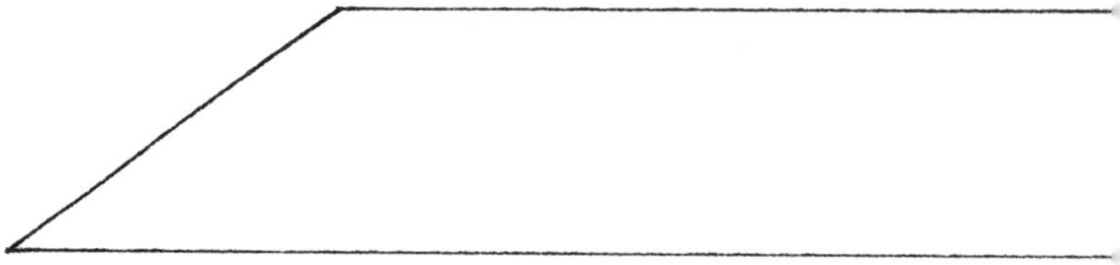

Practice Tip

Keep the hip of the elevated leg even with the hip of the standing leg and keep warrior III in the sagittal plane.

FUN FACT

This is where the Virabhadra, created by Shiva, places the decapitated head of Sati's father, the king, on a stake. No worries though. Once Shiva calmed down, he brought the king back to life and gave him the head of a goat so he would never forget the error of his ways.

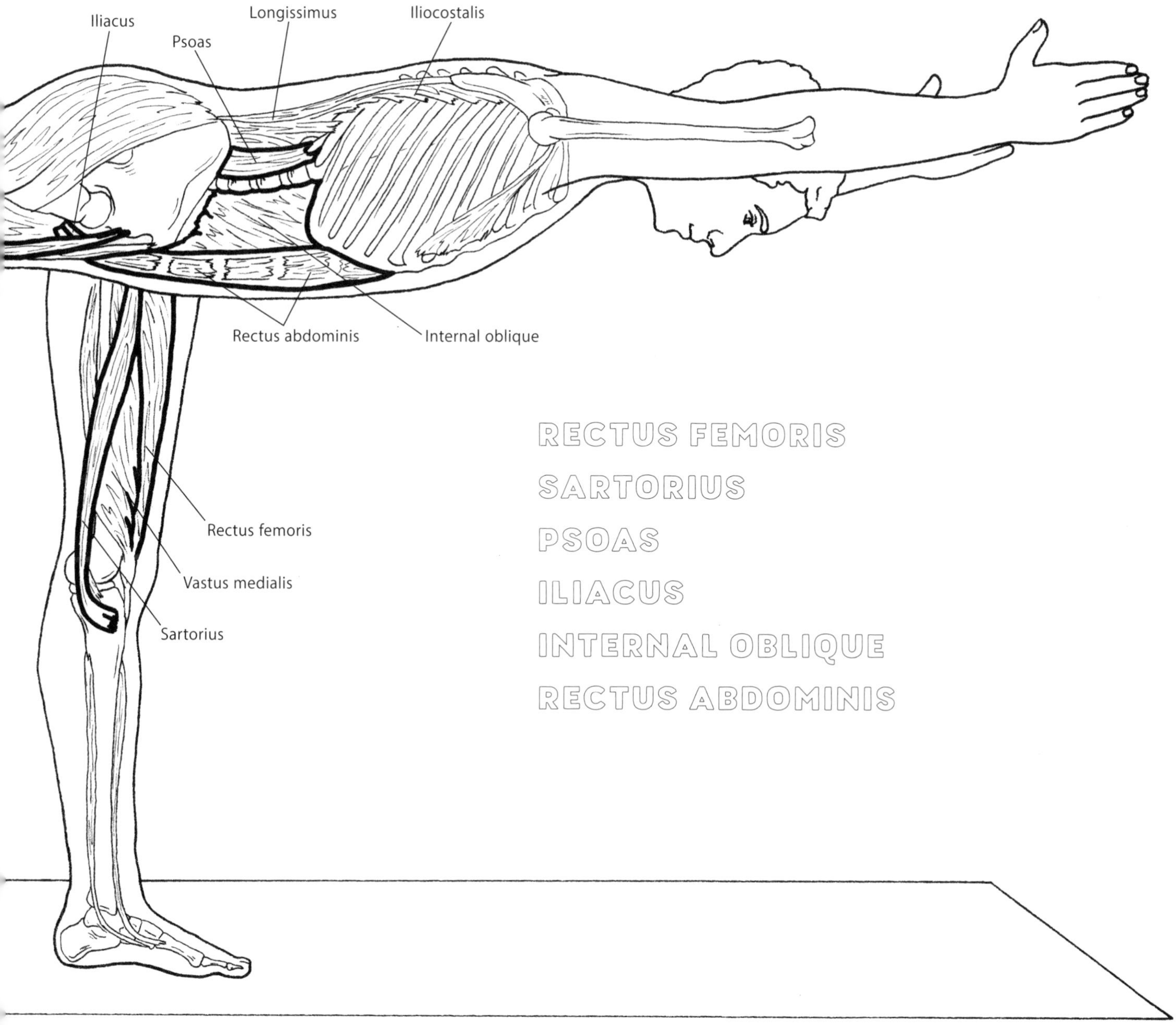

RECTUS FEMORIS

SARTORIUS

PSOAS

ILIACUS

INTERNAL OBLIQUE

RECTUS ABDOMINIS

Arm Balances

Arm balances are primarily strengthening postures. With all the weight ultimately coming to rest in your hands and/or forearms, you will need upper body strength, for sure. But as you start to tap in to the lifting energy of the body, they will become easier. At first, it may be necessary to muscle your way into these asanas, but don't forget that what we really want is balance. Always equally distribute your weight throughout the entire palmar surface of the hands. If you just dump it all into your wrists, you will pay a price. Remember the immortal advice from David Williams, an Ashtangi yogi with decades of yoga practice. He said, "If it hurts, you're doing it wrong." I think he's right!

Astavakrasana

ahsh-tah-vah-KRAH-sah-nah

Eight-Bends Posture

As with most arm balances, you're placing all of your weight in your hands. While some might think of these as great feats of strength, they are just another way to balance the body, and some may take less upper body strength than you think. As with all asanas, it's about getting your center centered.

Start seated on your mat. Place your knee behind your arm about midway between the shoulder and elbow as you bring that hand down on the mat, fingers spread wide. Keep the elbow slightly flexed and the knee relaxed so the foot can just hang, supported by the arm. Hook the ankle of the other leg on top of the leg supported by the arm as you place the other hand down, so both hands are shoulder-distance apart and ready to take weight. In a simultaneous action, lean your weight forward into your hands and out of your seat, bring your elbows into flexion, and send your heart center forward. As that is happening, your pelvis moves up and back as you rotate the spine to send the legs out to the side. The knees move toward extension, and the feet are in dorsal flexion and pronated. Keep adducting the hips and squeeze that arm.

Although you may get a stretch in the hamstrings as you extend the knees, and the gluteal muscles may feel some

EXTENSOR CARPI RADIALIS LONGUS

EXTENSOR CARPI RADIALIS BREVIS

EXTENSOR CARPI ULNARIS

EXTENSOR DIGITORUM

EXTENSOR DIGITORUM LONGUS

TIBIALIS ANTERIOR

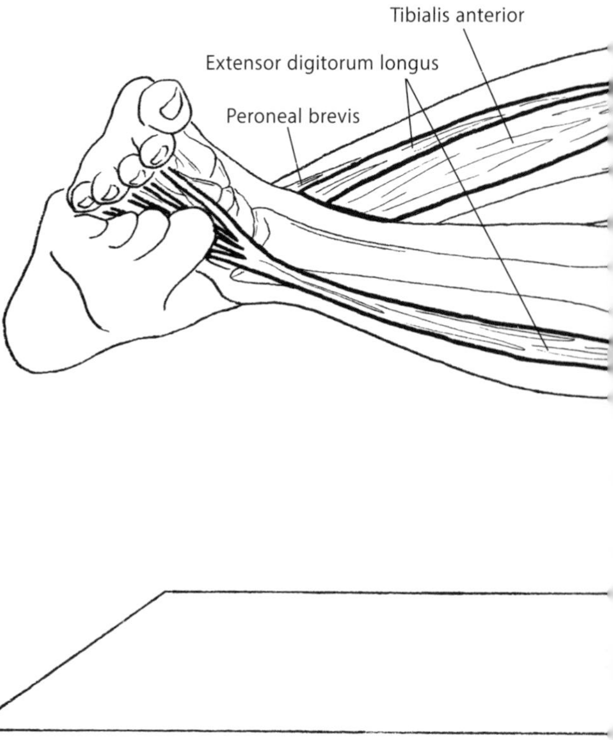

lengthening, we're going to focus more on what's working here. And there is a lot working.

UPPER BODY

The hands are taking all the weight, while the wrists are in deep extension. This is going to really work the extensor carpi radialis longus, extensor carpi radialis brevis, and extensor carpi ulnaris muscles with an assist from the extensor digitorum muscles. To maintain flexion in the elbows, the triceps brachii muscles are in eccentric contraction and resisting the pull of gravity. Your rotator cuff muscles are working hard here to keep the shoulders feeling strong as they support and send the weight down to the hands.

The spine will be in slight flexion and fairly deep rotation, with the exception of the cervicals, which will just be in extension as you try to gaze forward.

LOWER BODY

With the legs wrapped around the upper arm, the adductor muscles are working hard to pull the legs toward each other. The quadriceps muscles are also working pretty hard to extend the knees. Working your way down the legs, you will feel the peroneal muscles contracting to pronate the ankles. Extensor digitorum longus will help the peroneal muscles pronate the ankle and also assist the tibialis anterior to keep the foot in dorsal flexion.

FUN FACT

Astavakrasana is named after the famous yogic sage Ashtavakra. His mother attended her father's Vedic classes along with Ashtavakra's father while he was still in the womb. One day, from his mother's belly, he corrected his father's pronunciation of the Vedas. His father was so irate he cursed Ashtavakra to be born with eight bends in his body. Ashtavakra had the last laugh and became the most honored Vedic scholar in the land.

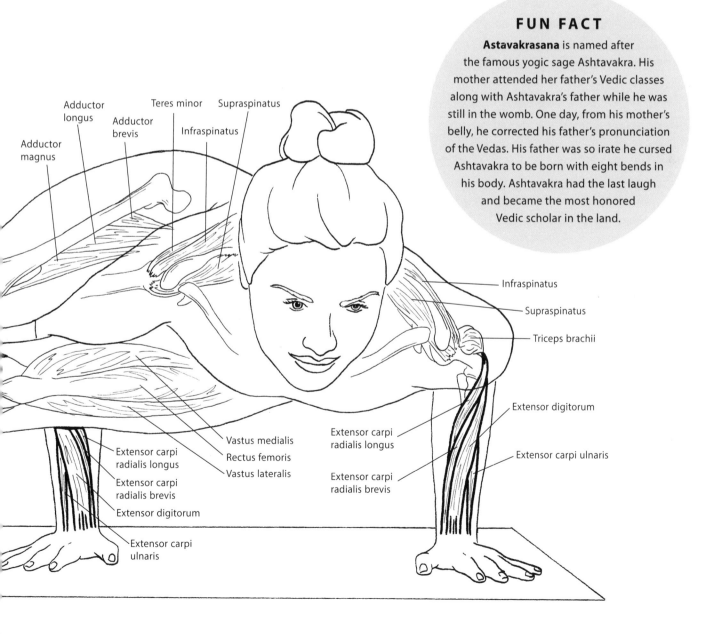

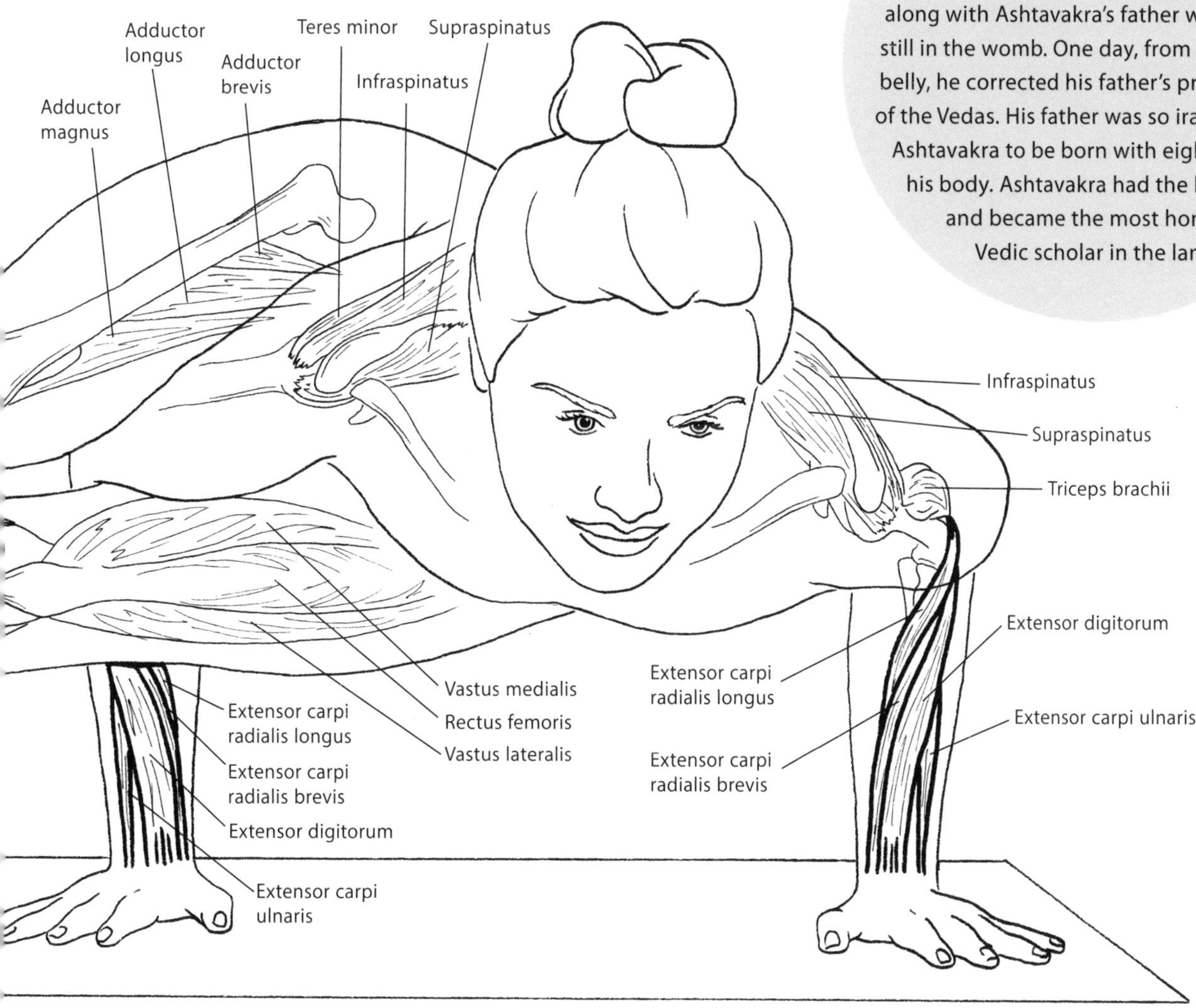

Parsva Bakasana

PARS-vah bah-KAH-sah-nah

Side Crow

Having a strong and stable **bakasana** (crow pose, in which both knees rest on the arms) is not a prerequisite for **parsva bakasana**; in fact, some find it easier (when modified) than the straight-on bakasana. Most of your spine will be in deep rotation, but your cervical spine will be in extension as you look forward. Obviously all the weight is in your arms, so a fair amount of upper body strength is necessary, but more than that is finding the balance. As it is in all aspects of yoga, we are looking for balance.

Most will first attempt **parsva bakasana** from a squat position. From a deep squat, rotate the spine to hook your upper arm outside the opposite knee/lower thigh (keeping the heels lifted will make it easier). Holding the twist, place the hands down along the side body, shoulder-distance apart, fingers pointing forward and spread wide. Keep the front leg connected to the upper arm and lean forward, taking weight out of the feet and into the hands, keeping the hips floating in the middle. Keep your knees and ankles stacked to avoid taking the rotation into your pelvis.

UPPER BODY

Like most arm balances, the wrists will be in deep extension, asking the wrist extensor muscles to work hard. On the other side, the flexors of the wrists will get a deep stretch. The biggest and most superficial of these are the flexor carpi radialis, flexor carpi ulnaris, and palmaris longus muscles.

Having most of your weight on one arm while the elbow maintains about 90 degrees of flexion is asking for a lot of strength from the biceps brachii, brachialis, and brachioradialis muscles. It will get some help from the flexor carpi radialis, flexor carpi ulnaris, and palmaris longus muscles as they cross over the elbow joint as well and will act as synergists during elbow flexion. Pay attention as you ask the distal end of these muscles to lengthen and the proximal ends to strengthen. If you can keep your center of gravity stable, these muscles will have to work less.

The shoulders are held in external rotation, strengthening the posterior deltoid muscles along with the two rotator cuff muscles that assist in internal rotation at the glenohumeral joint: the infraspinatus and teres minor muscles.

LOWER BODY

There is work to be done to keep the knees evenly stacked, one on top of the other. You will need to employ the gluteu maximus of the top leg to keep that top knee from creepin too far forward. Otherwise, the lower body is primarily supported by the strength of the upper body and your abili to keep your center over your hands.

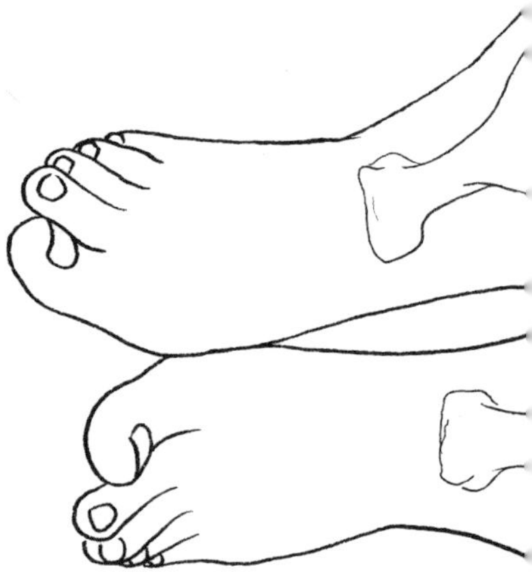

Practice Tip

To modify this posture and make it more accessible, place the lower hip on the elbow and use both arms to take the weight. As your upper body strength improves, you will be able to float your hips. As your balance improves, you will use less muscle. It will get easier!

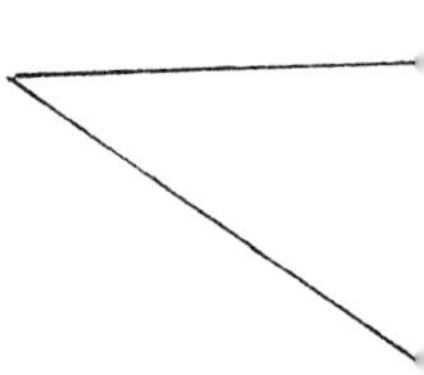

FLEXOR CARPI RADIALIS
FLEXOR CARPI ULNARIS
PALMARIS LONGUS
INFRASPINATUS
TERES MINOR
GLUTEUS MAXIMUS

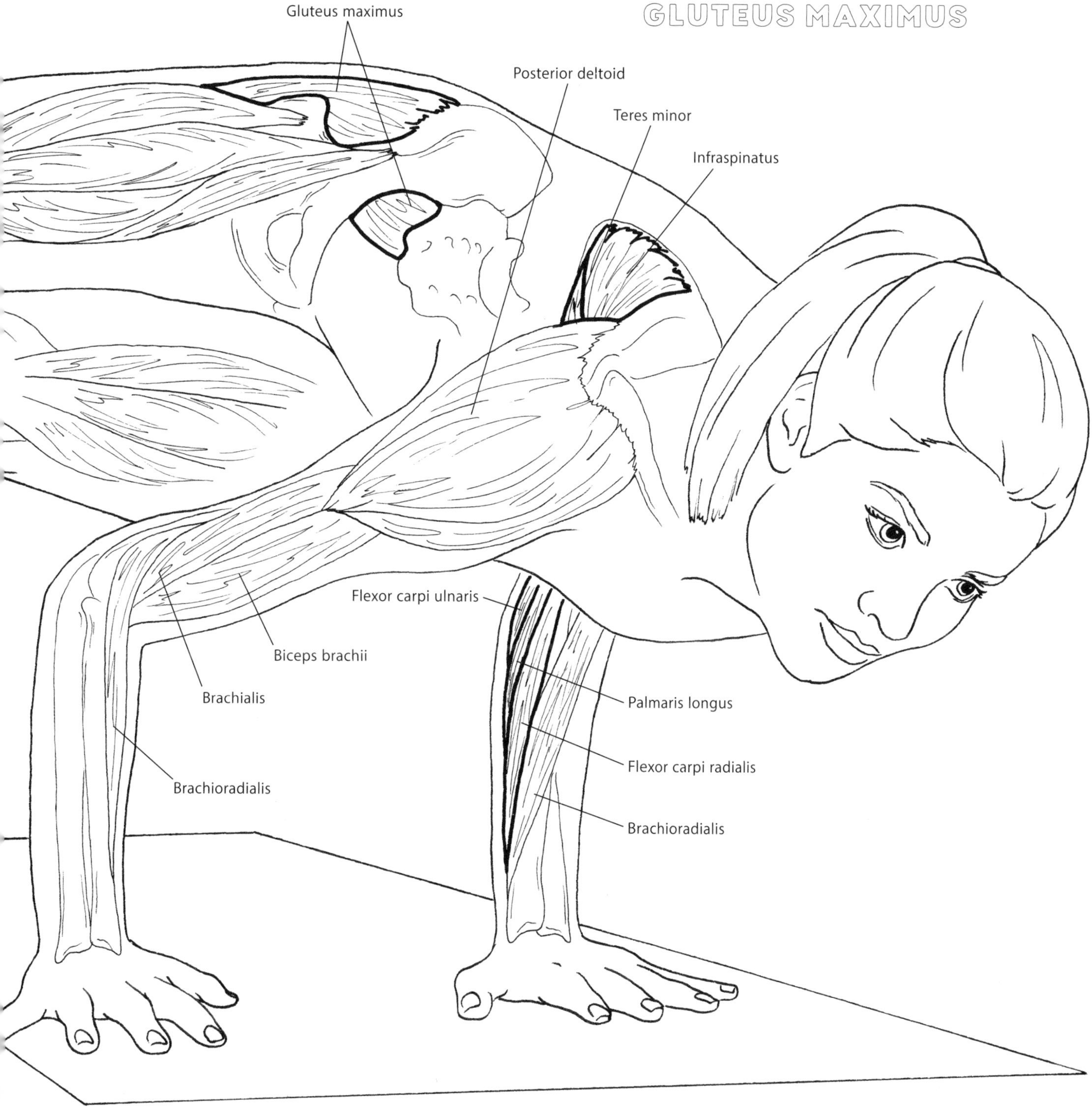

Kukkutasana

koo-koo-TAH-sah-nah

Rooster

Kukkutasana takes your lotus **(padmasana)** to a whole new level, literally. This asana can be dated at least as far back as the 15th century, as it is one of the asanas found in the *Hatha Yoga Pradipika,* the first text known to describe hatha yoga practices, including asana practice, written by Swami Svatmarama. This is an advanced asana as it requires a full padmasana and a fair amount of upper body and core strength.

Start seated on your mat and fold your legs into **padmasana**. Then slip your arms between the calf and thigh of each leg. Ground your hands evenly as you bring your center of gravity forward and take all the weight out of your seat and into your hands. I know it sounds so simple, but this will take great power and great control.

LOWER BODY

The hips will be abducted and in deep external rotation to maintain the lotus, and they will be brought into deep flexion as the legs lift up. Lotus pretty much holds itself together; the real work here is maintaining the hip flexion. Your biggest, strongest hip flexors, namely the psoas and iliacus, are working really, really hard here.

UPPER BODY

Adding to the challenge of this asana is keeping the rib cage and heart center forward and elevated, the proud chest of a rooster. The anterior, middle, and posterior scalene muscles of the neck will all be working here to keep the chest lifted even as the spine is drawn toward flexion. Because most of the spine will be flexed (your cervical spine will go into extension to face forward), the rectus abdominis and both the internal and external obliques will be called into action to keep the spine steady as you hold the asana.

The triceps brachii muscles in the arms will be strongly engaged to keep the elbows extended. To keep the elbows from going into flexion, the flexors of the elbow must maintain eccentric contraction. Brachialis is a strong elbow flexor and sometimes overlooked, literally, as it lies deep to the biceps brachii, a very showy muscle.

The muscles along the posterior back will not feel like they are getting much of a stretch here as they will be working hard in eccentric contraction so the torso can remain lifted and steady.

FUN FACT

The rooster is a symbol of ego in Hindu mythology. **Kukkutasana** will also challenge the ego and its sense of pride of accomplishment once you are able to express the posture. Kukkutasana reminds us to conquer the ego, not the asana.

Practice Tip

If the body is strong and flexible enough, sometimes the hardest part of **kukkutasana** can be slipping the arms between the thigh and calf. If you are sweaty enough, getting that sweat on your arms may be helpful to get them to slip right through!

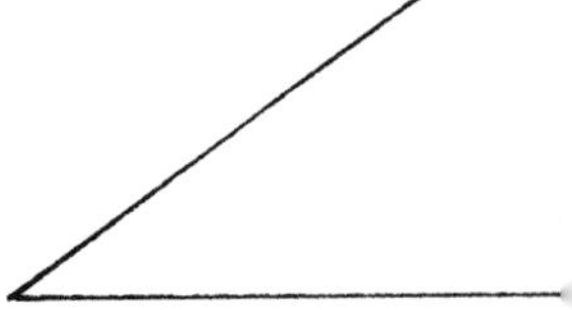

COLORING TIP

The psoas and iliacus muscles eventually come together and form the iliopsoas and attach with a common tendon. Blending the colors you choose for these muscles as they travel down toward the insertion site can help remind you of this.

PSOAS
ILIACUS
RECTUS ABDOMINIS
INTERNAL OBLIQUE
BRACHIALIS

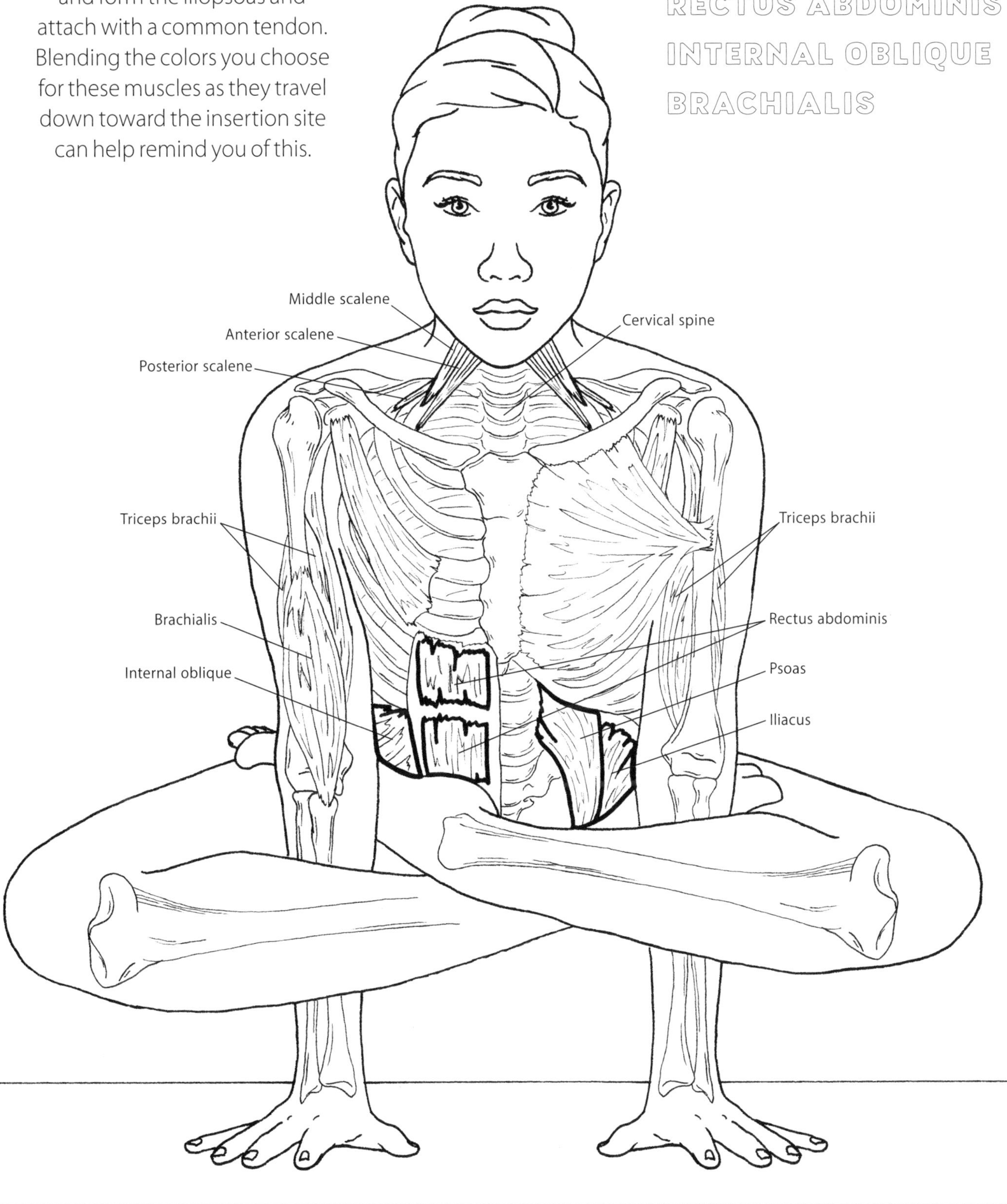

Eka Pada Bakasana

EK-ah PAH-dah bah-KAH-sah-nah

One-Legged Crow

Eka pada bakasana is an opportunity for your crow to take flight. This is a very advanced asana, which requires a strong and stable **bakasana** (crow pose, in which both knees rest on the flexed arms) first. Eka pada bakasana will ask for more strength, particularly in the hip that's extending the leg up and back. It is also asking for a strong center of gravity as you shift more weight to one side as the leg on the other side lifts off.

There are various ways to approach this asana. Some find it easier to start from **bakasana** and then send one leg back and up. For those with a solid tripod headstand, such as **sirsasana B**, you may find it easier to start there and bring one knee to the upper arm, keeping the other leg fully extended. Of course, now you have to lift the head and look forward. No matter how you get there, once you do get there, make sure to smile as this is a very accomplished asana.

UPPER BODY

With all the weight in your hands and your wrists in extension, pretty much all of the muscles along the posterior forearm and wrist will be called into the action. The biggest and most superficial of these are the extensor carpi radialis longus and extensor carpi radialis brevis muscles along with the extensor carpi ulnaris and extensor digitorum muscles. You will also feel the deeper extensor muscles of the forearm, including the extensor digiti minimi, extensor indicis, extensor pollicis longus, and extensor pollicis brevis muscles.

The elbows are held in flexion, keeping your biceps brachii, brachialis, and brachioradialis working hard in concentric contraction, while the triceps brachii muscles are working hard in eccentric contraction to keep the elbows stable.

LOWER BODY

As your hands support the weight of the body, the gluteus maximus will be working its butt off (pun intended) to keep the extended leg lifting high. It will get a lot of help from the hamstring muscles. The other leg will have an easier time of it as the upper body will support it.

FUN FACT

Stories have been told of crows that bring gifts to humans who feed them or treat them kindly. Feed this asana with practice and treat this asana kindly and you will receive gifts of strength, balance, and confidence.

Practice Tip

Placing strong, sturdy yoga blocks under the shoulders to help take the weight will make **eka pada bakasana** more available until you build up enough upper body strength to hold the asana in just your hands.

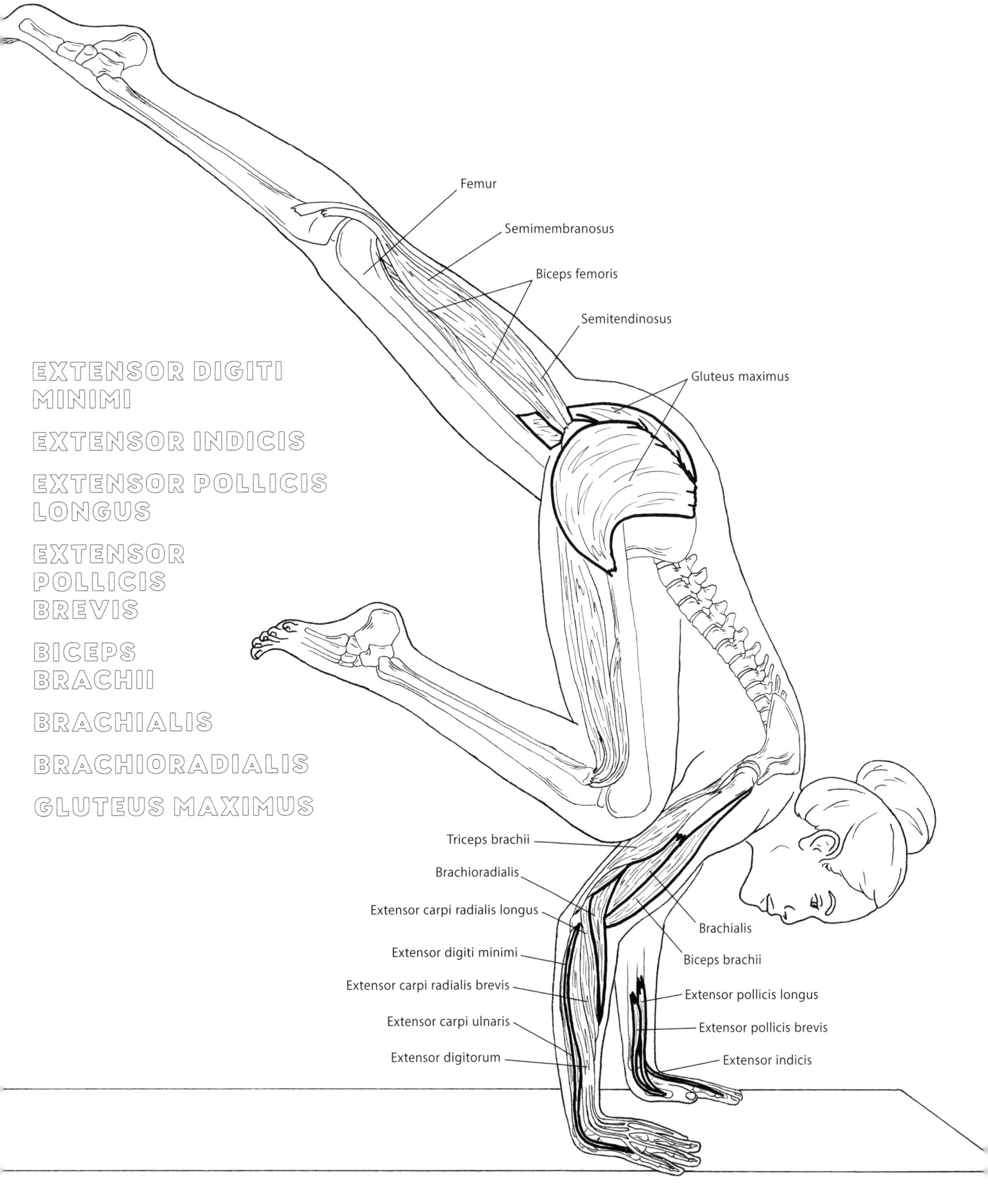
Femur
Semimembranosus
Biceps femoris
Semitendinosus
Gluteus maximus
EXTENSOR DIGITI MINIMI
EXTENSOR INDICIS
EXTENSOR POLLICIS LONGUS
EXTENSOR POLLICIS BREVIS
BICEPS BRACHII
BRACHIALIS
BRACHIORADIALIS
GLUTEUS MAXIMUS
Triceps brachii
Brachioradialis
Extensor carpi radialis longus
Extensor digiti minimi
Extensor carpi radialis brevis
Extensor carpi ulnaris
Extensor digitorum
Brachialis
Biceps brachii
Extensor pollicis longus
Extensor pollicis brevis
Extensor indicis

Adho Mukha Vrksasana

AH-doh MOO-kah vrik-SHAH-sah-nah

Downward-Facing Tree

I think of **adho mukha vrksasana** as a fundamental and foundational inversion and, all things being healthy, the first inversion I would teach a student. The reason for this is that it's the safest. There is no weight in the neck or head, and it's easier on the arms, though it's not easy. Anyone who had done this as a kid can usually get back up there pretty quickly as an adult; that is the beauty of muscle memory. For others approaching it for the first time, it may take a while.

Start on your mat in **adho mukha svanasana**. Ground your hands and externally rotate your shoulders as you move toward pronation in your forearms. Your shoulders should feel really strong here, and the weight should be evenly distributed throughout the hands. The creases in your wrists should create horizontal lines parallel to the front edge of the mat. The length of your hamstrings will determine how much effort you will need to pull your pelvis up and over your shoulders. At first, it's best to use your strongest leg to kick off the floor while the other leg sweeps up. Keep your spine neutral and pelvis even; focus on kicking the pelvis up and over the shoulders rather than getting the feet over the head. Using a wall at first is helpful. Knowing how to fall out of the handstand, if necessary, is imperative. Never rotate the spine if you fall out of your handstand. You're much safer either going backward and landing in **urdhva dhanurasana** (if you are confident you can) or the other way and landing on your feet.

UPPER BODY

Since all the weight is in the shoulders and down to the hands in this asana, that is where we will focus.

The shoulders, arms, and hands in **adho mukha vrksasana** are the same as in adho mukha svanasana. The serratus anterior muscles must work here both to keep the scapula pressed onto the posterior ribs and pulling inferiorly and away from the ears. The glenohumeral joint should be kept in external rotation as the forearm is held in pronation. The pronator teres and pronator quadratus muscles will do this for you with some help from the brachioradialis. As these muscles hold it together, other muscles in the forearm and palm will be active in keeping the balance by making corrections with your fingers. As with all asanas, you should make balance corrections with what's on the ground. In this case, your hands, and more specifically, your phalanges, or fingers. As your palms press into the earth, let your fingers negotiate the balance. Much the same way your toes correct your balance when you are standing.

LOWER BODY

The hamstring and quadriceps muscles are working hard to keep the legs strong. The iliopsoas also works really hard here to prevent the pelvis and spine from moving out of neutral and to keep your center of gravity. Everybody has a foot position that works for them. There are different ideas of what the feet should be doing. I think that whether you draw energy up through your heels, toes, or balls of your feet, do what gives you the strongest lift. Best of all, enjoy a view of the world from a different perspective and, as always, remember to breathe.

FUN FACT

As hard as you feel your fingers working, you don't actually have any muscles in the fingers. It is the thirty-four muscles of the palms and forearms that give your fingers strength.

SERRATUS ANTERIOR
PRONATOR TERES
PRONATOR QUADRATUS
BRACHIORADIALIS

COLORING TIP

The serratus anterior muscles insert along the anterior surface of the medial border of the scapula and fan out to their origin site at ribs 1 through 8. Coloring in the ribs to contrast will really show you the strength of these "superhero" muscles.

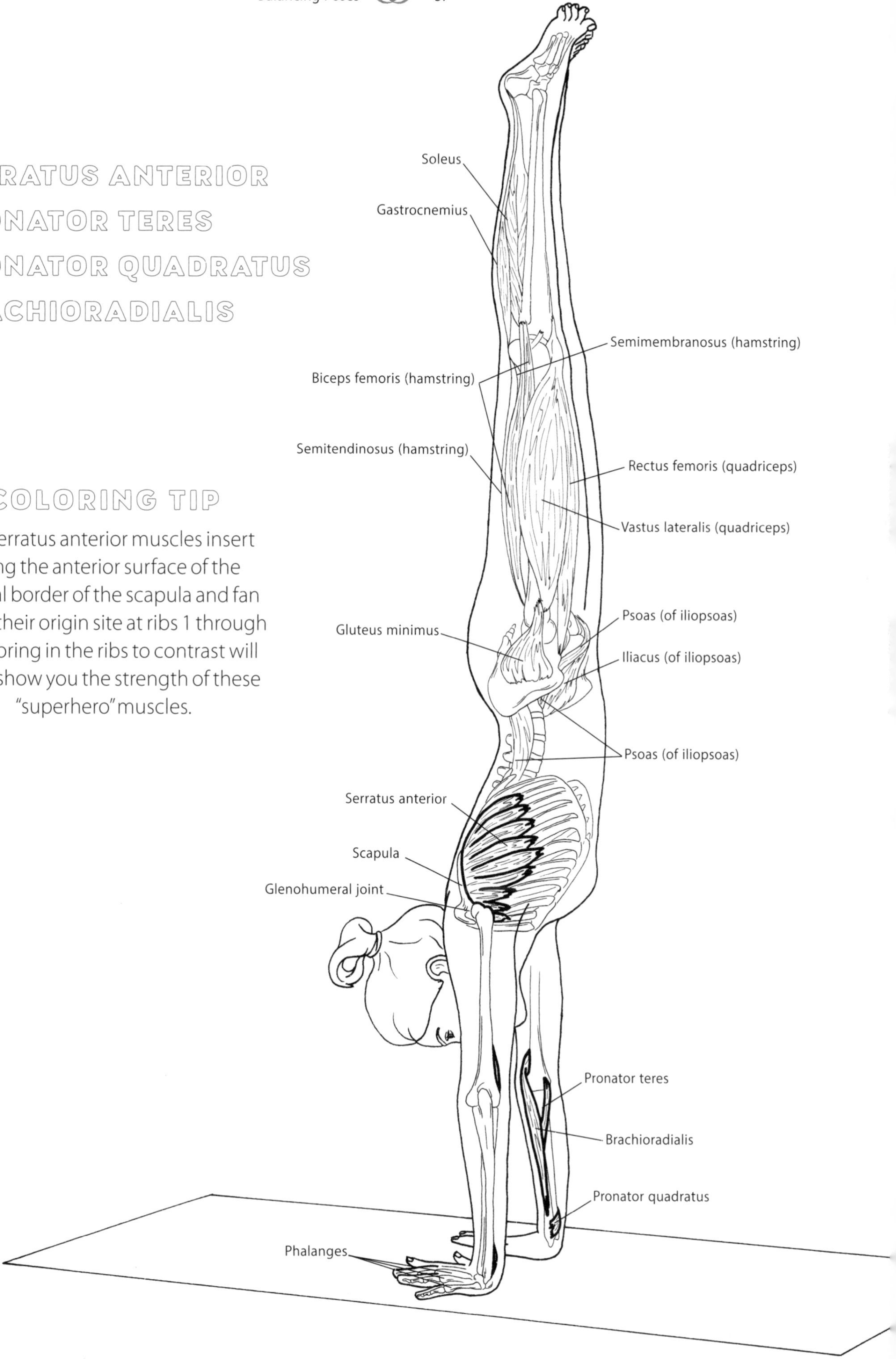

Pincha Mayurasana

PIN-chah my-ur-AH-sah-nah

Feather of the Peacock

Pincha mayurasana is often confused with its "sister" posture, **vrishchikasana,** or scorpion. When most practitioners first approach the forearm balance they are usually somewhere between these two asanas; not quite straight up and down, as in **pincha mayurasana**, but not quite in a full-on backbend like vrishchikasana either. Although they are both forearm balances, that is where the similarity ends. Pincha mayurasana is basically a headstand body, but the head is floating, by virtue of the forearms taking all the weight as your shoulders maintain deep flexion.

Starting on your mat in **adho mukha svanasana**, bring the forearms down on the mat, shoulder-distance apart and parallel to each other, fingers spread wide. As you kick your feet up, remember, the first goal is to establish the alignment of the pelvis over the shoulders. Once up, you are trying to establish a neutral body. Because you have just turned yourself upside down, this will take more effort than when you are the other way around. Again, using a wall in the beginning is helpful. Knowing how to safely fall out of the asana, if you need to, is imperative.

UPPER BODY

Since most of the action here is in the shoulders, that is where we're going to focus. All the shoulder flexor muscles are going to have to work hard here. That includes the anterior deltoid, the upper fibers of the pectoralis major, and the long head of the biceps brachii muscles. To complement this, the big extensor muscles of the shoulders have to really lengthen. Getting a good stretch here are the posterior deltoid, the lower fibers of the pectoralis major, the long head of the triceps brachii, latissimus dorsi, teres major, infraspinatus, and teres minor muscles. That's a lot of muscles getting to really open up.

The elbows are held in flexion at about 90 degrees, and the forearms are pronated. The biceps brachii are called into action to hold the elbows in flexion. It's getting a lot of help from the brachialis, brachioradialis, flexor carpi radialis, and palmaris longus muscles. To keep the forearms in pronation so the hands can firmly ground, you will also feel the pronator teres, which runs along the palmar side of the forearm (out of view here) and the pronator quadratus muscles working hard.

LOWER BODY

Like in **sirsasana** (headstand), ideally your lower body is energetically reaching up. This is not to say that those big muscles in the legs aren't engaged to keep the legs straight and maintain the posture, but that you should not forget to engage the energetic aspect of this and all the asanas.

FUN FACT

Peacocks are the national bird of India and associated with several Hindu gods and goddesses, including the goddess of wealth, Lakshmi. Peacock feathers are often kept in the home to invite wealth and prosperity into the household.

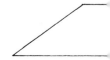

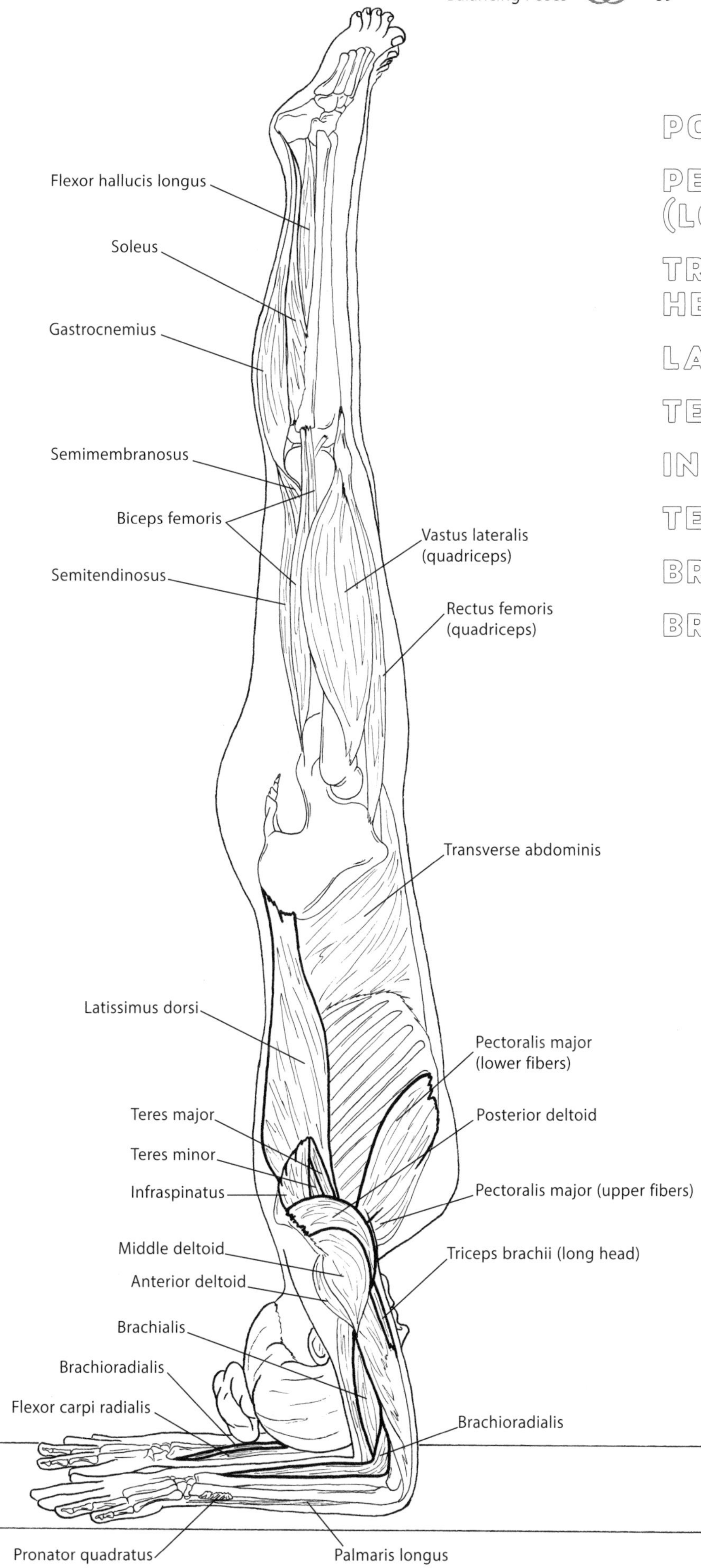

POSTERIOR DELTOID

PECTORALIS MAJOR (LOWER FIBERS)

TRICEPS BRACHII (LONG HEAD)

LATISSIMUS DORSI

TERES MAJOR

INFRASPINATUS

TERES MINOR

BRACHIALIS

BRACHIORADIALIS

Practice Tip

Don't let your elbows take all the weight here. Evenly distribute the weight throughout the forearm and ground the hands like crazy, right up to your fingertips.

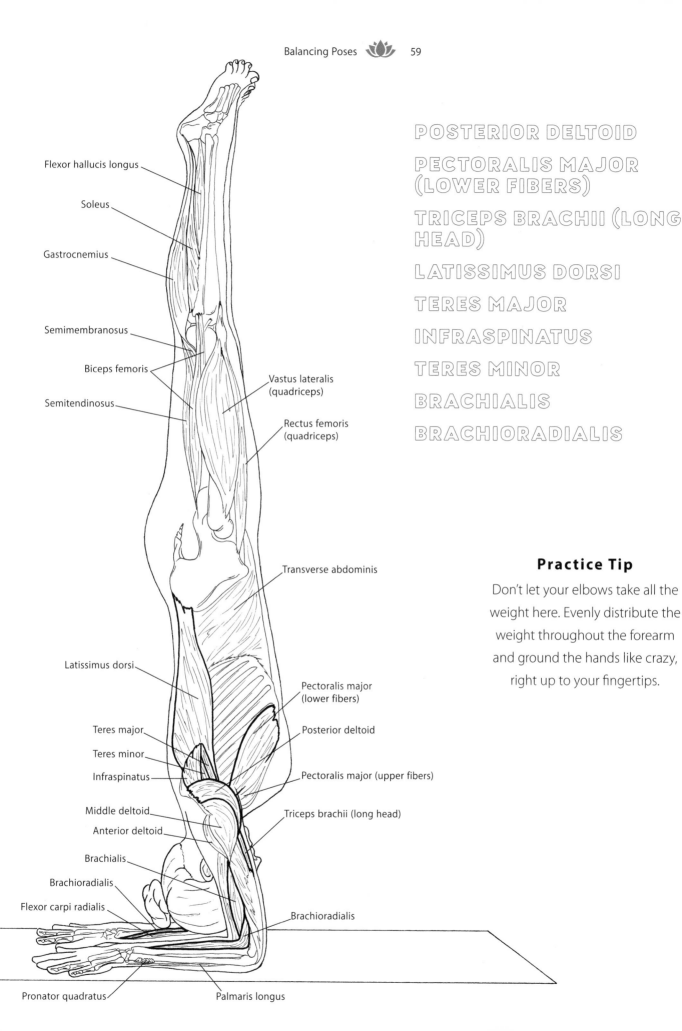

Inversions

Inversions give you the opportunity to turn your world upside down. Technically speaking, any posture that brings your head below your heart is an inversion, including some arm balances. We will explore two of the more common inversions, ***sirsasana B*** *and* ***salamba sarvangasana****, which is not typically considered a balancing pose but is included here.*

For some, going upside down can be a bit scary, but inversions have great health benefits and should be included in a well-rounded practice.

Salamba Sarvangasana

sah-LAHM-bah sar-vahn-GAH-sah-nah

Supported All-Limbs Posture

Salamba sarvangasana is named "all limbs" posture for a reason. It is asking a lot. As challenging as it is to accomplish, most practitioners can express this asana, though it may take a little (or a lot) of time to get the full expression. The idea is to get the body in a vertical line, with the spine in deep flexion around the junction of C7 and T1. The elbows are flexed and the shoulders are in deep extension and external rotation. When properly aligned, the shoulders should reach about 90 degrees in extension. This asana is asking a lot, but most folks can do it!

Start lying supine on your mat with your arms along your sides, palms down. Draw your knees toward your chest and send your feet to the sky, lifting your pelvis. Flexing the elbows, place the hands on the back with fingers pointing up. Try to keep your elbows no wider than your shoulders and get your hands as close to the shoulders as possible. As all the weight falls to the shoulders and neck, we are going to focus on what should be going on up there (or down there?).

UPPER BODY

Your infraspinatus, teres minor, and posterior deltoid will have to work double time to keep the shoulders externally rotated and in extension. The triceps muscles will be a big synergist here to maintain deep shoulder extension. What you lack in shoulder extension will be made up in deeper spinal flexion. Remember, the goal is to get your body as vertical as possible.

Your scapula should be retracted and in downward rotation. This is going to ask both rhomboid major and rhomboid minor muscles to contract along with the levator scapula muscles. Your scapula should provide a nice platform to take a lot of the weight of the body.

The neck is also taking weight as the cervical spine is in deep flexion. This will require the ligamentum nuchae, a very flexible ligament in your neck, to lengthen. Straining this ligament is perhaps the most common injury folks experience with this asana. Stabilizing your neck will ask the SCM muscle and the scalenes to hold steady and support the neck.

Don't forget that the upper arms, all the way to the elbows, should be grounded. If your arms feel light, you are putting more weight than you should in the neck and shoulders.

LOWER BODY

It's all about staying strong here. The big muscles of the upper and lower legs will all be working hard. You will feel all the quadriceps muscles working to keep the knees extended and all the hamstrings trying to pull the hips out of flexion. The gastrocnemius and soleus will be pulling the ankle toward plantar flexion. But up toward the toes you want to press the balls of the feet up and spread the toes wide.

TRICEPS BRACHII
RHOMBOID MAJOR
RHOMBOID MINOR
LEVATOR SCAPULA
LIGAMENTUM NUCHAE
ANTERIOR SCALENE
MIDDLE SCALENE

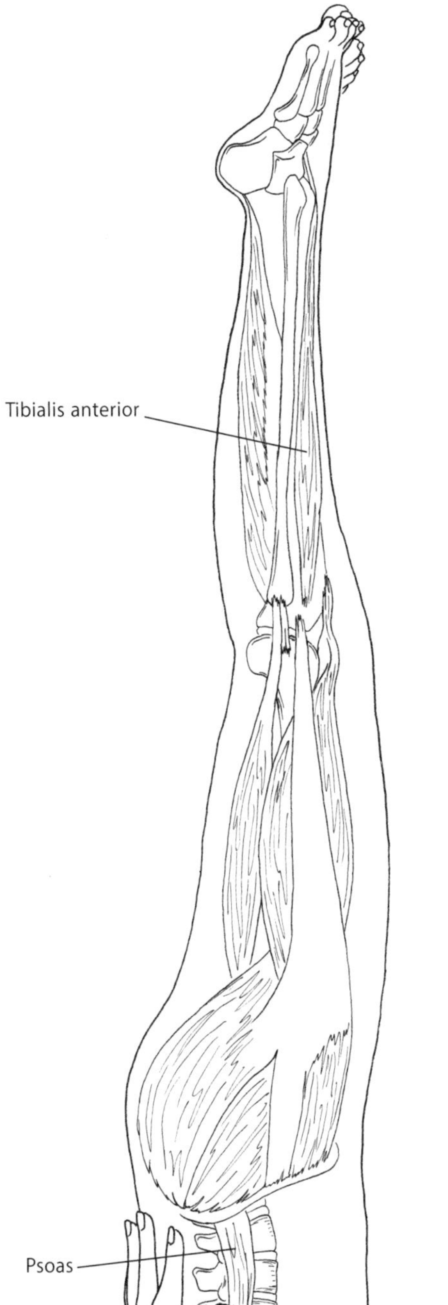

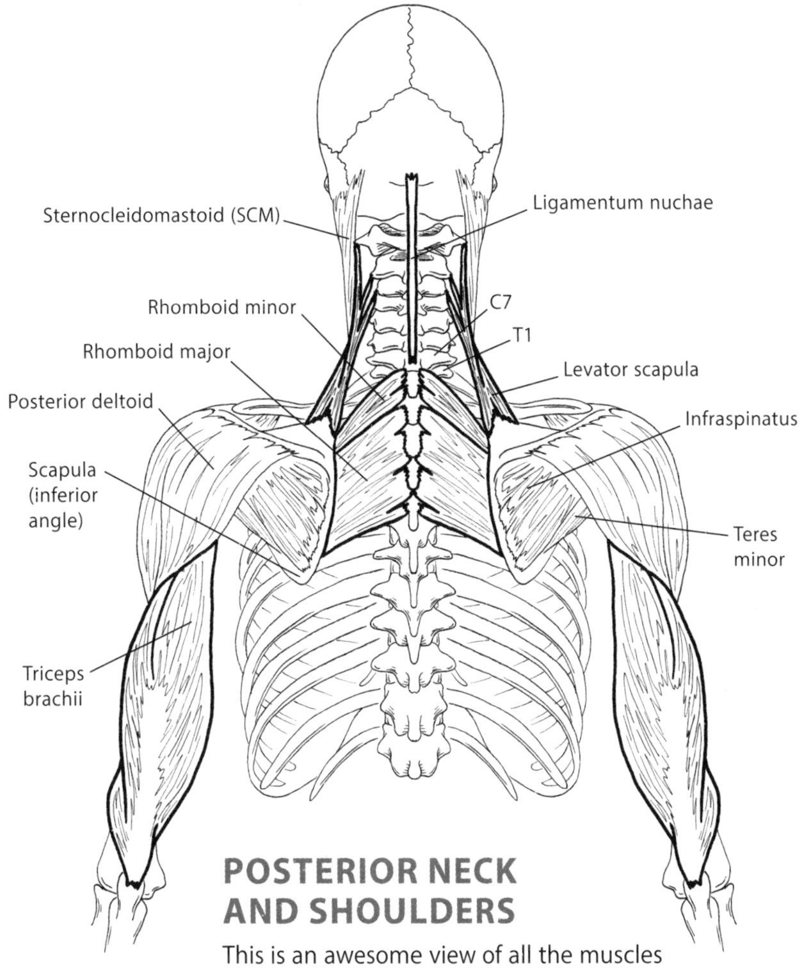

POSTERIOR NECK AND SHOULDERS

This is an awesome view of all the muscles in the posterior neck and shoulders that accommodate this pose. The ligamentum nuchae is a strong ligament running from the occiput to the C7 vertebra. This asana wants it to lengthen. We know that ligaments are not meant to stretch but to maintain stability. Don't ask for more than this ligament is willing to give.

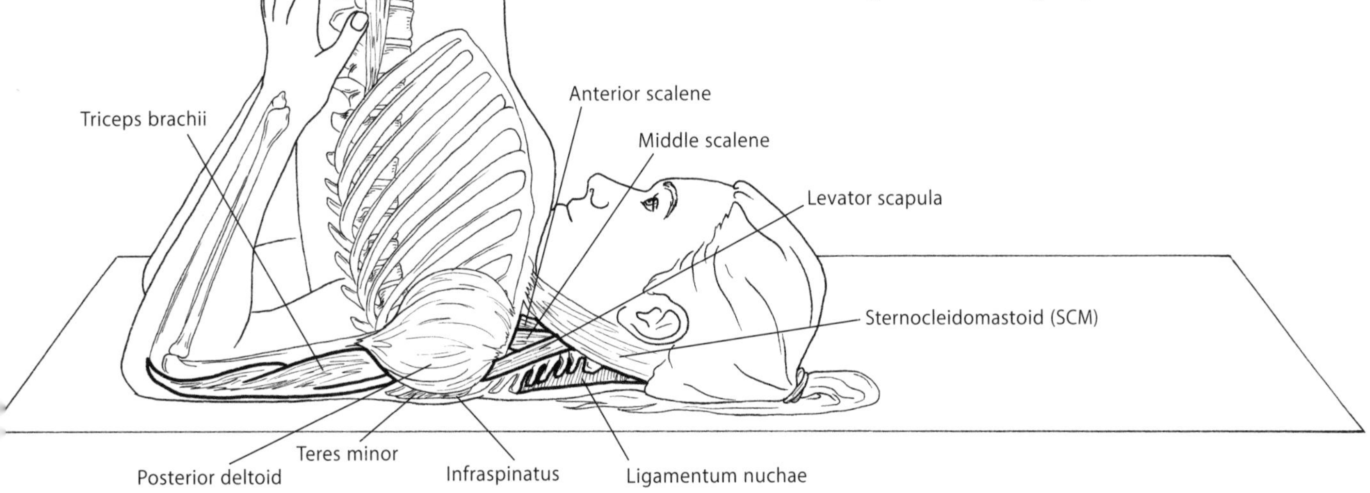

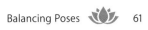

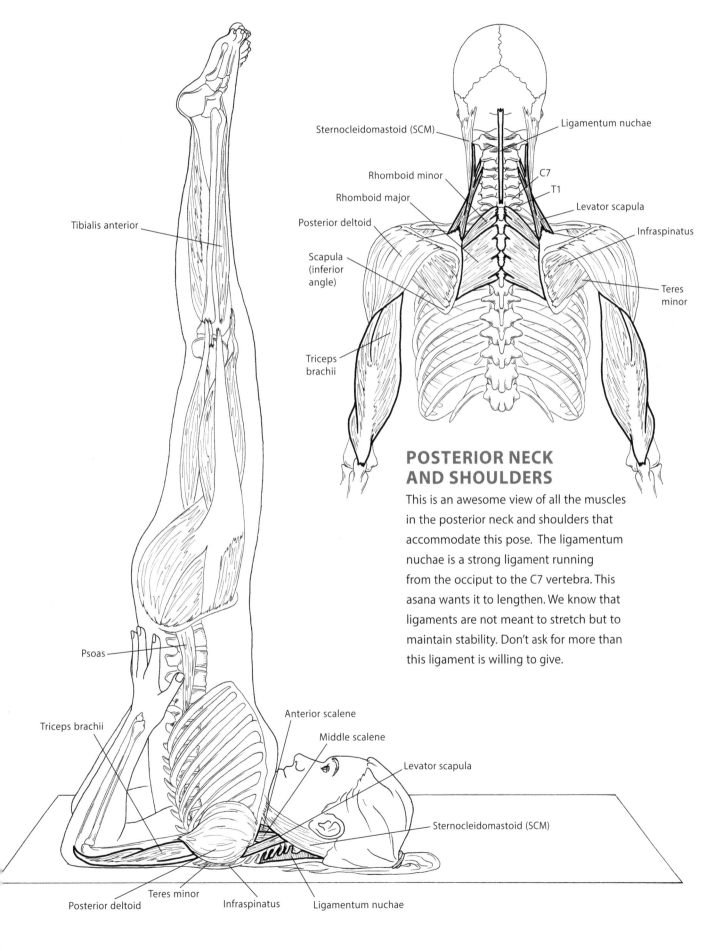

Sirsasana B

sheer-SHAH-sah-nah B

Tripod Headstand

If you tried a headstand as a kid, chances are this is the way you did it. If you have never done a headstand, this should not be the first one you try. This version of **sirsasana** requires very strong muscles in the neck to keep the cervical spine super stable. The hands will take some weight, but unless you have a really strong upper body, it's very difficult to regulate the amount of weight on the head. The hands are more for keeping the balance than supporting weight. The better you can align your body with gravity, the easier this asana will be.

There are many ways to approach this asana. This is just one of them. Start on your hands and knees with hands shoulder-distance apart and fingers spread wide. Place the top of your head in front of your hands, creating an equilateral triangle with the head and hands representing the angles. Elbows will be flexed 90 degrees and shoulder-distance apart. With toes tucked, lift your knees and hips as you would for **adho mukha savasana** (downward-facing dog) and walk your feet as close to your head as possible (without bending the knees!) getting the pelvis as high as possible. Then use your core strength and, if necessary, a little controlled kick off the floor to line the pelvis up over the shoulders. Extend your legs straight up and do your best to keep the best alignment you can as you try to find the path of least resistance.

UPPER BODY

As you maintain balance in the asana, all the muscles in the neck are working very hard to support all that weight and keep the spine, particularly the cervicals, stable. Deep in the posterior neck are the suboccipital muscles. They are a group of four muscles: rectus capitis posterior major, rectus capitus, posterior minor, obliquus capitis superior, and obliquus capitis inferior. These muscles form what is commonly referred to as the suboccipital triangle. Longissimus capitis, splenius capitus, and levator scapula, though more superficial than the suboccipital muscles, are also deep stabilizing muscles of the posterior neck.

Deep in the anterior neck are the rectus capitis anterior, longus capitis, and longus colli muscles, which are also working very hard to maintain stability. They will get a lot of help from the bigger scalenes and the even bigger sternocleidomastoid (SCM) muscles, which are more superficial and are located along the lateral neck.

LOWER BODY

You are doing your best to maintain neutrality in your hips as you keep the legs fully extended, lining up the knees and ankles with the hips.

THE NECK MUSCLES

The full illustration of **sirsasana B** gives you a good view of the suboccipital muscles. Here we can see the bigger, stronger, more superficial muscles of the neck, which will be working to support most of the weight of body. As these muscles strengthen, you can move on to even more challenging versions of sirsasana.

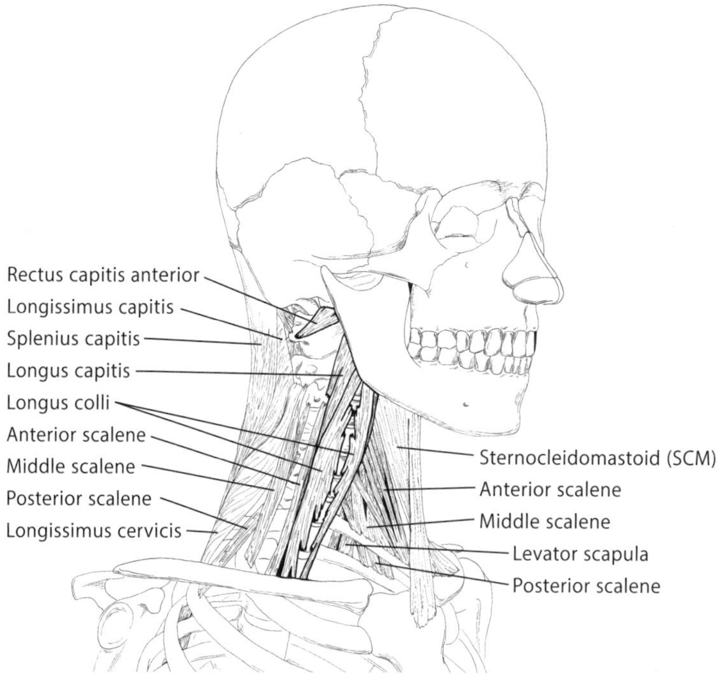

LONGUS CAPITIS

LONGUS COLLI

RECTUS CAPITIS ANTERIOR

RECTUS CAPITIS POSTERIOR MINOR

RECTUS CAPITIS POSTERIOR MAJOR

OBLIQUUS CAPITIS SUPERIOR

OBLIQUUS CAPITIS INFERIOR

FUN FACT

According to the *Guinness World Records*, on December 3, 2017, in Gujarat, India, 2,945 people stood on their heads to set the record for the most people performing a headstand at one time.

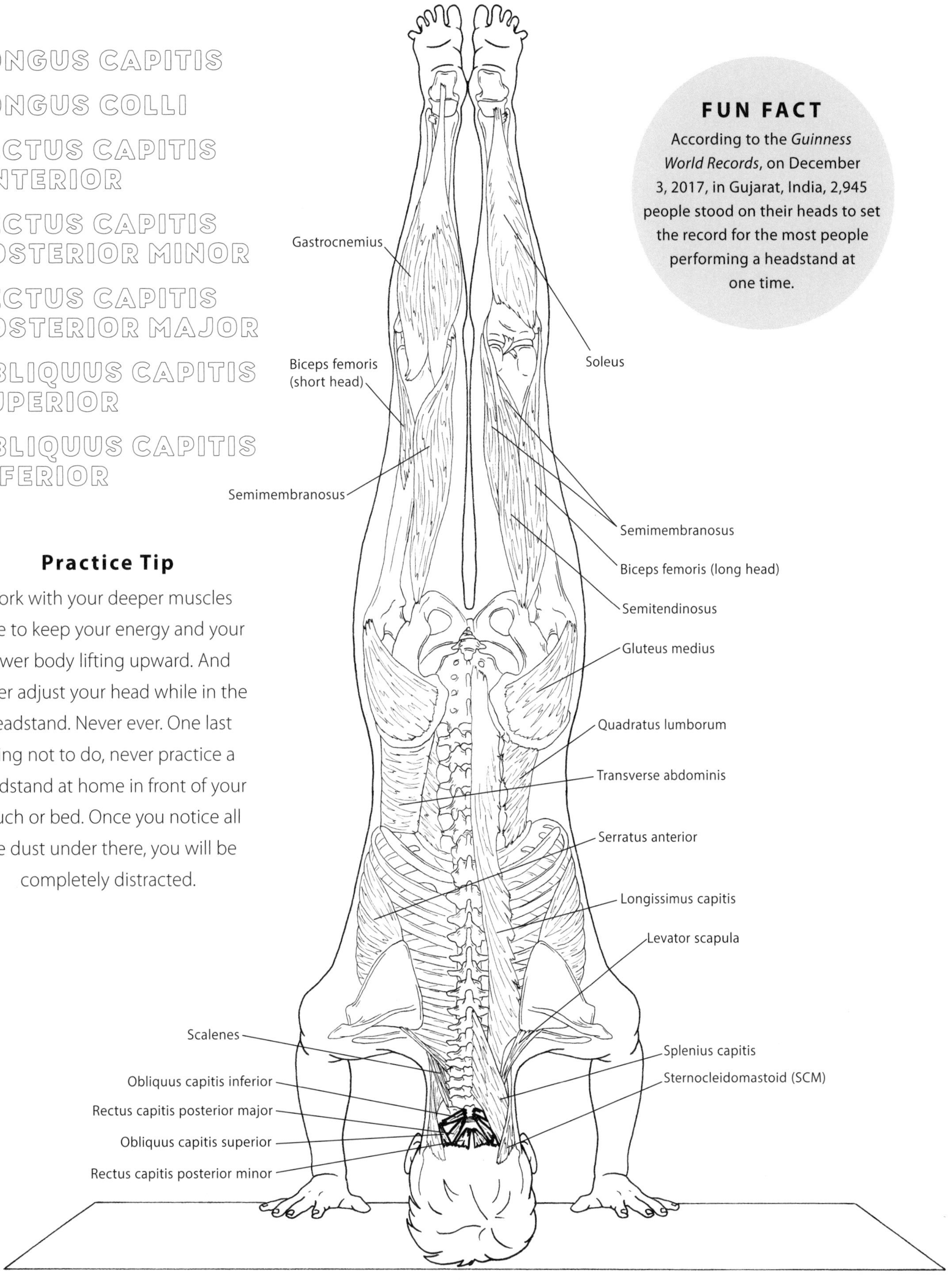

Practice Tip

Work with your deeper muscles here to keep your energy and your lower body lifting upward. And never adjust your head while in the headstand. Never ever. One last thing not to do, never practice a headstand at home in front of your couch or bed. Once you notice all the dust under there, you will be completely distracted.

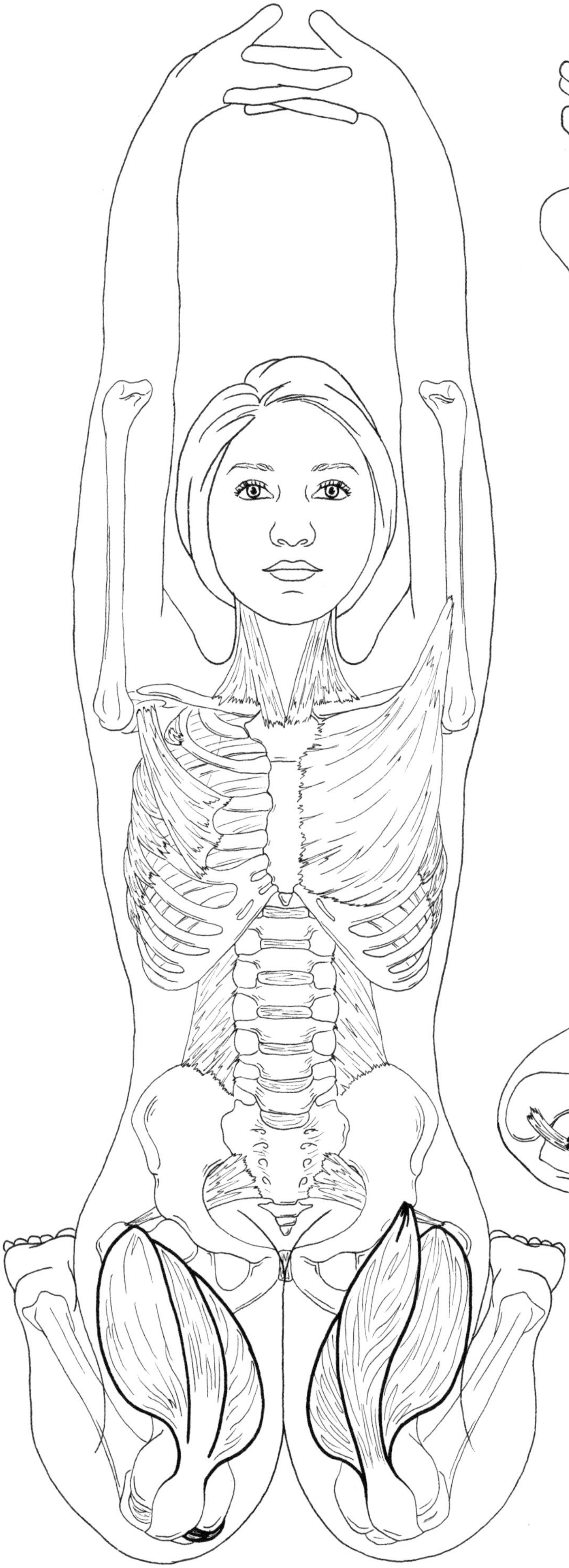

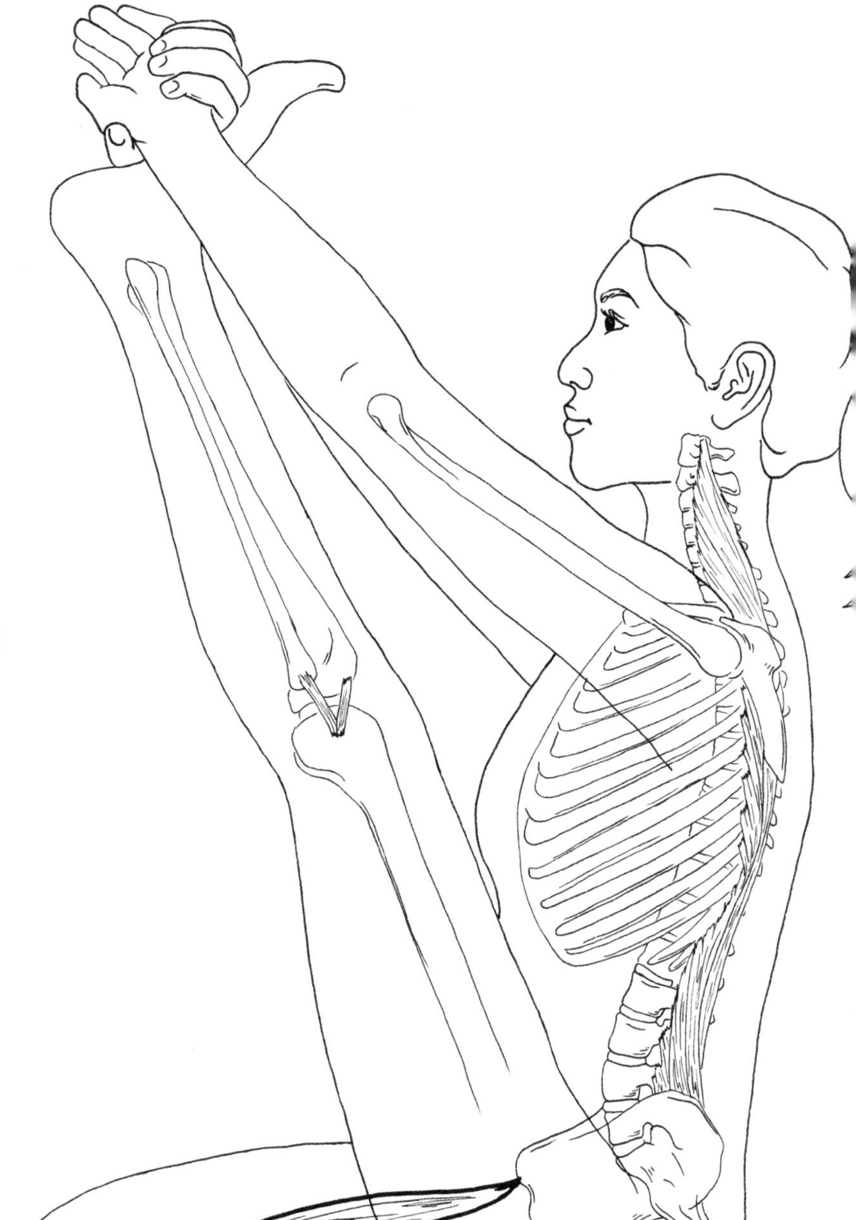

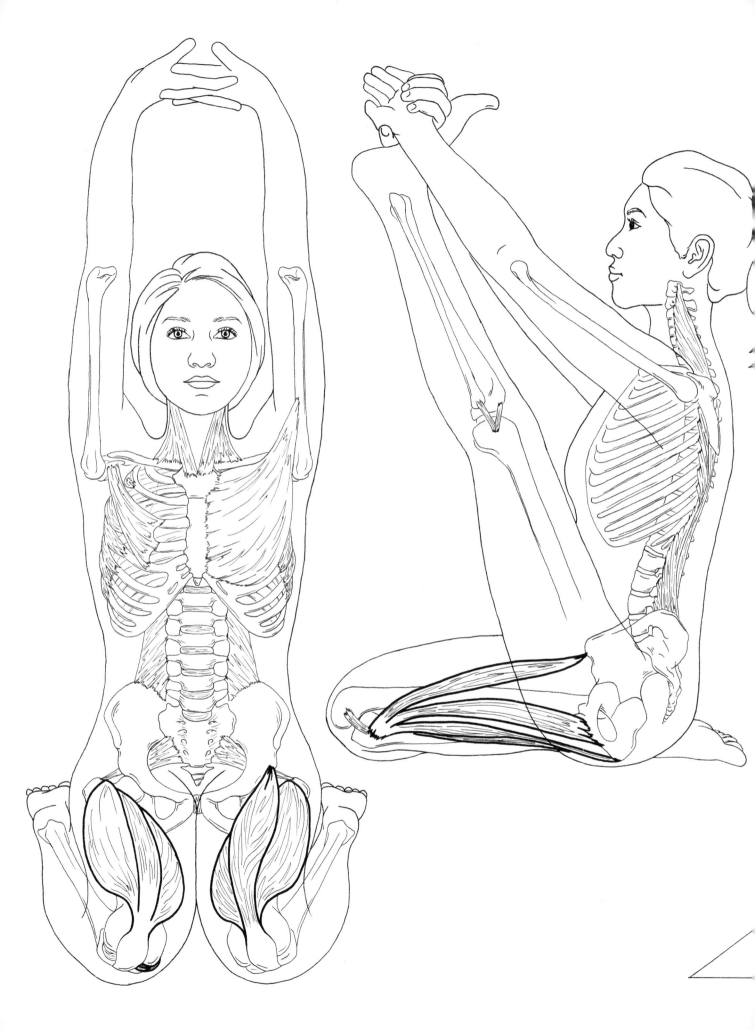

PART 3

Seated Asanas

This section includes seated forward bends, twists, and other asanas that are basically done on the mat. They're a little harder to categorize, so I have grouped them here under "other seated asanas."

These postures tend to be thought of more as a test of flexibility rather than strength, but that doesn't mean you aren't going to be using some muscle. Even in a basic seated bend, what do you think is going to pull your upper body toward your legs? Your core muscles of course! In a twist, there are a lot of muscles in the torso that have to work to rotate your spine. Again, it is about balancing strength and flexibility.

Please take your time to work up to the more challenging postures. If **sukhasana** (easy seated posture) isn't easy yet, don't move on to postures that will challenge your hips and knees even more. Remember, although we usually find asanas challenging, we should never find them painful.

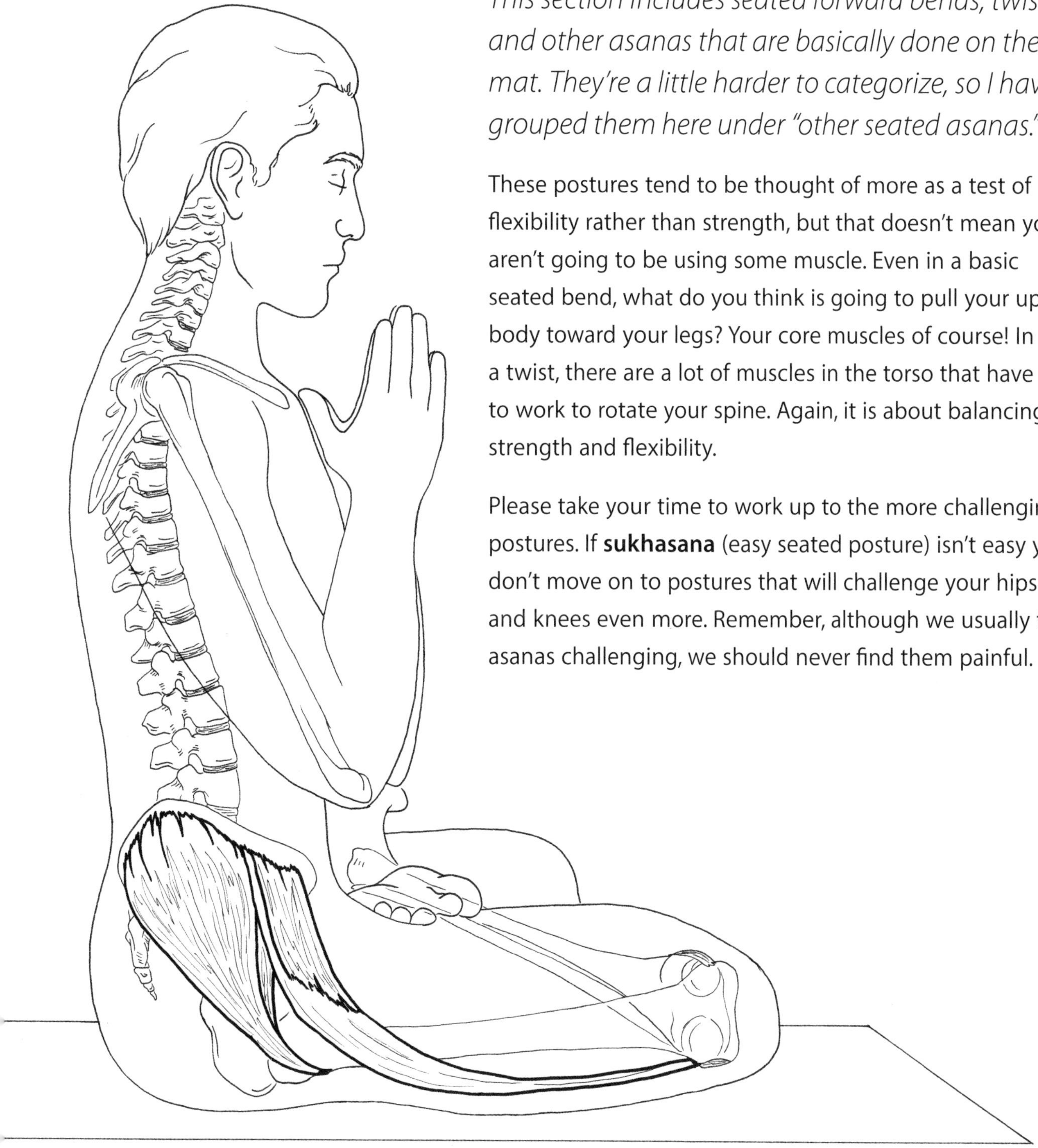

Seated Forward Bends

Seated forward bends are found in basically every yoga tradition. Most forward bends move the body through the sagittal plane; however, there are some that may involve rotation and/or lateral flexion moving the upper body through more than one plane of movement. This is also where a lot of yogis cheat the asana. Most seated forward bends ask that you bend at your hips (the acetabulofemoral joint) to bring the upper body closer to the legs. When they run into resistance from the hamstring muscles, most folks flex at the spine to bring the upper body closer to the legs. Don't do that; it will take the stretch out of the hamstrings. Bend the knees and keep the spine neutral. The only time your spine should flex is when you are so deep in the forward bend that you simply run out of room.

Paschimottanasana

POS-chee-moh-tahn-AH-sah-nah

Seated Forward Bend

Paschimottanasana is the quintessential seated forward bend and a fundamental, foundational yoga asana. Improving in this asana will improve all the other seated forward bends you practice. The object is to not touch the hands to the feet, though eventually that will happen. The idea here is to lengthen the muscles along the posterior leg. There should be no doubt where you should be feeling the stretch.

As with all the seated forward bends going forward in this section, first get proper alignment before going for your stretch, and, once established, don't ruin it!

Sitting up straight with a neutral spine, extend the legs as much as possible, straight out in front of you. Dorsal flex at your ankles and keep both your patella and phalanges (kneecaps and toes) pointing straight up, with toes spread wide. Establish this first. Then bring the hips through the full range of hip flexion and reach toward your toes. Use a strap until you can reach your feet, and bend the knees rather than the back to keep the hamstrings happy in the stretch.

LOWER BODY

As you flex at the hips, your three hamstring muscles—the biceps femoris, semitendinosus, and semimembranosus—will have to lengthen to bring the upper body closer to the legs. Remember, your hamstrings attach at the ischial tuberosities (sit bones), and you should not feel the stretch there. That's asking for trouble as it's the most common point of tendonitis and tears of the hamstrings. The more you try to pull the sit bones back, the longer your hamstrings have to get, so pay attention and don't overdo it. Keeping your ankles in dorsal flexion and the knees extended will also stretch the gastrocnemius muscles and the deeper soleus muscle in the lower leg.

UPPER BODY

You will notice that practitioners who can get their upper body all the way down to their legs end up with some degree of spinal flexion. This is as it should be as you simply run out of room. Until the upper body is all the way down to the legs, keep your heart center pulling forward and your shoulders drawing back. It may feel like you are moving toward spinal extension, but you won't end up in a backbend—you are just preventing spinal flexion. So keep it simple and keep the spine just as you set it up before you started flexing your hips. Just move from the hips. Period.

FUN FACT

Paschimottanasana was first described way back in the 15th century in the *Hatha Yoga Pradipika,* the first text to ever describe the asanas and a sacred text among hatha yoga practitioners.

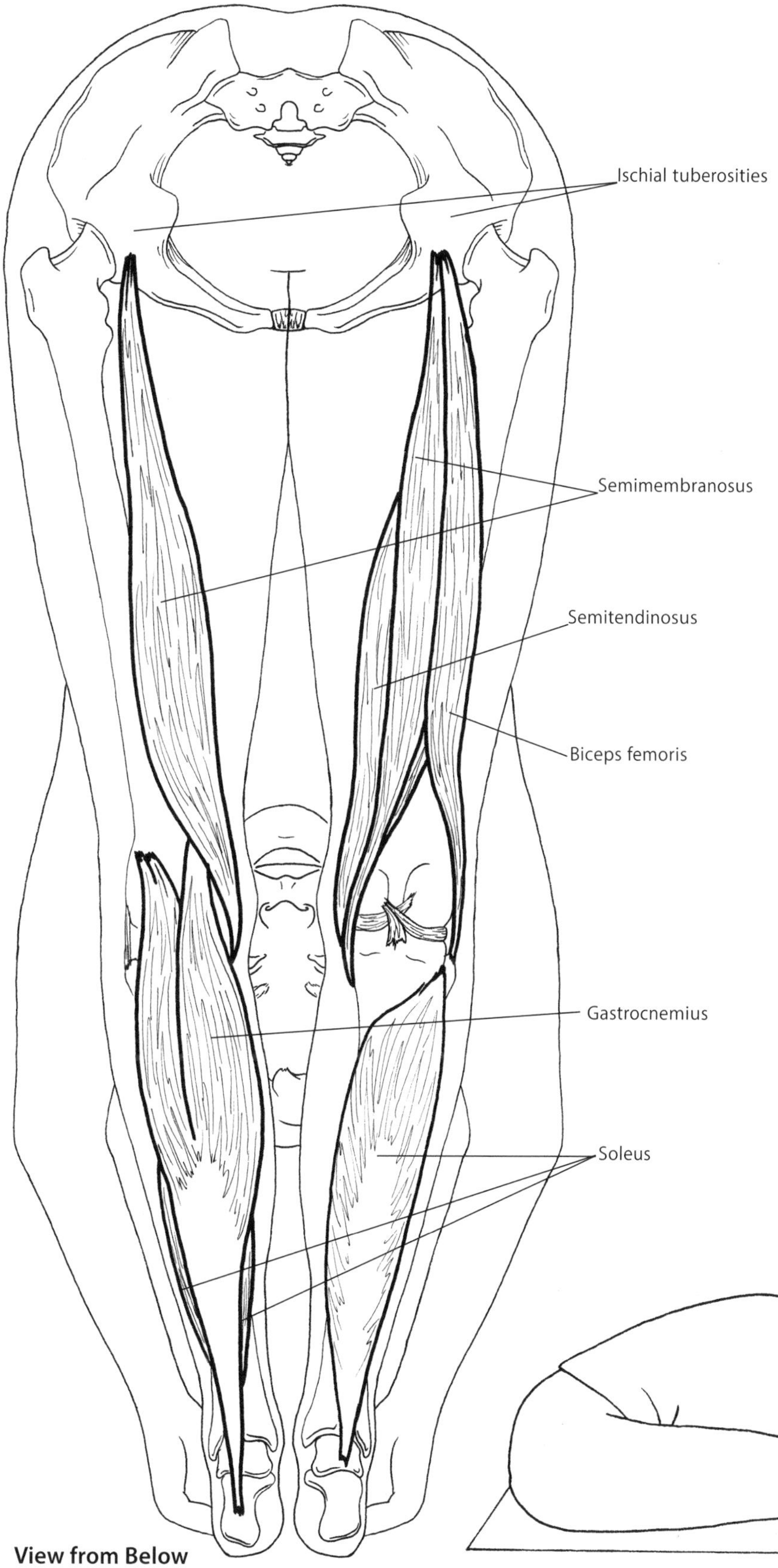

View from Below

Practice Tip

Sit up on a blanket or bolster to make neutralizing the spine easier, and use a strap to connect to the feet. This will give you the room you need to prevent your back from rounding and pulling your pelvis the opposite way, toward posterior tilt. As stated above, it is the pelvis and hips that move here, not the spine.

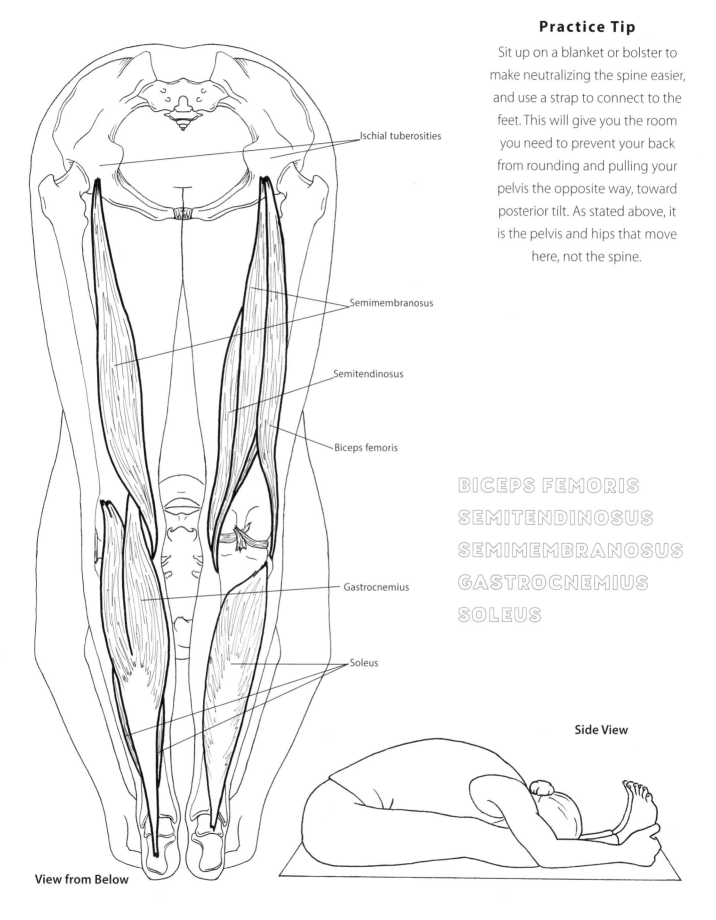

BICEPS FEMORIS
SEMITENDINOSUS
SEMIMEMBRANOSUS
GASTROCNEMIUS
SOLEUS

Side View

Upavishta Konasana

oo-pah-VEESH-tah koh-NAH-sah-nah

Wide-Angle Seated Forward Bend

Upavishta konasana is done by most people in phys ed class as a warm-up stretch before sports activities or as just a way to stretch out, way before they ever stepped foot into a yoga class. Where **paschimottanasana** focuses on stretching the muscles in the back of the legs, the focus here is clearly on the muscles along the inner thighs—the adductor muscles. These are big, strong muscles you're trying to stretch here. Go slowly and take time to find that first deep stretch. Give the muscles time to respond. Hang out with it, and then maybe go a little deeper. They will usually let you know if you have overstayed your welcome (i.e., the stretch doesn't feel so good anymore). As you pay more attention to what you're doing, you will become more sensitive to how you feel and know when to say when.

Start by sitting up straight with your legs as abducted (wide) and as extended (straight) as you can comfortably get them. If you are unable to sit up straight, prop under the sit bones and/or bend your knees. Keep your toes and knees pointing straight up to avoid the hips from going toward external rotation. For some, just getting the proper alignment setting this up is enough of a stretch. The only thing you want your hips to do is stay in deep abduction, and then flex the hips forward through their fullest range of motion.

LOWER BODY

You will feel a deep stretch along all five muscles that make up your adductors. They are the pectineus, adductor brevis, adductor longus, adductor magnus, and gracilis. The semimembranosus and semitendinosus, the most medial of your hamstring muscles, will feel a deep stretch here as well. Your quadriceps muscles should be held in concentric contraction to keep the knee in extension and maintain a strong foundation for the asana.

UPPER BODY

As you flex the hips, be careful not the let the curve in the thoracic spine get exaggerated and cause the upper back to round and, in turn, collapse your chest. Keep your heart leading the way by pulling the proximal ends of your clavicles up, lifting the sternum and dropping the 1st pair of ribs. This will give the subclavius muscles that run along the clavicles a nice stretch and that feels good whether you need it or not... and most of us need it!

Practice Tip

If you find it challenging to keep your back from rounding, place the hands behind the hips or interlace the fingers behind your back to bring the scapula closer together and to keep the chest from collapsing.

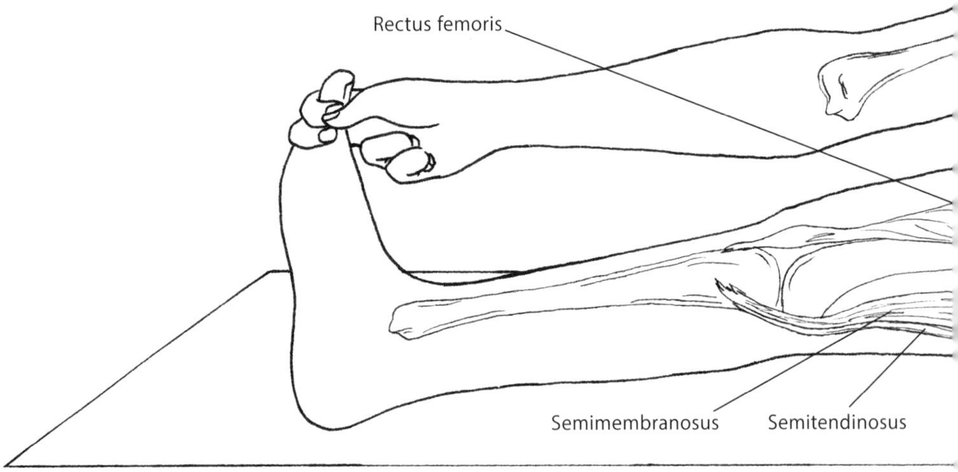

FUN FACT

As you get deeper and deeper in hip abduction, this asana becomes **samakonasana**, or even-angle posture. Nowadays gymnasts refer to this as the middle split.

COLORING TIP

The semitendinosus muscle has an extremely long tendon (probably why it's right there in the name). The tendon starts about mid-thigh and inserts at the per anserinus, that little bump toward the medial side of the superior aspect of the shin. Coloring the tendon a lighter shade than the muscle will really give you an idea of its length.

PECTINEUS
ADDUCTOR BREVIS
ADDUCTOR LONGUS
ADDUCTOR MAGNUS
GRACILIS
SUBCLAVIUS

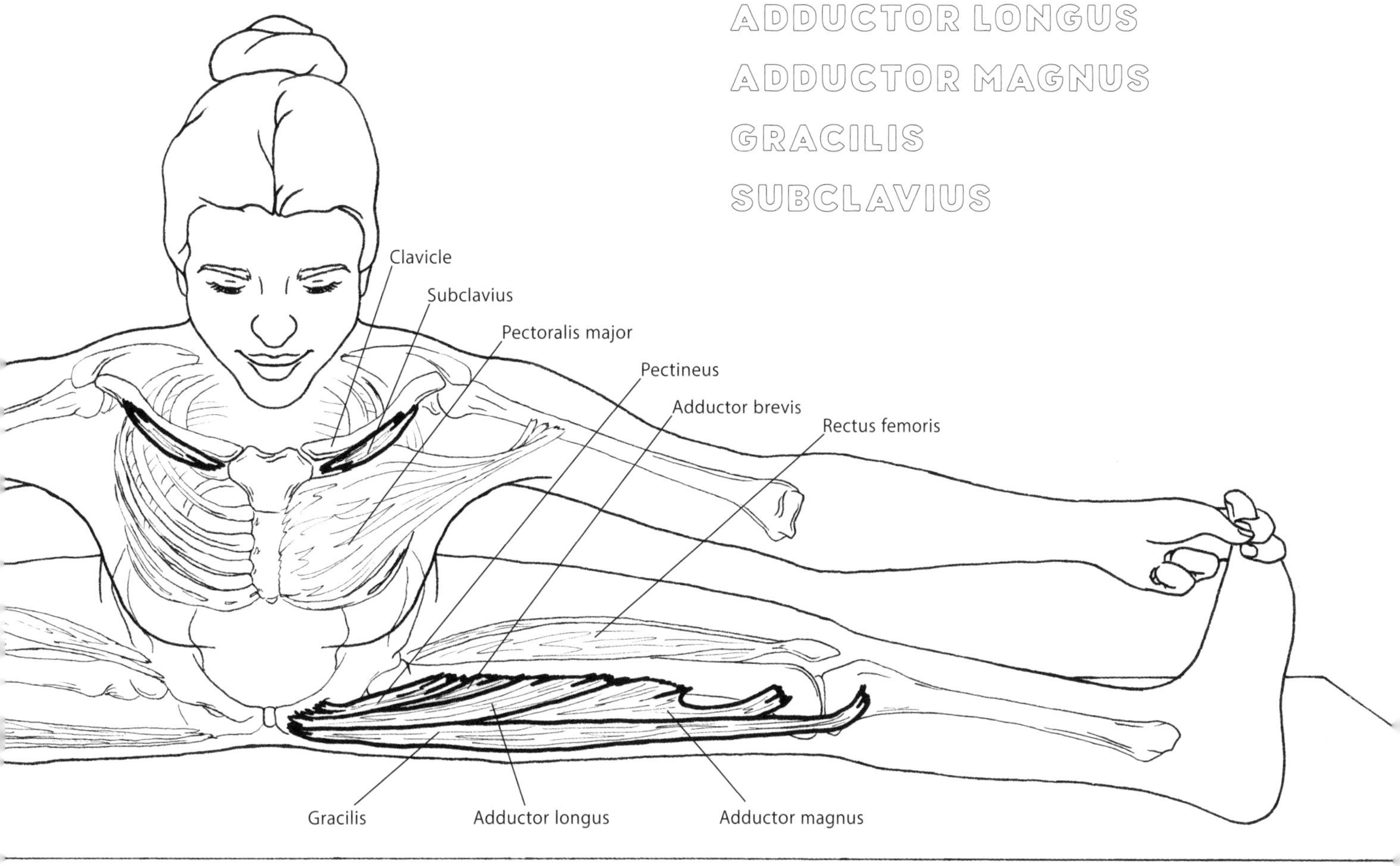

Baddhakonasana

bah-dah-koh-NAH-sah-nah

Bound-Angle Posture

Baddhakonasana is a fundamental yoga asana and available to most practitioners. It is a favorite among many yogis because of the nice stretch along the inner thighs and the deep stretch felt in all the gluteal muscles.

Sitting up straight, flex the knees as much as possible and abduct at the hips as much as possible, bringing the soles of the feet together and the heels as close to the pelvis as you can without rounding the back. The more you can flex your hips and bring the body toward a forward bend, the deeper the stretch along the inner thighs and gluteal muscles.

LOWER BODY

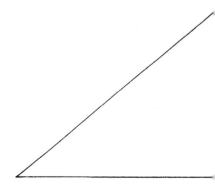

Deep flexion in the hips will allow the gluteus maximus to get a nice stretch. The hips are also externally rotating, stretching the other two gluteal muscles—the gluteus medius and gluteus minimus (anterior fibers)—along with the tensor fasciae latae (TFL) muscle. Four out of the five adductor muscles are all lengthening to accommodate the deep abduction of the hips, just as in **upavishta konasana**. They are the adductor magnus, adductor longus, adductor brevis, and pectineus. Gracilis, the "other" adductor, crosses the knee and, since the knee is flexed, really doesn't get much action here.

The hips in **baddhakonasana** are moving through all three planes of movement. I think that's what makes it feel so delicious.

UPPER BODY

Your psoas will have to work to pull your hips into flexion, but some folks will also wrap the first two fingers and thumb of each hand around the big toe (the "yogi toe hold") to help pull the hips into deeper flexion. Keep the spine neutral along with the shoulders and heart center open. Do not try, do.

Practice Tip

Baddhakonasana asks you to flex your knees as much as possible. Some practitioners like to use the elbows to press the knees closer to the floor. Do this as long as it feels good! For some, the knees may feel vulnerable. Putting blocks under the knees for support can make this asana more available.

COLORING TIP

The psoas muscle originates along the vertebrae and transverse processes of the lumbar spine. Using different colors for the tendons of the muscle where they originate will really show how strong this attachment is.

GLUTEUS MAXIMUS

GLUTEUS MEDIUS

GLUTEUS MINIMUS (ANTERIOR FIBERS)

TENSOR FASCIAE LATAE (TFL)

PSOAS

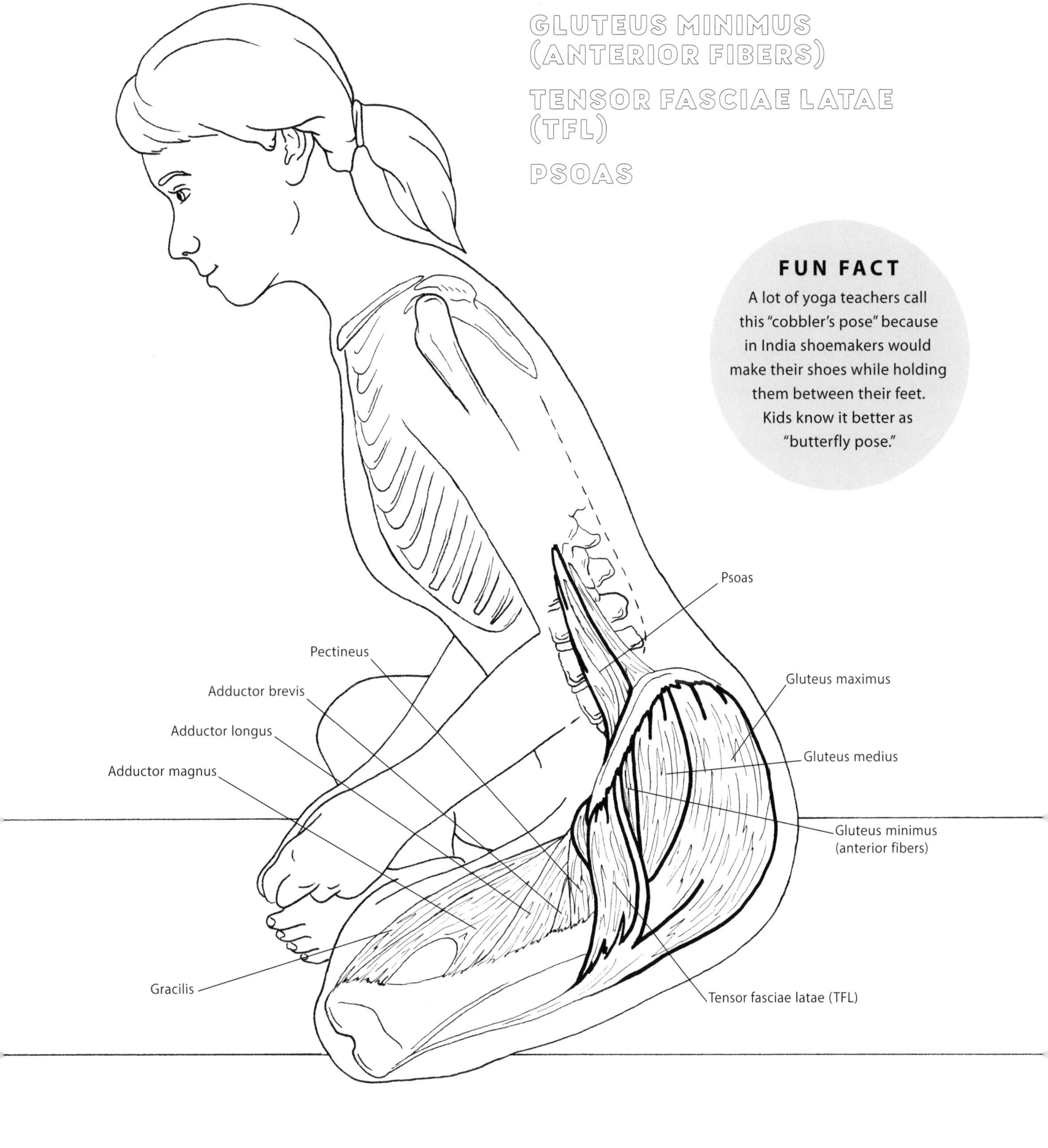

FUN FACT

A lot of yoga teachers call this "cobbler's pose" because in India shoemakers would make their shoes while holding them between their feet. Kids know it better as "butterfly pose."

Janu Sirsasana

JAH-noo sheer-SHAH-sah-nah

Head-to-Knee Posture

Janu sirsasana, even though it translates as head-to-knee pose, does not want you to aim your head for your knee. You should aim your sternum toward your knee. This asana combines the extended leg stretch of **paschimottanasana** and the inner thigh stretch of **baddhakonasana** and adds a spinal rotation, making this a very efficient asana with a lot to offer.

As always, get set up first. Sit up straight and bring one leg fully extended out in front of you, bending the other leg out to the side to form a 90-degree angle between the thighs, or as close to that as you can get. Because of the positioning of the legs, the hip of the bent leg will be farther back than the hip of the extended leg. In order to face forward, you will have to rotate your spine slightly toward the extended leg. Then, as in most seated forward bends, flex at the hips. Once you have a deep forward bend happening, keep the hip of the bent leg grounding like crazy, and emphasize spinal rotation toward the extended leg, trying to line up your sternum with your patella.

LOWER BODY

As you hold the forward bend, the hamstrings in the extended leg will get a deep stretch. Keep the ankle of the extended leg in dorsal flexion with toes pointing straight up. As the calcaneus (heel bone) moves away from the knee, the tibialis anterior muscle will have to concentrically contract, and the tibialis posterior muscle will get a chance to lengthen. Also lengthening here is the Achilles tendon. As with all tendons, it will give you just a little stretch. The adductor muscles of the bent leg will keep a stretch with the hip in abduction. Trying to externally rotate the hip of the bent leg as you keep the hips flexed will give your gluteal muscles a juicy stretch.

UPPER BODY

Keeping the hip of the bent leg grounded as you rotate the spine toward the straight leg will give your quadratus lumborum, that deep back muscle that originates along your iliac crest and inserts at the lumbar spine, a nice, deep stretch as the ribs spiral away from the hip. Most of your spine should be in pure rotation. The cervical vertebrae of the neck, however, should be neutral. Part of the fun is trying to isolate the cervical spine from the rest of the spine so your gaze is forward, rather than over your shoulder.

THE KNEE STABILIZERS

It is the deep ligaments in the posterior compartment of the knee that connect the femur to the bones of the lower leg—the fibula and tibia. Their main job is to keep the knee stable, such as in **janu sirsasana**. We usually refer to these ligaments by their initials: the MCL (medial collateral ligament), the LCL (lateral collateral ligament), the ACL (anterior cruciate ligament), and the PCL (posterior cruciate ligament).

Posterior View

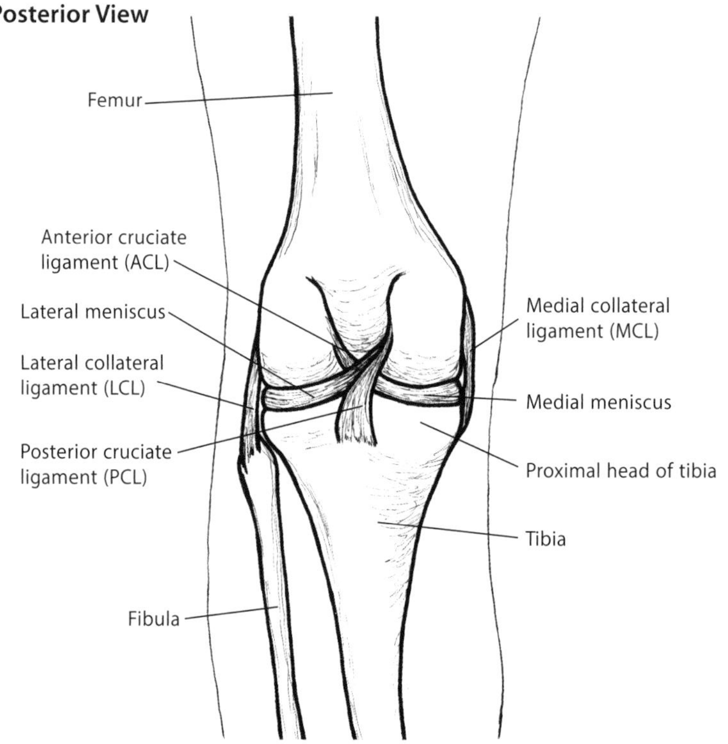

Practice Tip

Use a strap to make a connection between the hands and the foot of the extended leg and give yourself enough slack to keep your heart in front of your shoulders.

FUN FACT

Even Derek Jeter of the New York Yankees was often spotted practicing **janu sirsasana** before games!

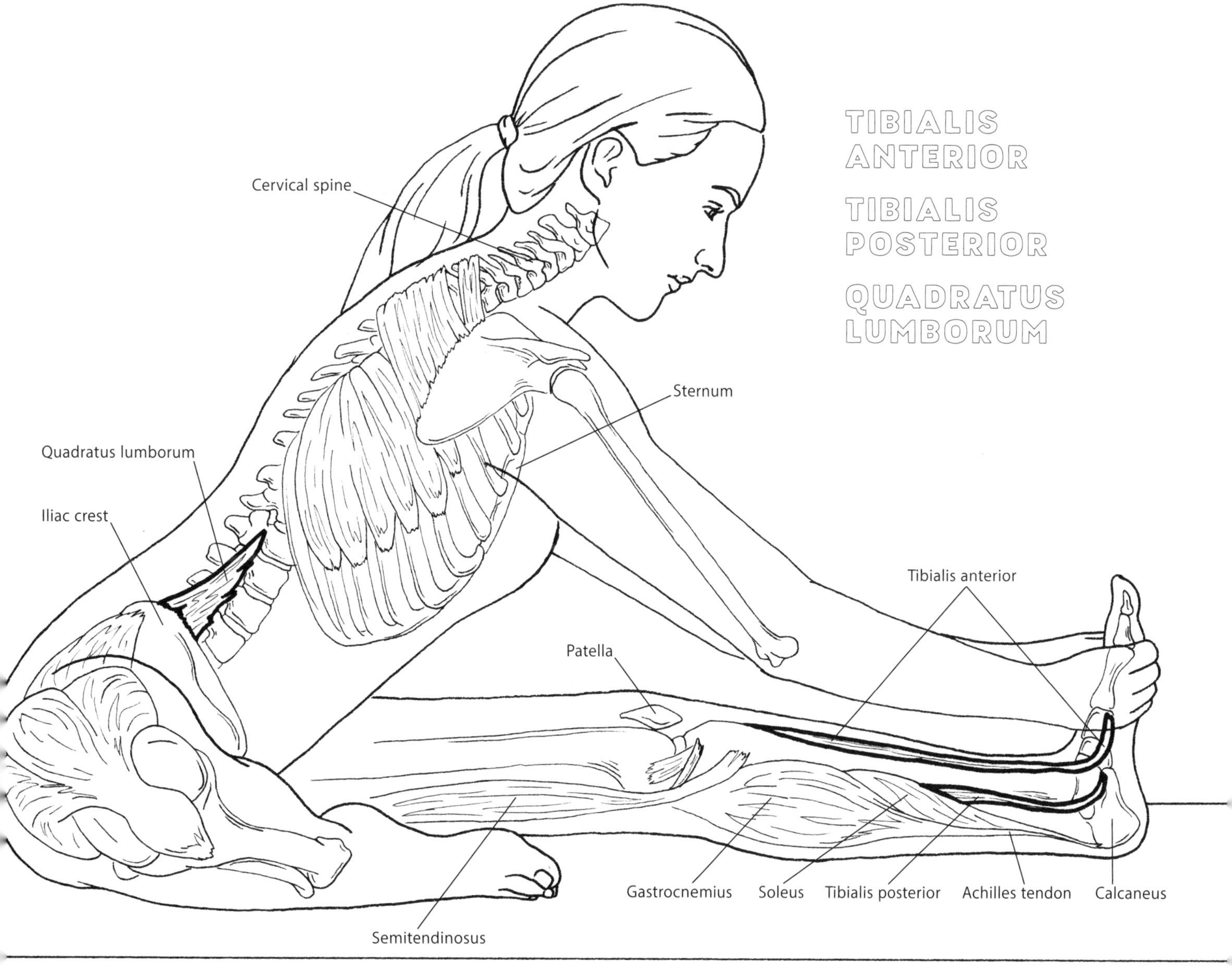

Ardha Baddha Padma Paschimottanasana

ARD-ah BAH-dah PAHD-mah POS-chee-moh-tahn-AH-sah-nah

Half-Bound Lotus Forward Bend

Ardha baddha padma paschimottanasana is an advanced forward bend. All the big joints in the lower body have to be okay with this one. Both hips are flexed, of course, but the hip of the leg in **ardha padmasana** (half lotus, in which one foot rests on the opposite hip with the knee fully flexed) will also have to be in deep external rotation. The knee is flexed fully and the ankle is in deep plantar flexion as well. A lot of practitioners will have to work up to this one, but it's worth it!

This posture is entered very similar to **janu sirsasana**, except that the bent leg is now in **ardha padmasana** and the arm on that side is wrapped behind the back, reaching for the lotus foot.

LOWER BODY

All the gluteal muscles will get a deep stretch here; the gluteus maximus because the hips are flexing and the gluteus medius and gluteus minimus by virtue of the deep external rotation in the hips inherent in **ardha padmasana.** You must be able to externally rotate the hip enough and not apply any pressure to the knee to get the leg in a half lotus. Many overzealous yogis have suffered injury to their medial meniscus by forcing a lotus before it is ready. To maintain deep flexion in the knee, the vastus lateralis, vastus intermedius, vastus medialis, and the lower fibers of rectus femoris, otherwise known as the quadriceps muscles, will have to lengthen here. The tibialis anterior will also get a deep stretch as the ankle in the lotus leg holds the foot in deep plantar flexion. The hamstrings in the straight leg will get a stretch if you can flex your hips deep enough with everything else going on.

UPPER BODY

Whichever leg is in **ardha padmasana**, the arm on that side is going to try to wrap around the back and reach for the foot. This is going to ask for a lot of internal rotation at the shoulder. The subscapularis is your strongest rotator cuff muscle and the strongest internal rotator of the shoulder. It gets a lot of help from the teres major and a little more help from the latissimus dorsi and pectoralis major. You will be asking the infraspinatus and teres minor to lengthen here; be careful you don't ask too much!

Practice Tip

If you're able to get your half lotus all the way there but can't reach the big toe with your wrap, put a small loop in the end of a long strap to encircle the lotus foot and hold on to that to keep the lotus leg in position. If you're unable to reach the foot of the straight leg with your other arm, use the rest of the strap to wrap around the foot and hold with your other hand. Some people refer to this as "yoga bondage." (Or maybe that's just me!)

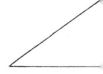

COLORING TIP

Here are three of your four quadriceps muscles. (The fourth, the vastus intermedius, is hidden under the rectus femoris.) These muscles come together to form a common tendon. Blending the three colors you choose for these muscles as they approach the knee will form the quadriceps tendon that attaches to the patella, your kneecap.

GLUTEUS MEDIUS
GLUTEUS MINIMUS
VASTUS LATERALIS
VASTUS MEDIALIS
RECTUS FEMORIS

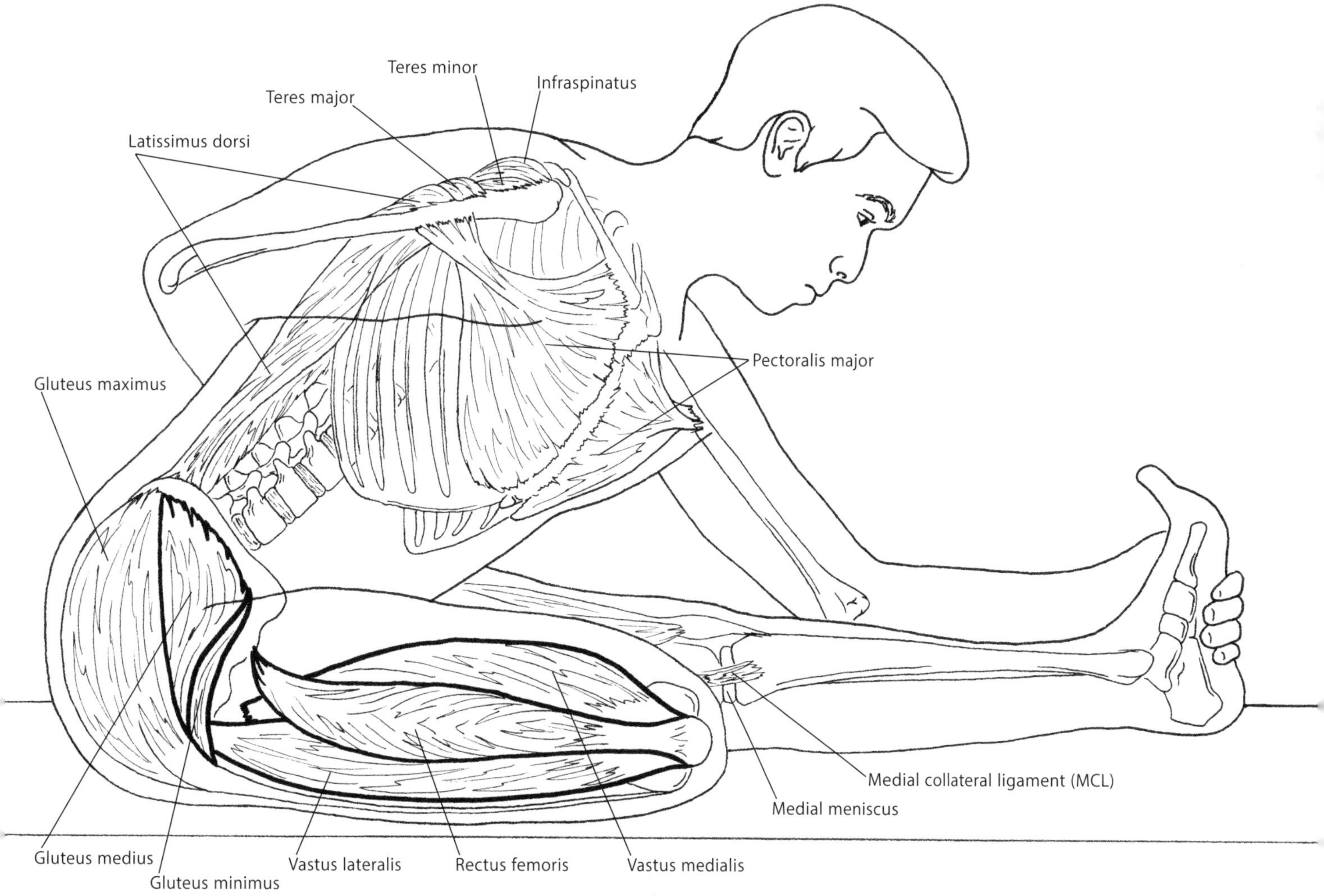

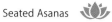

Triang Mukha Eka Pada Paschimottanasana

TRI-ahng MOO-kah EK-ah PAH-dah POS-chee-moh-tahn-AH-sah-nah

Three-Limb-Facing One-Leg Forward Bend

This asana is another fairly advanced forward bend, though maybe more accessible than **ardha baddha padma paschimottanasana** with the use of props. It requires great flexibility in the lower body, and the knee joint has got to be on board for this.

Seated on your mat, bring one leg into **ardha virasana** (half hero, in which one knee is fully flexed with the foot alongside the hip, plantar side up and toes pointing back) and fully extend the other leg straight out in front of you. Keeping your pelvis evenly grounded, flex at the hips toward the forward bend and reach for your foot.

LOWER BODY

The hips are in deep flexion, but here it can be a little more challenging to pull yourself into the forward bend. The psoas muscle along with the iliacus (iliopsoas) are our strongest hip flexors, and you will need them here. In addition, the rectus femoris, sartorius, gluteus minimus, and tensor fasciae latae (TFL) are also very strong and act as synergists when you flex your hips. All of these muscles need to be in concentric contraction to create and hold deep hip flexion in this asana. These are not the only muscles that are pulling the upper body closer to the legs, the adductors help to some extent as well. Getting a nice stretch up here in the hips is the gluteus maximus.

The knee of the straight leg is in full extension, if possible. The quadriceps muscles keep the leg straight. They should be engaged and held in concentric contraction. This will, of course, stretch the hamstrings, gastrocnemius, soleus, and tibialis posterior—aka, the bigger muscles along the back of the leg. The ankle of the straight leg is in full dorsal flexion. This means your tibialis anterior muscle must concentrically contract and hold. The extensor digitorum longus and extensor hallucis longus keep the toes pulling back. (Hallucis is your big toe. I know I am adding to your anatomy lexicon, and I am not sorry.) It feels like giving the bottom of your foot, the plantar surface, a big stretch. Keep these muscles in concentric contraction and don't let your foot just flop.

The knee of the bent leg is in full-on flexion and very, very, very slight medial rotation to bring the heel alongside the hip with the plantar surface of the foot facing up. The quadriceps will have to lengthen to accommodate this and the quadriceps tendon that encases the patella (knee cap) must be on board. Be very mindful of any discomfort in the knee and back off at the slightest hint of pain. The ankle of the bent leg is in full plantar flexion. This is going to ask your tibialis anterior muscle to really stretch. Note that the bent leg is being held in place by the floor, gravity, and your own body weight. There is no need to "work" to keep the position, just be mindful of the pressure on your joints.

UPPER BODY

As you reach for the foot, be careful not to collapse your chest, and keep the shoulders pulling back. Try to let your heart lead the way. Try to avoid spinal flexion here, and do your best to keep your spine neutral.

FUN FACT

Learning a few root words in Sanskrit can help make what seems like a mouthful make sense. "Tri" means three, "ang" limb, "mukha" face, "eka" one, "pada" foot, "paschim" west or back, "ottan" intense, and, of course "asana" means posture. So this is "three-limb-facing one foot intense back posture."

Practice Tip

Use a block to raise *both* sit bones evenly to help the bent leg find the posture. To take pressure off the ankle of the bent leg, put a small prop, like a rolled-up towel, under the ankle.

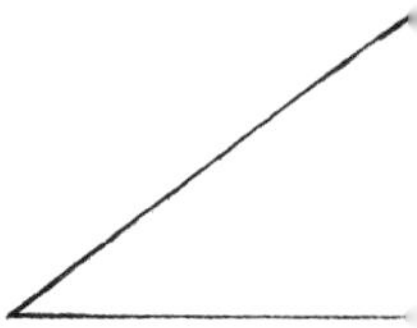

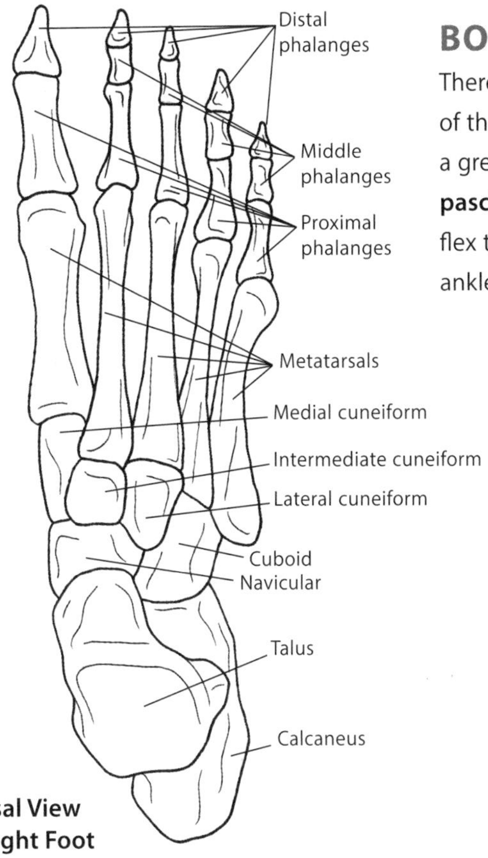

Dorsal View of Right Foot

BONES OF THE FOOT

There are 26 bones that make up just one foot/ankle. That's about one-eighth of the total number of bones in the entire body! This affords the foot and ankle a great deal of movement. In most forward bends, like **triang mukha eka pada paschimottanasana**, we want the foot in dorsal flexion, but you can also plantar flex the foot, invert and evert, pronate and supinate, and abduct and adduct the ankle. That's a lot of movement, and for that, you need a lot of bones!

RECTUS FEMORIS

SARTORIUS

GLUTEUS MINIMUS

TENSOR FASCIAE LATAE (TFL)

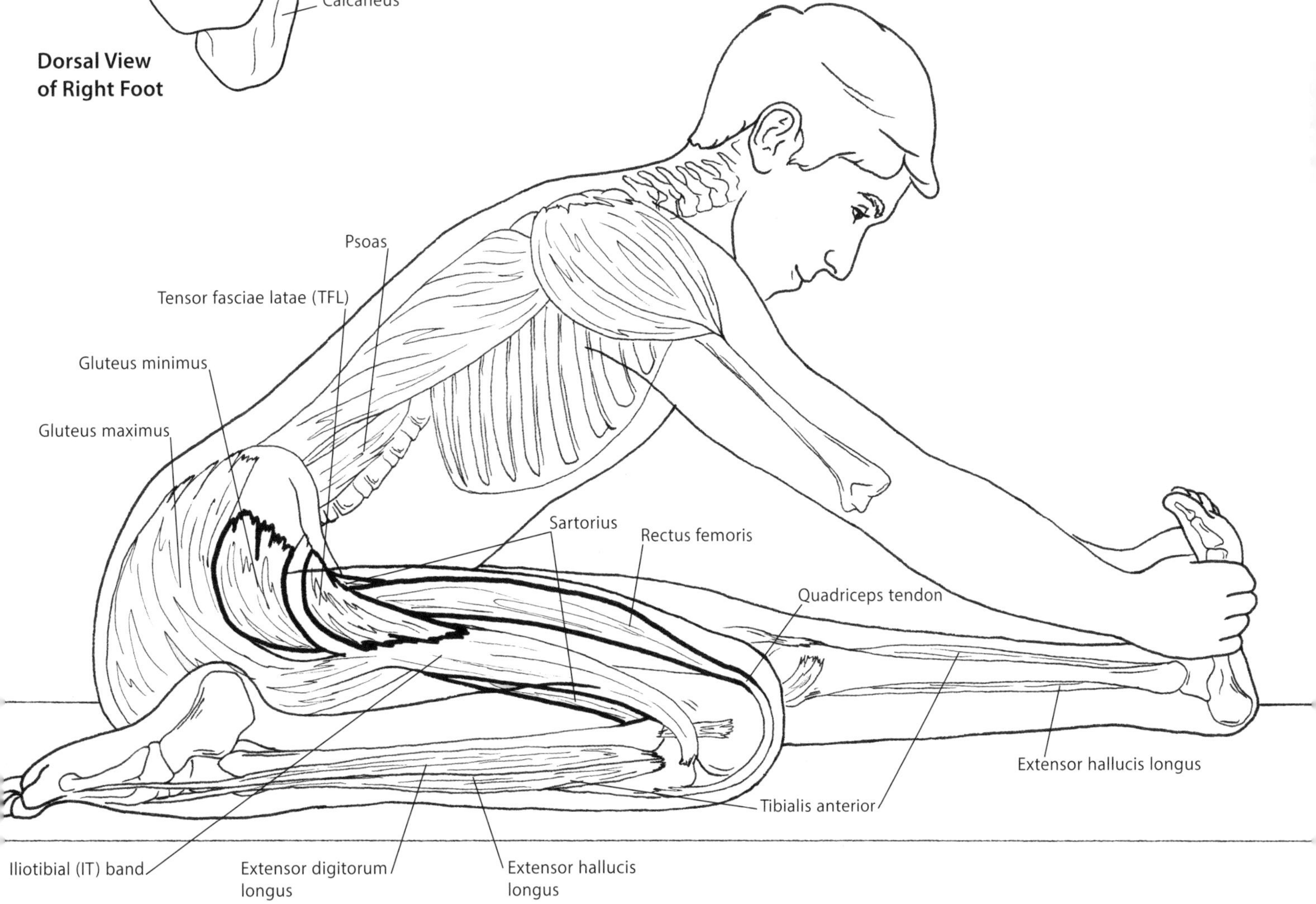

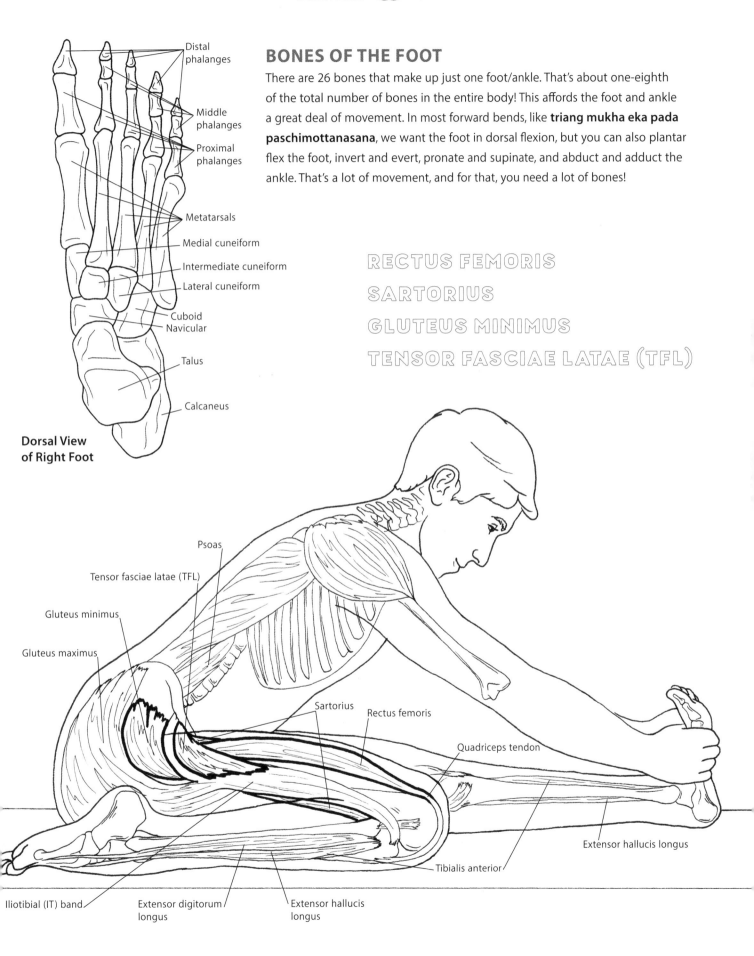

Marichyasana A

mar-ee-chee-AH-sah-nah A

Marichi's Pose A

This is where yoga asanas can get a little pretzel-like. **Marichyasana A** makes a forward bend very challenging because of the leg positioning and the wrap of both arms behind the back. This is a much easier wrap (not that it is easy!) however than what **ardha baddha padma paschimottanasana** asks for from just that one arm. At least here you have two arms to cover all that ground. But you do have to work your way around that leg as well.

Sitting on your mat, extend one leg straight out in front. Bend the other leg, a lot, to get that foot as close to the outside of the hip as you can. Internally rotate both shoulders, wrap the arm on the side of the bent leg around the leg as the other arm reaches for the other side. Then, flex at the hips and enter the forward bend.

LOWER BODY

Your hip flexors (the muscles that flex the hips; e.g., the psoas and rectus femoris) are going to work like crazy here to try to pull your upper body closer to the extended leg. There is no way to get around some core work here.

The knee of the bent leg should be fully flexed with the foot placed outside the hip and the knee hugging in. The deeper you go with that flexed knee and the farther back along the hip that you can take that foot, the easier the wrap of the arms will be. This is going to put the quadriceps muscles in a deep stretch. The quadriceps tendon and patella tendon, which attach your quadriceps to the tibia at the tibial tuberosity, will lengthen a little here as well. Be mindful and remember, although tendons will give a little, they are really not meant to stretch. Avoid any stress on the knee. Keep your toes pointing forward.

The hamstrings in the extended leg will have to lengthen, and your foot should be held in dorsal flexion. The tibialis anterior, extensor digitorum longus, and extensor hallucis longus must be held in concentric contraction to keep that foot flexed.

UPPER BODY

To achieve a deeper wrap, get that shoulder as far in front of the bent leg as possible, and then internally rotate the shoulder like crazy. Bring the upper arm in front of the lower leg and reach your hand behind your back as far as you can. The other shoulder on the side of the straight leg is going to do the same thing, but you can cover more ground with this arm because you won't have a leg to wrap around. This is going to ask your infraspinatus and teres minor (two of your rotator cuff muscles) to stretch. If possible, hold the wrist of the arm wrapped around the bent leg. If not, get a hold of whatever you can, even if that means using a strap. Don't push your shoulders. In time, you will get a hold of yourself.

Your spine will rotate slightly much in the same way as in **janu sirsasana,** trying to center the upper body over the straight leg.

Practice Tip

Press the upper arm into the shin of the bent leg to help keep that sit bone grounded.

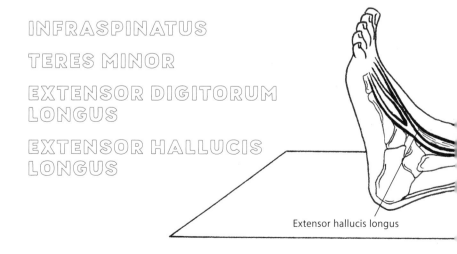

INFRASPINATUS

TERES MINOR

EXTENSOR DIGITORUM LONGUS

EXTENSOR HALLUCIS LONGUS

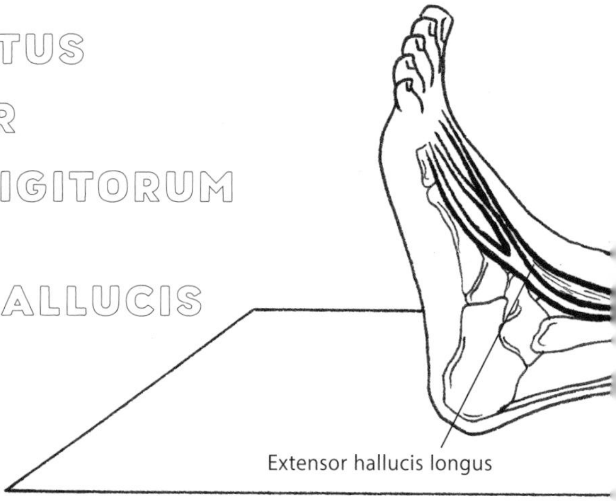

Posterior View

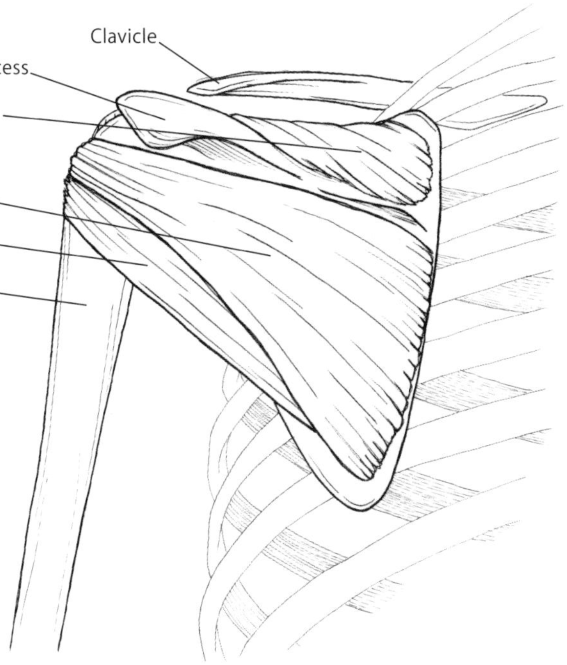

ROTATOR CUFF MUSCLES

The infraspinatus and teres minor muscles basically do the same thing, externally rotate the shoulder. This is why they get a good stretch when the shoulder is in internal rotation, as it is when you're wrapping your arms behind your back in **marichyasana A.** But, make no mistake, the main job of all the rotator cuff muscles is to keep your arm attached to your body.

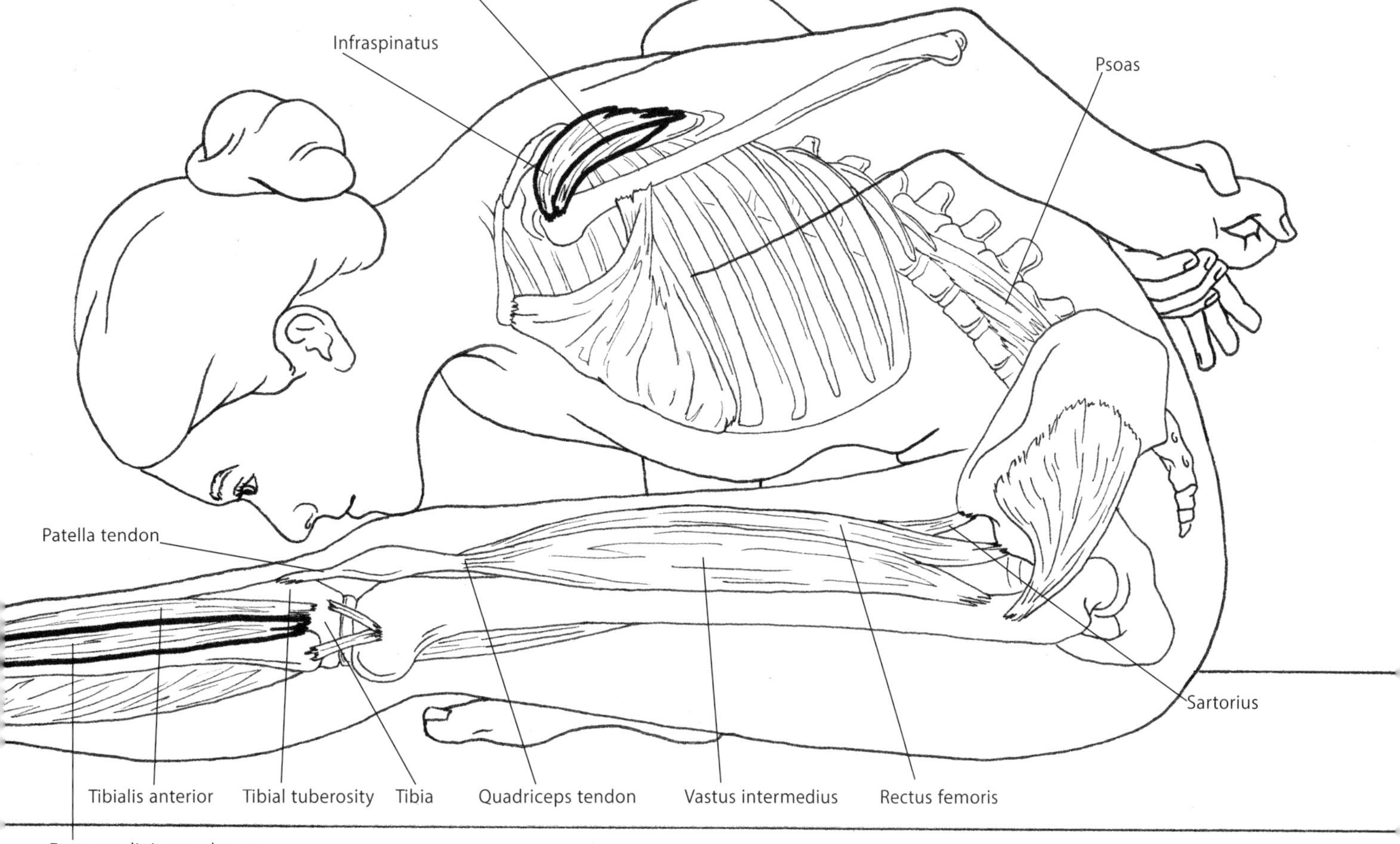

Seated Twists

Seated twists are meant to emphasize spinal rotation and move the upper body through the transverse plane. Of course, what the legs and arms are doing is important, too. Trying to get the legs and/or arms in a certain position can really mess with the spine and pull it toward flexion, extension, or lateral flexion. Most seated twists want you to start sitting up straight with the spine neutral. Have the leg and arm position accommodate a neutral spine.

Ardha Matsyendrasana

ARD-ah MOTS-yen-DRAH-sah-nah

Half Lord of the Fishes

Ardha matsyendrasana is a foundational and fundamental seated twist that will prepare you for more challenging twists to come. There are many variations to this twist to make it a little easier, such as extending the bottom leg with the foot flexed, or harder, such as wrapping the arms under the top knee and behind the back.

Sitting on your mat, bend one knee in front, bringing the foot alongside the opposite hip with the knee centered and down on the mat. Plant your other foot outside the bottom knee with the toes pointing forward and your knee pointing toward the sky. Sitting up straight, rotate your spine toward the side of the top knee, hooking the opposite elbow outside that knee. Keep that forearm vertical and palm open. The other arm reaches behind the pelvis, grounding the hand.

LOWER BODY

The hips are flexed because you're sitting up straight. The hip of the top knee more so by virtue of flexing the knee and grounding the foot. While both hips are adducted, the hip of the top leg is in slight internal rotation, while the hip of bottom leg is in slight external rotation. The internal rotation of the hip on the top knee results in a great stretch for the gluteus maximus and all of the deep 6 lateral rotators of the hips. The piriformis is by far the biggest and strongest of the six, but you will also feel the deeper gemellus superior, gemellus inferior, obturator internus, obturator externus, and quadratus femoris muscles. A lot of folks will also get a good stretch along the iliotibial (IT) bands. Remember, keep both sit bones evenly grounded. If you feel like you're going to tip over, straighten that bottom leg. Grounding comes first.

Both knees are fully flexed, which will need the quadriceps muscles to lengthen. The foot of the bottom leg that is folded back is supinated, in other words, the foot is turned inward lengthening the lateral side of the ankle.

UPPER BODY

The spine is in pure rotation, from the lumbar vertebrae all the way up to the cervicals. Ensure that you do not extend, flex, laterally flex, or otherwise mess with it. Simply sit up straight and rotate. The lumbar spine will give you a little rotation, about 15 degrees. The vertebrae are very big down there as the lumbar spine's main job is to support the body. The thoracic spine will give a little more rotation, about 40 degrees, as the vertebrae are somewhat smaller than the lumbar vertebrae. The cervical spine on its own, gives you about 90 degrees. That is mainly because these vertebrae are much smaller (only having to support the head). The cervical vertebrae have a fair amount of muscles working unilaterally to get you the deepest rotation here. The biggest of them is the sternocleidomastoid (SCM) muscle that, when brought into concentric contraction, will rotate the head to the opposite side. The splenius capitis, splenius cervicis, and longissimus capitis will all concentrically contract to rotate the head to the same side. As all of these muscles work to rotate the head to one side, their paired muscles on the other side will enjoy a nice stretch.

Practice Tip

If you can't hook your elbow without rounding your back, place your forearm or hand on the outside of the knee instead.

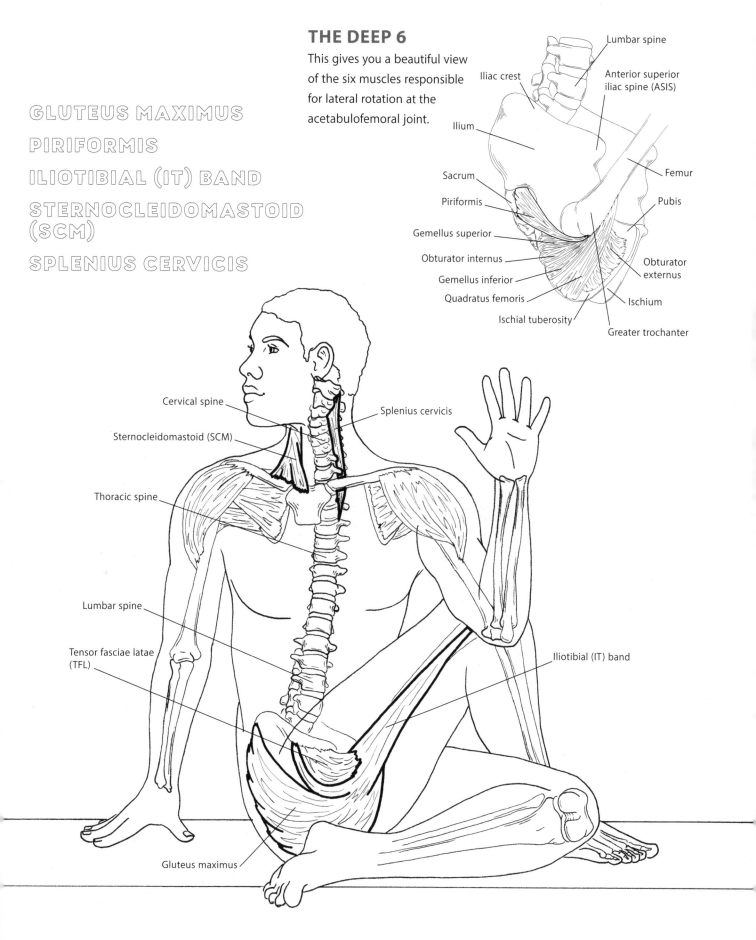

GLUTEUS MAXIMUS

PIRIFORMIS

ILIOTIBIAL (IT) BAND

STERNOCLEIDOMASTOID (SCM)

SPLENIUS CERVICIS

THE DEEP 6

This gives you a beautiful view of the six muscles responsible for lateral rotation at the acetabulofemoral joint.

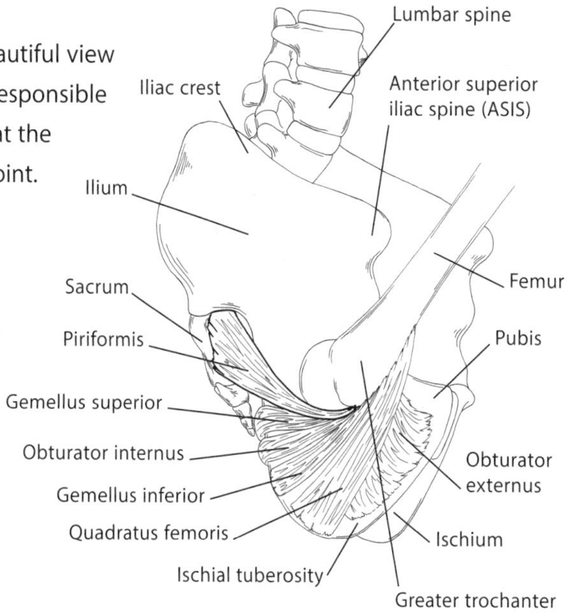

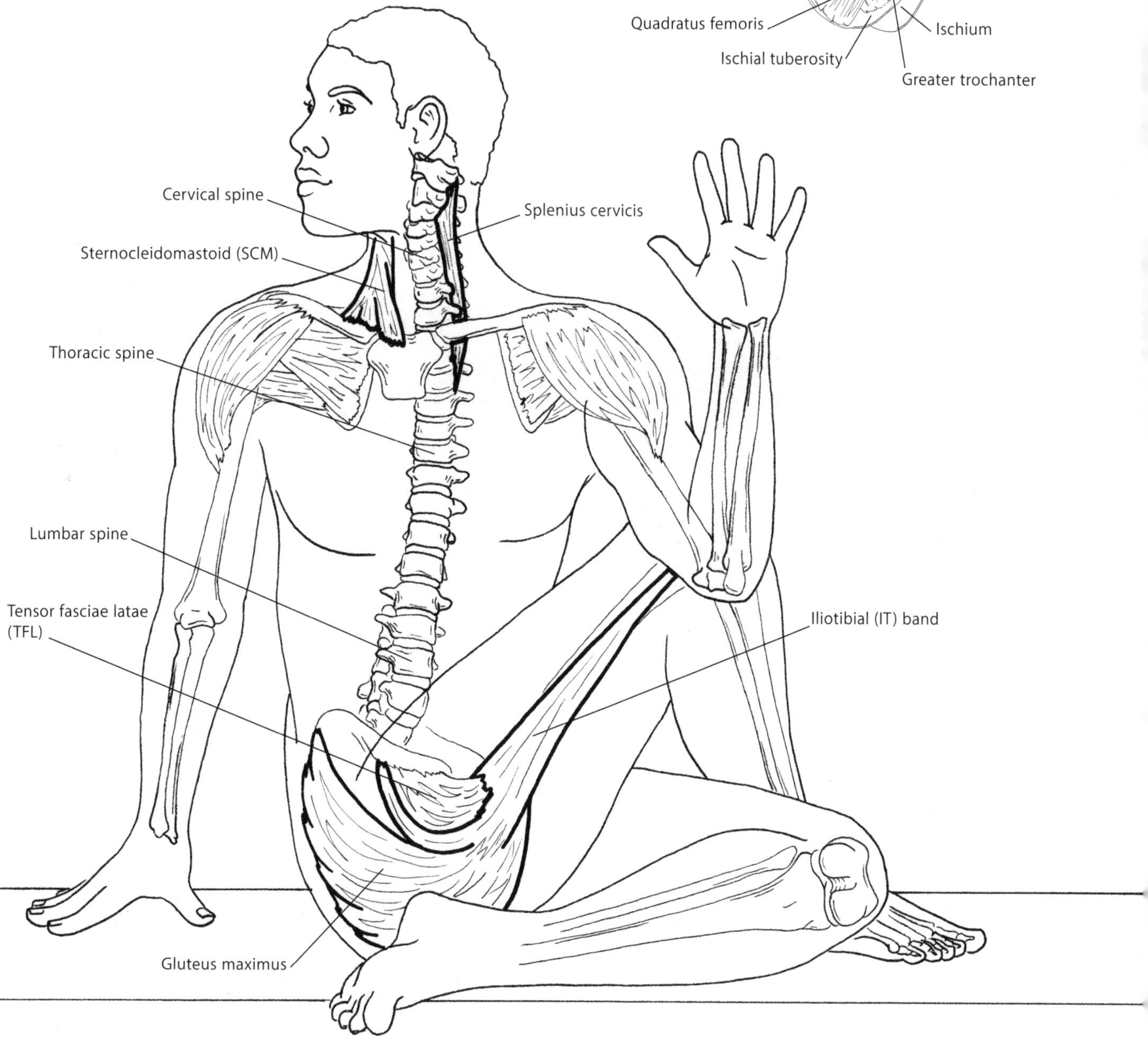

Marichyasana C

mar-ee-chee-AH-sah-nah C

Marichi's Pose C

Marichyasana C is a deeper variation of **marichyasana A**. The legs are the same and you still want to wrap your arms behind your back, only this time you do it with a twist. The less you can twist, the more this is going to ask of your shoulders. As your spinal rotations deepen and your shoulders start to increase in range of motion, this asana will become more available, maybe even comfortable one day!

Set this up the same as you did for **marichyasana A**, sitting up straight with one knee bent, foot placed outside the hip, toes forward; the other leg is extended straight out in front, with the foot in dorsal flexion. Then, twist as deeply as you can toward the bent leg and try to hook your opposite elbow outside the knee. If this works, start to slide the arm down to get the shoulder outside the knee. Then, deeply internally rotate at the shoulder and flex the elbow to bring the upper arm in front of the lower leg with the hand reaching behind the back. The other arm will do the same, internally rotating at the shoulder and reaching behind the back, but this arm has an easier time with no leg in the way.

LOWER BODY

The most important thing for the hips and legs here is to stay aligned and grounded. Don't let all your attention go toward the twist and forget to keep the extended leg active and the foot of the bent leg grounded. Too often I see students with a

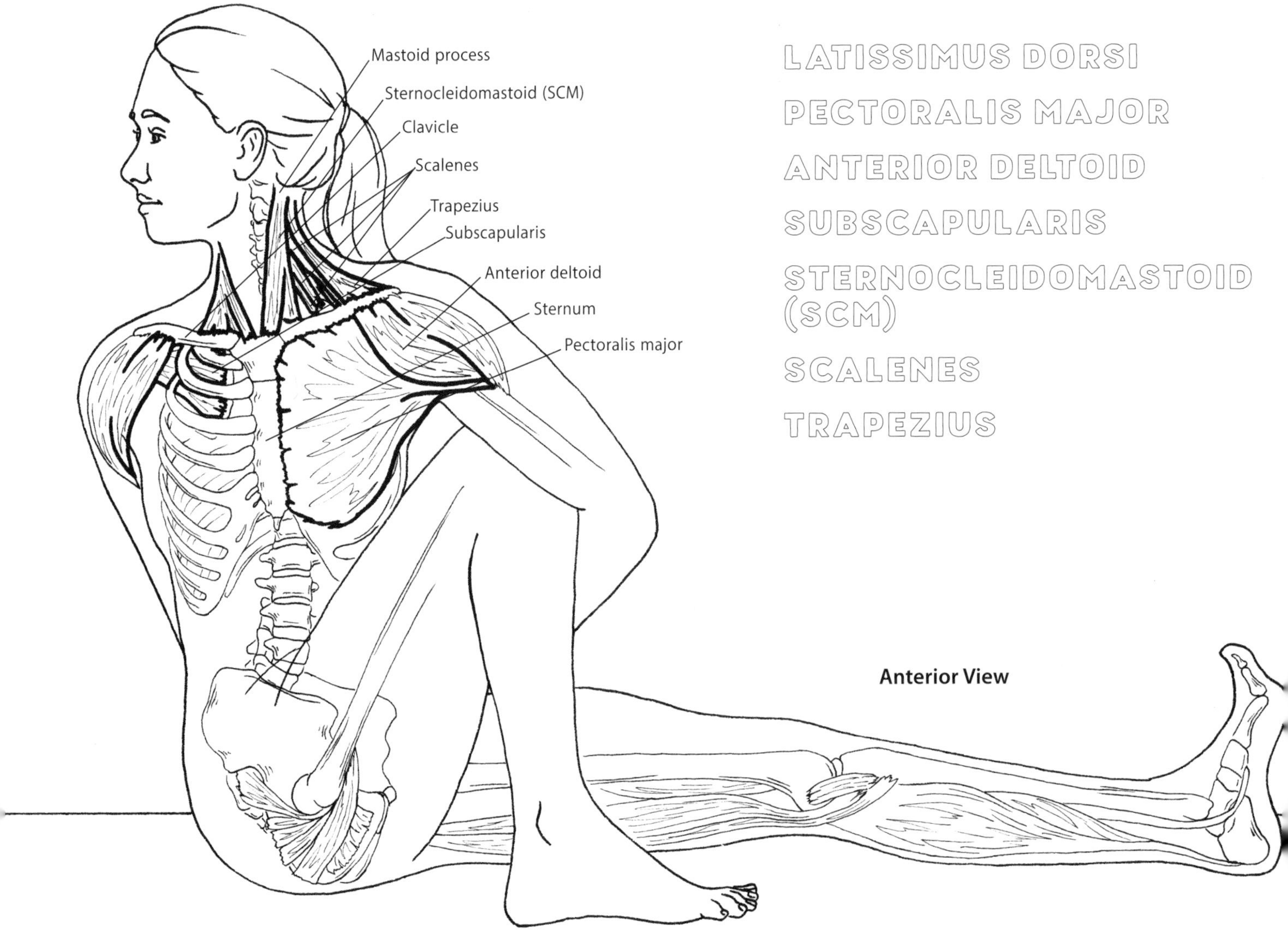

LATISSIMUS DORSI
PECTORALIS MAJOR
ANTERIOR DELTOID
SUBSCAPULARIS
STERNOCLEIDOMASTOID (SCM)
SCALENES
TRAPEZIUS

Anterior View

nice deep twist but also with a useless, forgotten straight leg and the foot of the bent leg peeling up off the mat.

UPPER BODY

The shoulder has some very strong internal rotators; the very big and powerful latissimus dorsi and, as always, its partner the teres major; all the fibers of the pectoralis major muscle; and the anterior deltoid muscle, along with the strongest rotator cuff muscle, the subscapularis. Because this asana calls for such deep internal rotation, the muscles that externally rotate the shoulder must stretch, a lot. These muscles include the smaller infraspinatus and teres minor muscles, two more of your rotator cuff muscles, and the posterior deltoid. Don't let your bigger muscles or your ego overpower the smaller, weaker external rotators.

Your spine is in full rotation all the way up the cervical vertebrae. The sternocleidomastoid (SCM) muscle is a strong and quite showy neck muscle. As you rotate your neck, the sternocleidomastoid on one side will contract while the other side gets a big stretch. You can see it bulging under the skin as it travels from the mastoid process behind the ear down toward the sternum and clavicles. All three scalene muscles and the upper fibers of the trapezius muscle are also strong cervical rotators. All of these muscles work unilaterally to rotate the head to the opposite side. But they are not alone. There are more muscles that could be listed here. It takes a lot to keep that big smart brain of ours up where it belongs.

Practice Tip

This is a very deep twist; make sure that wherever you take it, it doesn't take your breath away. Every asana should be breathable. If you can't breathe, you should try to change your environment. On and off the mat.

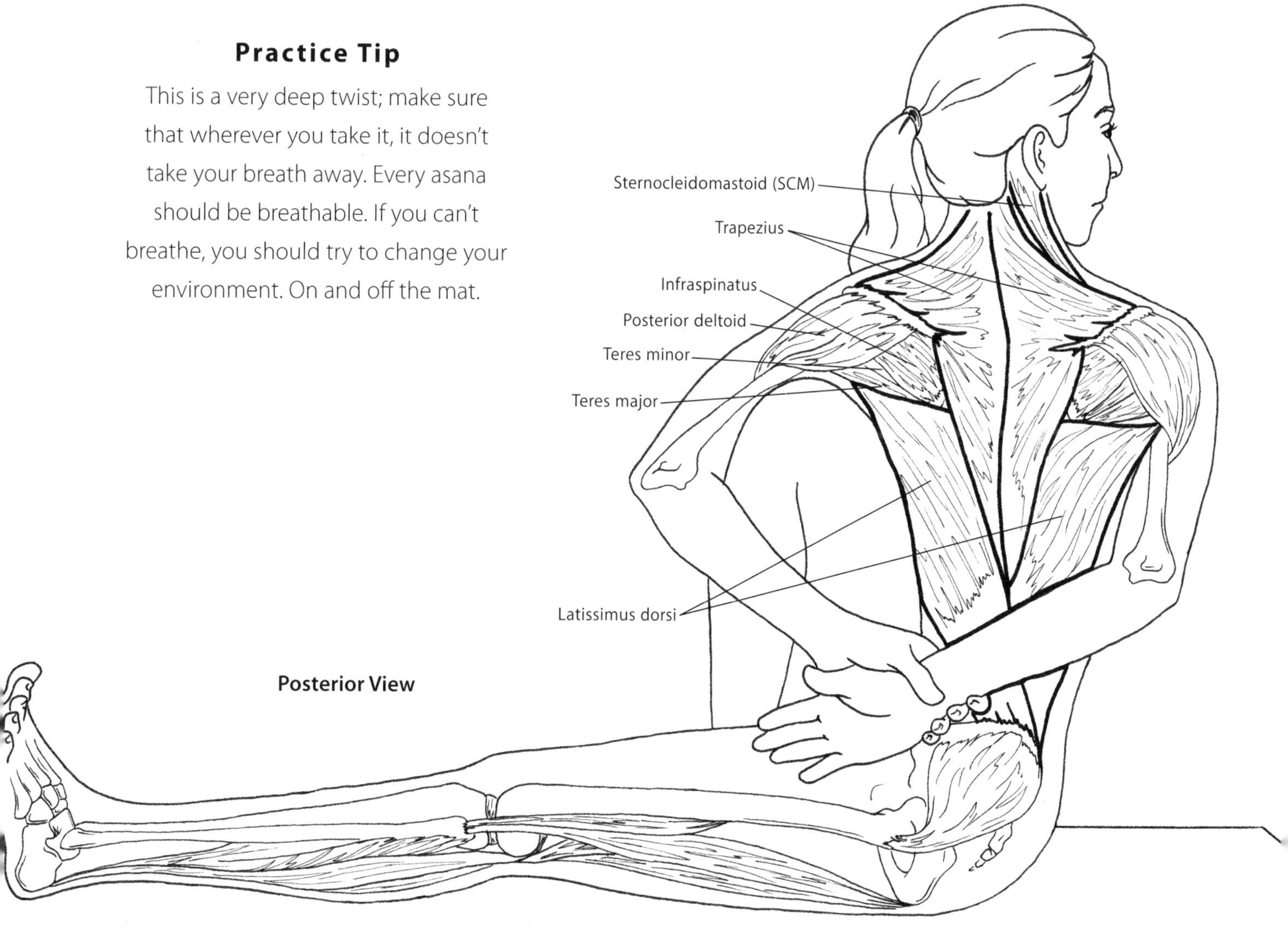

Posterior View

Bharadvajasana

bah-rah-dva-JAH-sah-nah

Bharadvaja's Twist

This is one of the twists you have been preparing for. Not only is it asking for deep spinal rotation, but it wants you to do it while in a half lotus and half hero posture, respectively, with your legs, as one arm wraps behind the back and the other tucks under the opposite knee.

Sitting on your mat, fold one leg back in **ardha virasana** (half hero), and then fold the other leg into **ardha padmasana** (half lotus). Keeping your sit bones evenly grounded, rotate toward the ardha padmasana leg, bringing the arm on that side behind your back reaching your hand for your lotus foot. The other arm crosses the front of the body and the hand tucks under the knee, palm down.

LOWER BODY

This would be a very long section if we covered everything going on in the pelvis and legs; fortunately, postures that require the legs to be in **ardha padmasana** and **ardha virasana** are covered elsewhere in the book. Remember, your legs, particularly your knees as they pertain to this asana, are your friends, and nothing you do in this or any other asana should hurt them.

UPPER BODY

We are going to focus on some of the smaller, deeper muscles that rotate the spine and all those muscles getting a big stretch in the arms. The multifidi and rotatores muscles are small in size, but great in number. The multifidi muscle originate at the sacrum and at each transverse process. They make their way up the spine all the way through the cervicals. They may skip a few vertebrae before inserting into the spinous process of the vertebra above. The rotatores are deep to the multifidi. They first originate at the transverse processes of the lumbar spine and, like the multifidi, continue up to the cervicals, but are most prominent in the thoracic spine. The rotatores, however, may only skip one vertebra, at most, before inserting at the spinous process of the vertebra above. These muscles are deep rotators of the spine and when contracted will rotate the spine to the opposite side. They work unilaterally, so while one side is working, the other side gets a good stretch.

The forearm of the arm in front is supinating, and the wrist is in deep extension. The pronator teres muscle will have to lengthen to bring the forearm into supination. The shoulder (glenohumeral joint) of the back arm is internally rotating, and the wrist is also in slight extension while the fingers hold on to the big toe. The flexor carpi radialis, flexor carpi ulnaris, and palmaris longus, the most superficial of your wrist flexors, will all get a good stretch.

FUN FACT

Bharadvaja may be the only sage to decline Shiva's invitation to heaven. He declined because he wanted to keep experiencing the joy of teaching yoga here on earth for a few more lifetimes.

Practice Tip

Don't make getting the wrap more important than keeping the alignment of the spine. Use a strap to pick up the slack until you can get a grip!

MULTIFIDI
ROTATORES
FLEXOR CARPI RADIALIS
FLEXOR CARPI ULNARIS
PALMARIS LONGUS

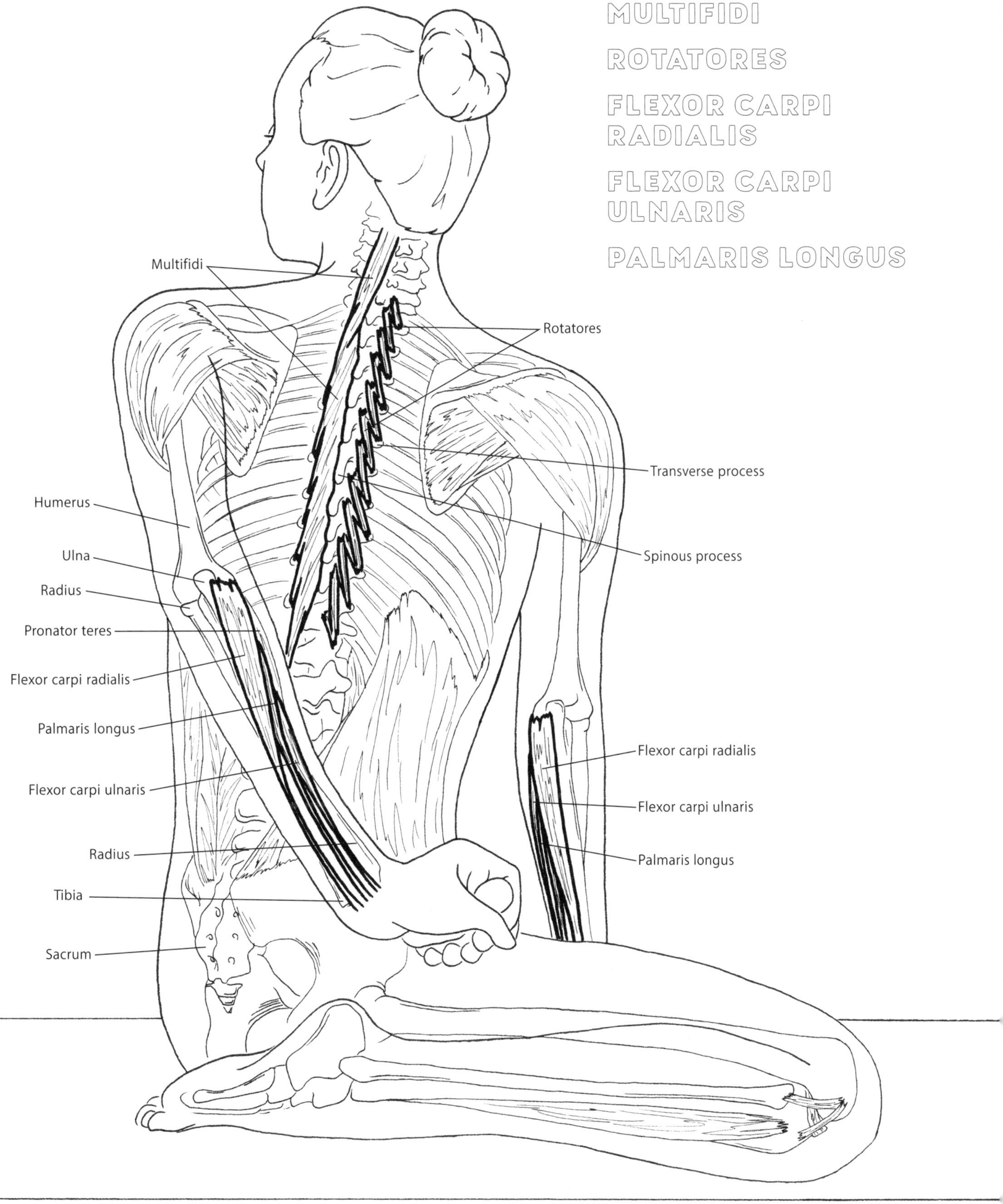

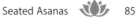

Pasasana

pah-SAH-sah-nah

Noose

Of all the twisting asanas, I find **pasasana** to be one of the deepest and most challenging. It is asking your torso to rotate about 90 degrees. That's a lot. On average, the lumbar and thoracic spine together rotate about 55 degrees. A lot of practitioners will cheat this by rotating the pelvis to make up for what they can't get out of the spine. You will know you're doing this if you can't keep your knees evenly aligned with each other.

First thing is getting into a deep squat, keeping the heels down. Next, twist as deeply as you can and hook an arm outside the opposite knee. Then, deeply internally rotate that shoulder, and wrap the arm around the front of both legs (yes, both legs) as the other arm also reaches back. Clasp your hands together behind your back and hold on.

LOWER BODY

The lower body has a lot of work to do here. It is in a deep squat. The hips are in deep flexion, and the legs are pressed together. To keep the hips from rotating along with the spine, you should engage the psoas of the leg you're twisting toward and the gluteus maximus of the leg you're twisting away from. This will help keep your hips evenly flexed and help to even out your knees. To keep the legs together, your adductors should be working hard until that wrap can hold it all together. **Pasasana** is asking for all of this while you keep your feet, particularly your heels, firmly grounded. Your ankles will be in deep dorsal flexion, working your tibialis anterior muscle like almost no other asana can. Careful not to overdo it here and cause the ankle to stay flexed deeper than it should.

UPPER BODY

Your biggest rotators of the spine are your external obliques and the deeper internal obliques. These muscle groups both work unilaterally to rotate your torso to one side. When your external obliques contract, they pull the trunk to the opposite side; whereas, when the internal obliques contract, they pull the trunk toward the same side. Because they are working unilaterally, the other side of these muscles will, of course, get a good stretch. The smaller, deeper rotatores and multifidus muscles are also actively rotating the spine. If you are fortunate enough, or have practiced long enough, you can hook your shoulder outside the opposite knee and wrap your upper arm around both legs.

The wrap of the arms here asks a lot of your shoulders. Because the arm is leveraged against the leg, you must be careful not to overdo it. The shoulders will be in deep internal rotation and extension as you try to reach your arms behind your back. Your posterior deltoid must lengthen to internally rotate the shoulder, but also must work to pull the shoulders into extension. The same is true for the infraspinatus and teres minor muscles. Negotiate this very judiciously and keep your shoulders happy!

Practice Tip

Prop up the heels, giving your feet a feeling of being in high heels, or as some of my students like to say "Barbie feet," to keep your ankles healthy until they are ready to go all the way down to the mat.

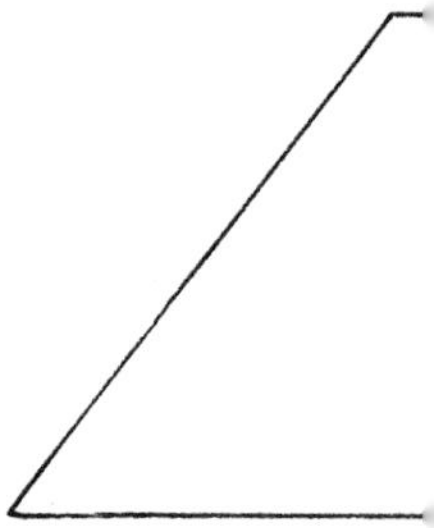

EXTERNAL OBLIQUE
INTERNAL OBLIQUE
POSTERIOR DELTOID
INFRASPINATUS
TERES MINOR

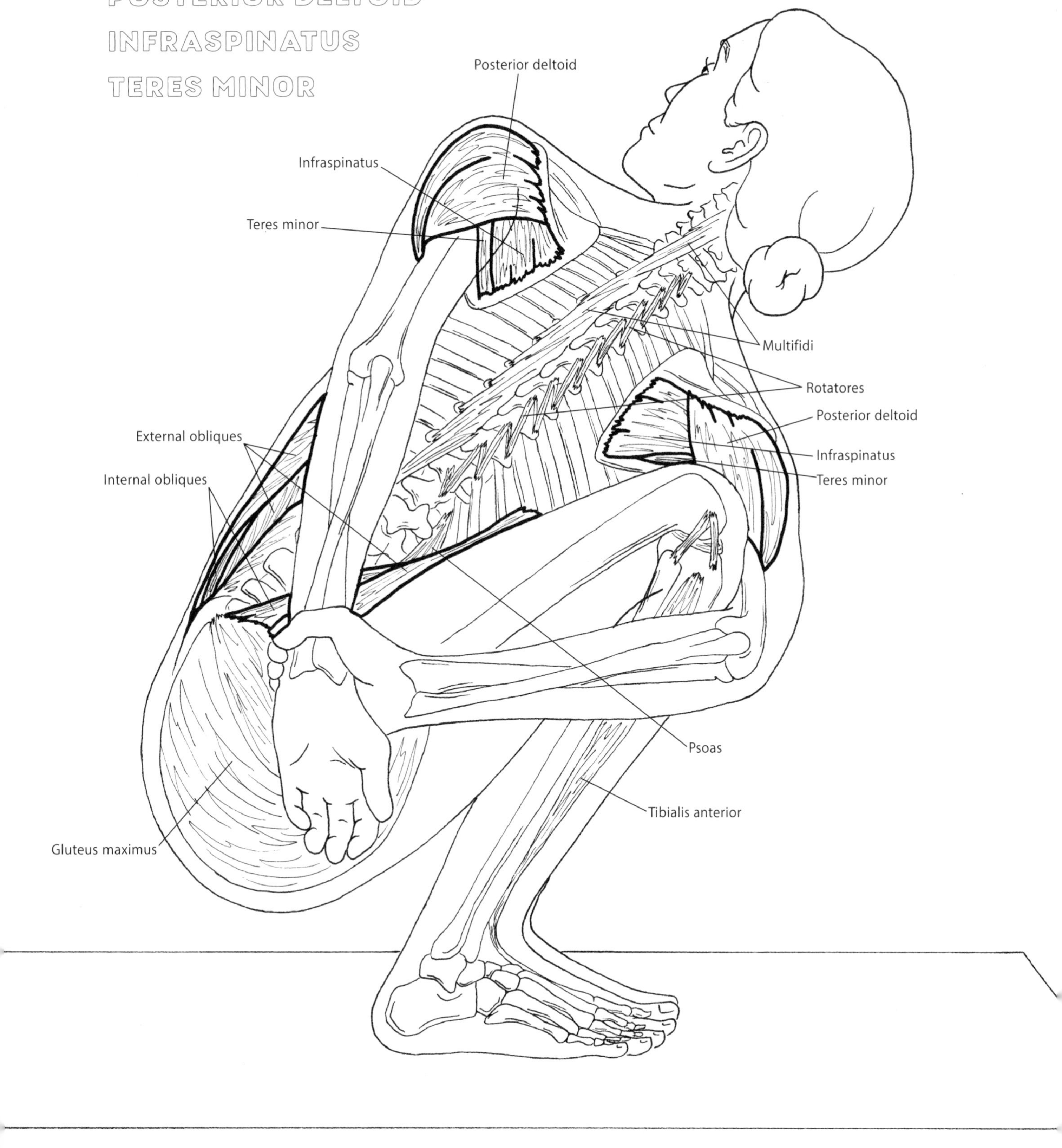

Other Seated Asanas

The other seated asanas in this section are not quite forward bends and not quite twists, although some do call for hip flexion and spinal rotation. One will even ask you to balance on just your sit bones. All of these postures are done on the mat and range from easy to challenging. Of course what's easy and what's challenging is relative to the body that is practicing the asanas. We start easy, with **sukhasana**.

Sukhasana

soo-KAH-sah-nah

Easy Seated Posture

You gotta love an asana with "easy" right in the name. Most of us just think of this as sitting cross-legged. For those who are less flexible, this "easy" seat should get comfortable before the more challenging ones are attempted. Learning how to sit up straight and what it really feels like to be properly aligned in your upper body will serve you well for the rest of your life. This asana will engage the core muscles to stabilize the hips as you sit up tall. It will also start to lengthen the bigger muscles in the hips and legs. What you do with your hands is more of a personal choice, although it should not interfere with keeping your shoulders aligned and relaxed.

Seated on your mat, cross one leg in front of the other, placing the foot under the opposite knee. Then sit up straight with hands rested. That's it. Perhaps the biggest thing here is what you're not doing. The shoulders should be relaxed. Your shoulders should line up right over your hips, and your ears should line up right over your shoulders. Too often, folks keep their shoulders lifted and rounded forward and the head too far forward.

LOWER BODY

This is going to ask your hips to maintain hip flexion and externally rotate. Your psoas and iliacus muscles, working together as the iliopsoas, are your strongest hip flexors and will have to maintain concentric contraction to keep the hips flexed, stabilized, and centered. While the definition of core muscles may vary, for yoga, we all hail the mighty psoas.

UPPER BODY

The transverse abdominis muscles are also strong core muscles and are needed here to help stabilize the pelvis. A weak core may cause the pelvis to fall into posterior tilt. This should be avoided. Relax the levator scapula muscles to drop the shoulders. Pull your scapulae closer together to lengthen to pectoralis major muscles and get your shoulders over your hips. Pull your head back to get your ears over your shoulders and allow the sternocleidomastoid (SCM) and upper portion of your trapezius muscles to return to their original length.

FUN FACT

While **sukhasana** may be easier for most people to practice, because the knees are lifted and all the weight is in the seat, it is harder to hold for longer periods of time than the more challenging padmasana, which allows the knees to help support the posture since they are down on the mat.

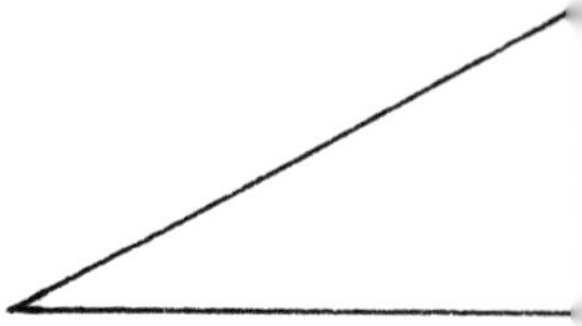

PSOAS

ILIACUS

TRANSVERSE ABDOMINIS

Practice Tip

Prop up your hips to make it easier to sit up straight. If the knees feel vulnerable, place blocks under your knees. The closer you put the blocks to your hips, the more support you will get.

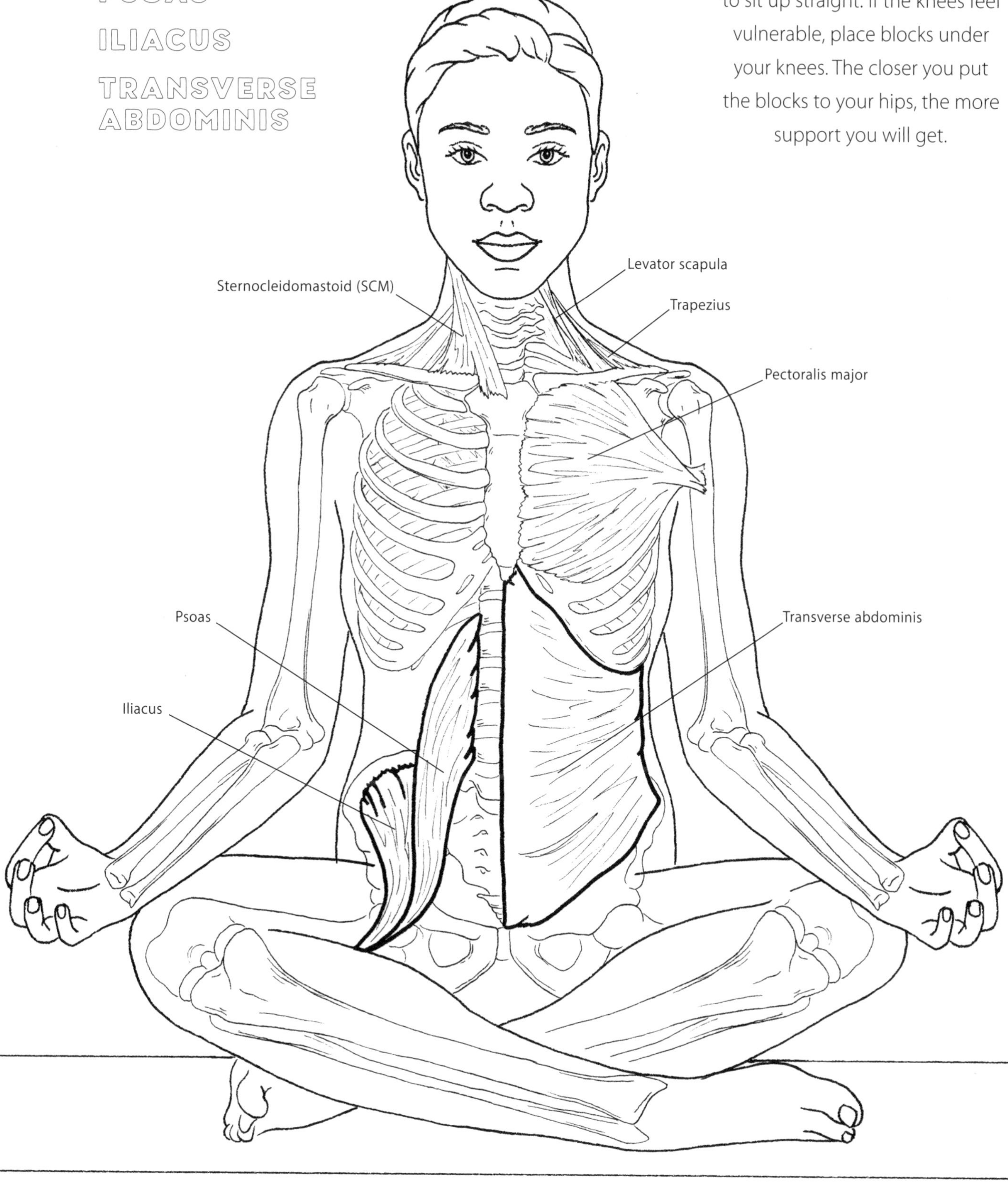

Padmasana

pad-MAH-sah-nah

Lotus

Padmasana is a goal asana for many yogis. It is often viewed as the ideal asana for meditation and is a great posture to work on. For most, this asana may not be attainable at first. The hips must be sufficiently open to externally rotate enough to place your foot on the opposite hip. If the hips are tight, practitioners will all too often let their knee pick up the slack. And that is a mistake. Knees should just be flexed and not rotated in any way. Once the lower body is agreeable to this asana, sitting up straight will become a lot easier. With your knees falling below the hips, the hip flexion is less than other seated asanas, requiring less effort to keep the hips centered and stable. Sitting up straight actually feels pretty easy once **padmasana** is realized.

LOWER BODY

Getting deep enough external, or lateral, rotation of the hips is key here. It's not that the lateral rotators have to work so much; it's more the internal, or medial, rotators of the hips that have to lengthen, a lot. The biggest of these includes the gluteus medius, gluteus minimus, and the tensor fasciae latae (TFL) muscles. It would be wise to warm up these muscles first with less-challenging asanas. If you try to force the foot to the opposite hip, your knee is sure to suffer. The knee will rotate, causing the lateral collateral ligament (LCL) to get really taut. The LCL originates at the lateral condyle of the femur and inserts at the head of the fibula. Asking too much here can permanently lengthen this ligament, causing instability in the knee. In addition, you may "crunch" the medial meniscus. Crunch is not a technical term, but you get the idea. Far too many yogis have forced a lotus or just held it for way too long and ended up injuring that precious cartilage that cushions the space between the femur and the tibia.

For a lot of folks, the ankles start off in deep plantar flexion, again, making up for the hips. If this is happening, chances are you have some knee rotation. The foot should feel rather comfortable up there on the hip, and the ankles should be rather neutral.

UPPER BODY

The upper body should feel tall and the spine should maintain neutrality. This will require the deep postural muscles along the spine to work for you, but they're used to it as they keep you sitting and standing up all day! As the hips evenly ground, your shoulders should line up over your hips, and your ears should line up over your shoulders. The body can, and should, relax and literally hang off the strong central support of the spine.

FUN FACT

In India, this is not considered an advanced posture. Most folks grow up with this, so it is almost expected that this asana is easy for most people and not really such a big deal as it is in the West.

Practice Tip

Be mindful and give this one time. Even though this is considered the "ideal" posture for meditation, just because you can't get this asana yet, or you can't hold it for more than a few seconds, doesn't mean you can't meditate. We often see asana translated as "posture." It literally means "seat." Just find your seat!

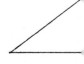

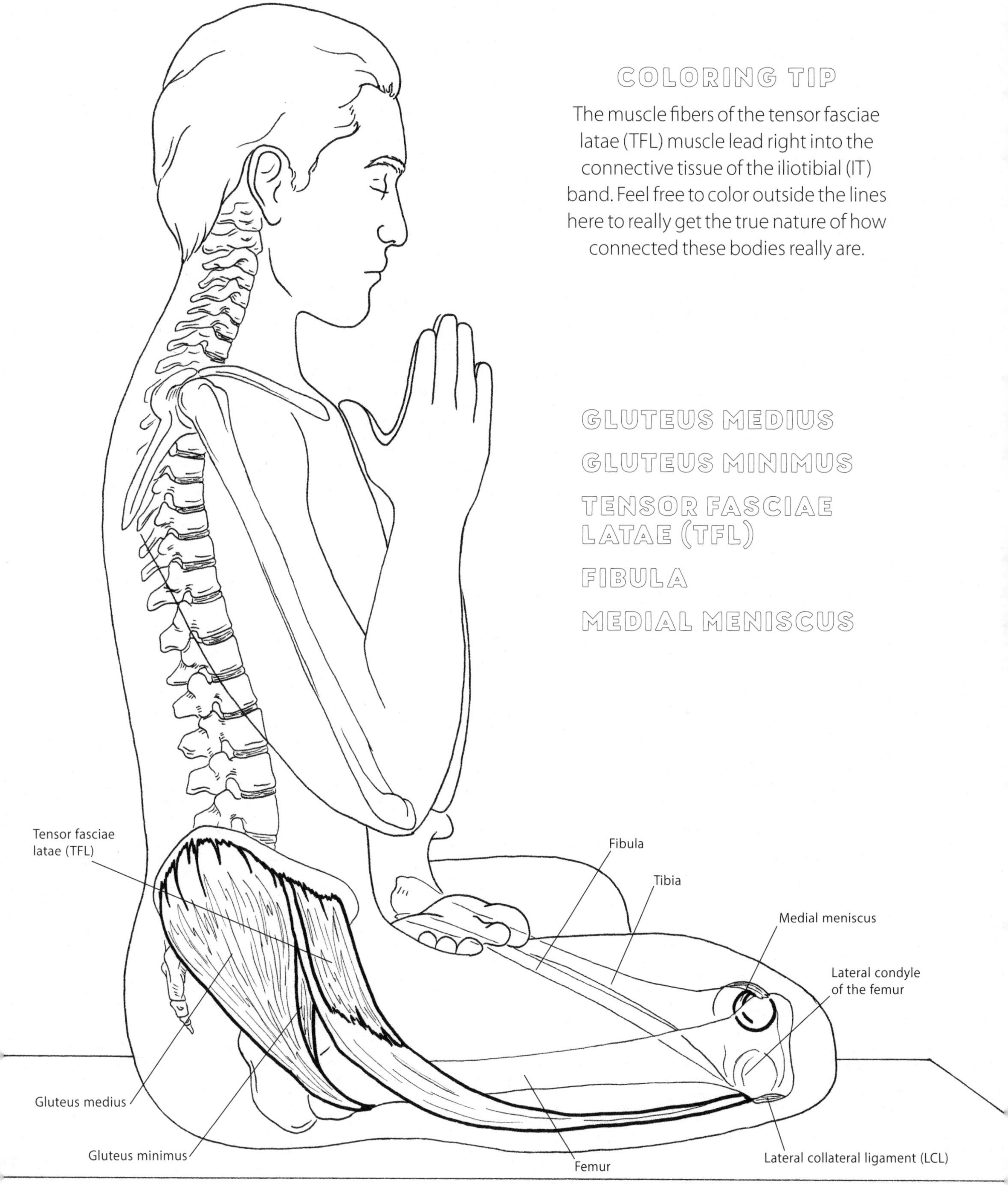

COLORING TIP

The muscle fibers of the tensor fasciae latae (TFL) muscle lead right into the connective tissue of the iliotibial (IT) band. Feel free to color outside the lines here to really get the true nature of how connected these bodies really are.

GLUTEUS MEDIUS

GLUTEUS MINIMUS

TENSOR FASCIAE LATAE (TFL)

FIBULA

MEDIAL MENISCUS

Virasana

veer-AH-sah-nah

Hero

I find **virasana** to be one of the most misunderstood postures. I can't tell you how many times I have heard students say that they were told never to do this because of the damage it would do to the knees. Like most things, there is a right way, and a wrong way. Done correctly, this pose can actually be very good for the knees. Done incorrectly, you will be setting yourself up for trouble.

Sitting on your mat, flex both knees to bring the tops of your feet on the mat alongside the hips with toes pointing straight back. Raise up the arms if you like.

LOWER BODY

The hips here are clearly flexed with the core muscles engaged to maintain flexion. What may not be so clear is the deep internal rotation required of the hips as well. It is the hips that should be rotating here; they are a ball-and-socket joint and built for that. The piriformis muscle, along with the other five lateral rotators of the hips have to give you some room and lengthen. It is this action, along with very, very slight rotation in the knee, that will allow the feet to hug the outside of the hips. If you force this asana and there is not enough rotation in the hips, the knees may try to rotate too much. This is a mistake. The knees are basically a hinge joint and not meant to give you very much rotation. Get the rotation from the hips! You should adduct the hips to keep the knees together, or at least no wider than your hips.

Keeping the knees happy is paramount here. The knees are in very deep flexion, more than if you were just sitting on your heels. This is going to stretch your quadriceps a lot. Since the vastus medialis, vastus intermedius, and vastus lateralis (three of your four quadriceps) all originate at the top of the femur and then travel along the front of the thigh to finally insert at the top of the tibia, the knee positioning here is asking for a lot of length from them. Rectus femoris, the strongest of the group and the only one that crosses the hips, will still get a nice stretch, even with the hips flexed. In response to the internal rotation at the hips and placement of the feet alongside the hips, the space between the medial condyle of the femur and the corresponding medial condyle of the tibia will have to increase somewhat. Holding that knee together on the medial side is your medial collateral ligament (MCL) and your medial meniscus. The MCL connects the femur to the tibia and stabilizes the knee. It should not be stretched. The medial meniscus cushions the space between the condyles and almost seamlessly attaches to the MCL. If you ask the knee for too much space here you run the risk of not only a tear to the MCL, but to the meniscus as well. There should be no pain in the knees. If it feels sketchy, back off.

Your ankles are in pure plantar flexion. The tibialis anterior is undeniably getting a big stretch here. Pointing the toes and feet out to the sides will increase the space in the medial knee and will almost certainly cause damage to the MCL and medial meniscus. Don't do that.

UPPER BODY

The glenohumeral joint, another ball-and-socket joint, and usually referred to as the shoulder, is in deep flexion and internal rotation. The pectoralis major is a huge muscle and its upper fibers are some of the strongest flexors of the shoulder. The pectoralis minor muscle will work to help keep the scapulae pulling down the back and in retraction. Be mindful to stay tall with the spine neutral and the chest feeling broad.

FUN FACT

Virasana is another asana named in honor of the brave hero Hanuman, who is often referred to as "Vir" Hanuman. This is a posture honoring not Hanuman's great strength, but his humility, faith, loyalty, and devotion to Rama, who to him, is God.

VASTUS MEDIALIS

VASTUS INTERMEDIUS

VASTUS LATERALIS

RECTUS FEMORIS

MEDIAL COLLATERAL LIGAMENT (MCL)

MEDIAL MENISCUS

Practice Tip

Prop up the sit bones if the knees will not accommodate this yet. Just sitting on something here can make what was an otherwise unattainable posture available. As the quadriceps lengthen and your hips open, the height of the prop will lessen until one day, it may no longer be necessary.

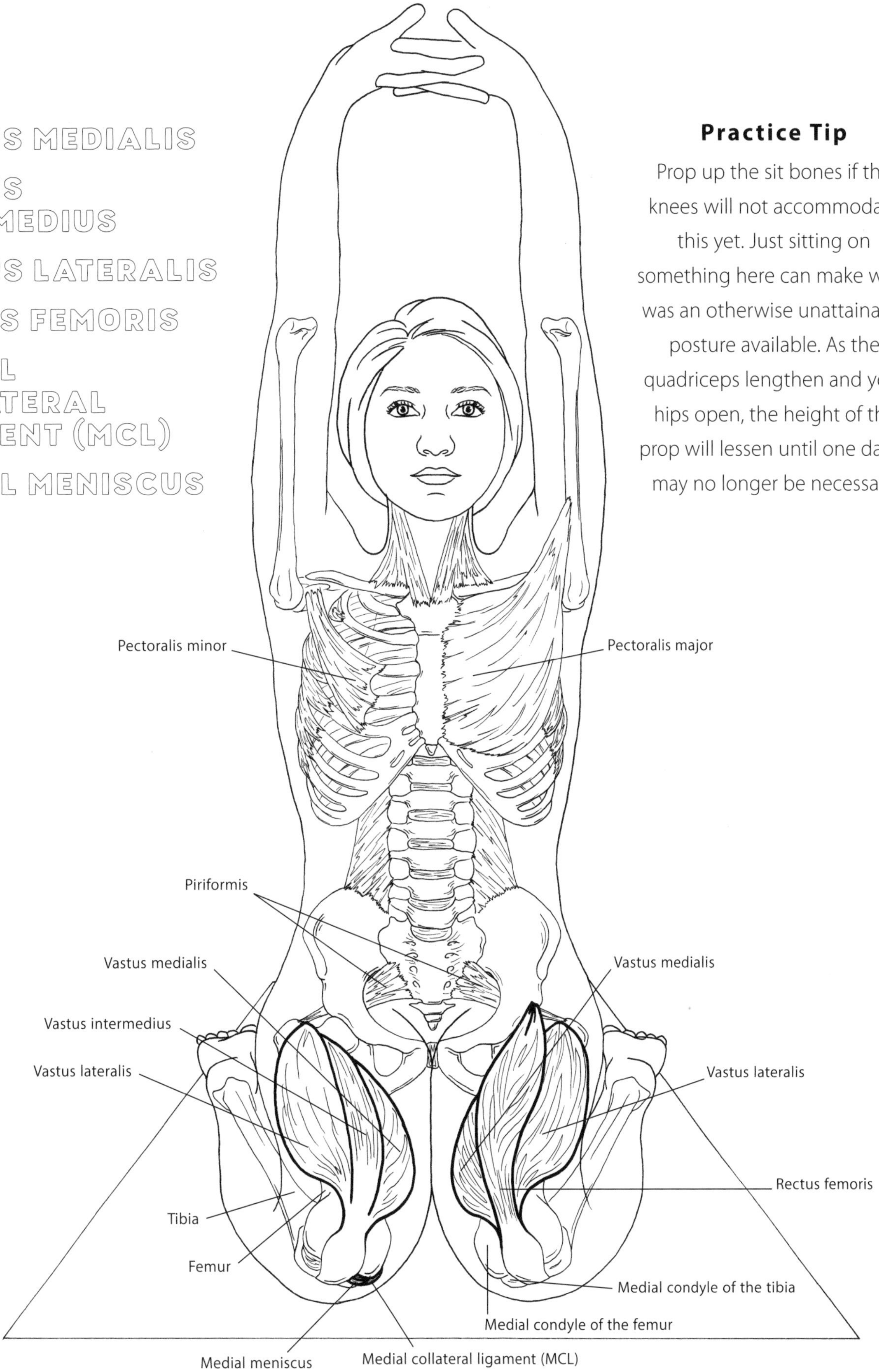

Parighasana (Iyengar)

pah-ree-GAH-sah-nah

Gate

Different yoga asana traditions have different takes on what they consider a proper **parighasana**. Iyengar yoga has you in a kneeling position, whereas the Ashtanga Vinyasa style performs this asana from a seated position. Either way, it's going to give you a juicy side bend. It is the challenge of the leg positioning where these two styles of yoga part ways. Because of the very different expressions this asana can take, I thought it would be worthwhile, and fun, to explore both.

Most folks will find the Iyengar version of **parighasana** more achievable than the Ashtanga version. You start kneeling on your mat with your hips lined up over your knees, facing forward. Abduct one hip to bring the leg straight out to the side with the toes pointing out to the same side in deep plantar flexion. (Some folks like to dorsal flex the foot here; I am not sure if Iyengar would like that!) The arm on the same side of the extended leg will stack on top of that leg with the palm up. Abduct the other arm at the shoulder to line it up with the ear, and then, keeping your hips fixed, laterally flex the spine to bring the top hand toward the bottom hand. Rotate the spine only at the neck to look up.

UPPER BODY

The facet joints of the spine will articulate with each other up and down the spine as you pull the spine into lateral flexion. The strongest muscles that will laterally flex your spine are the erector spinae muscles, the quadratus lumborum, and both the internal and external obliques.

The erector spinae muscles basically run vertically from the pelvis to the occiput (the bone at the base of the skull), branching into three distinct groups of muscles: the spinalis muscles, which are the most proximal to the spine; the longissimus, which runs lateral to the spinalis; and the iliocostalis muscles, which are the most distal from the spine of the group, and the strongest to pull the spine laterally. Since gravity always plays a role, notice that the quadratus lumborum muscle will be in eccentric contraction as it resists gravity while the spine is moving into lateral flexion. The transverse abdominis will get a big opening stretch here along the opposite side of the bend. It's like your waist gets a chance to breathe.

It is only the top shoulder that is really working here, and you're going to need every one of your deltoid muscles to deeply abduct that shoulder to get that top hand as close to the bottom one as possible.

LOWER BODY

The hip of the straight leg will be in abduction and the knee should be full extended. If you choose to dorsal flex the ankle, you will feel a nice stretch in the lower leg; whereas, if you choose to go with the foot flat on the mat and toes pointing forward, that will bring the ankle into supination, giving the lateral side of the lower leg a nice stretch. Keeping the toes pointing laterally, in true Iyengar fashion, will give the anterior ankle a big stretch.

Practice Tip

Remember, with all asymmetrical postures, and because most muscles are paired, whatever is really working on one side, will get a good stretch on the other side, and vice versa. Always practice both sides of an asymmetrical asana, maybe spending a little more time on the side you find more challenging.

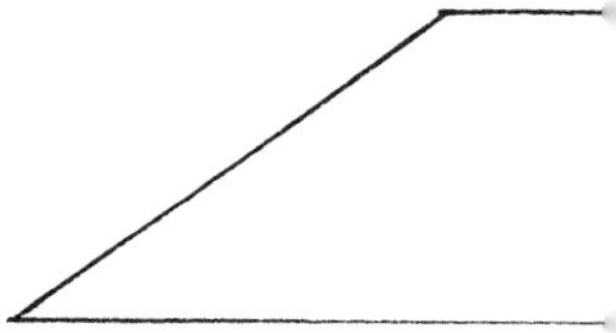

SPINALIS
LONGISSIMUS
TRANSVERSE ABDOMINIS
POSTERIOR DELTOID
MIDDLE DELTOID

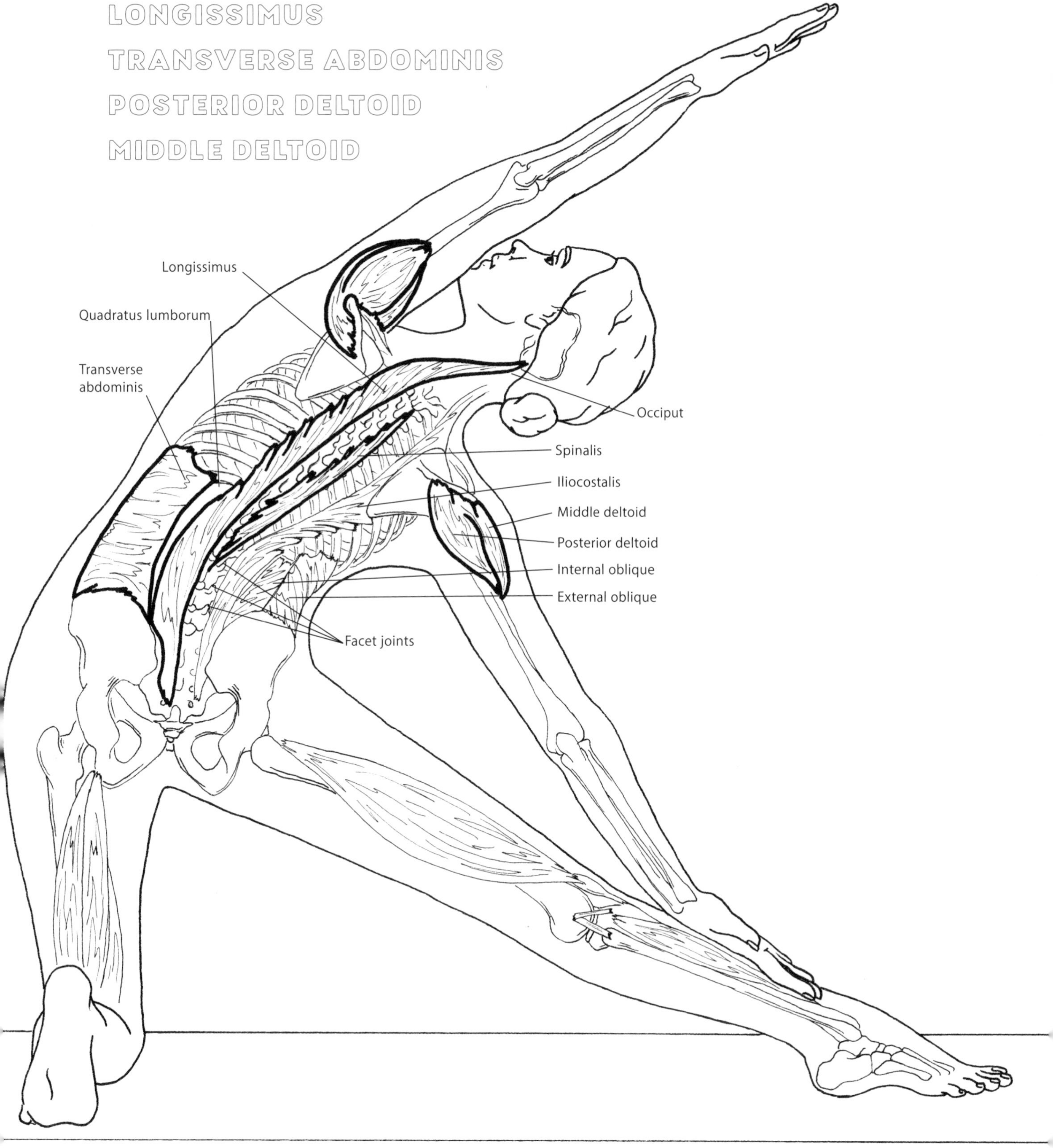

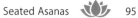

Parighasana (Ashtanga)

pah-ree-GAH-sah-nah

Gate

The Ashtanga Vinyasa version of **parighasana** asks everything from the spine and top shoulder that the Iyengar style calls for, and more. First, get seated on your mat and bring one leg straight out in front of you with the other leg bending back in **ardha virasana** (half hero), keeping about a 90-degree angle between the thighs. Laterally flex the spine toward the straight leg, bringing that bottom shoulder as close to the medial side of the knee as possible. Reach that arm along the medial leg and grab your foot, as you bring your spine into rotation, turning the chest toward the sky. Abduct the shoulder of the top arm and bring it alongside that top ear, trying to get this hand to the foot of the extended leg as well.

UPPER BODY

It is the rotation, added to the deep lateral flexion of the spine, that "helps" make this version a lot more challenging. You are calling into action all the muscles you need to laterally flex the spine and adding the multifidus and rotatores muscles to rotate the spine. The external obliques on one side are working double duty here to both laterally flex and rotate the spine to the opposite side, while the other pair of these muscles on the other side will enjoy a nice stretch. The internal obliques, although working for the lateral flexion, must give a little to allow for the rotation and vice versa on the other side. It's an interesting negotiation.

The deeper action in the shoulders adds some spice here as well. Whereas the Iyengar version only asks for abduction in the top shoulder, this version adds to that. At first, you need to horizontally abduct that bottom shoulder to snuggle it down inside the knee. Then externally rotate and abduct the shoulder to reach the hand for the foot. At first, the anterior deltoid is going to work a little to bring the shoulder into horizontal adduction; but when you externally rotate and abduct the shoulder, it will get a big stretch. The anterior deltoid of the top arm is at work here. Also getting a deep stretch are the pectoralis major and the subscapularis. The latissimus dorsi and teres major on the "top" side of the torso will also enjoy a nice stretch, but these muscles will be working on the "bottom" side of the torso to help with lateral flexion in the spine.

LOWER BODY

Depending on how deeply you can abduct at the hip will determine how much stretch you feel in the adductor and hamstring muscles of the straight leg. Be careful not to overdo it and end up lifting the sit bones of the bent leg off the mat. Even though each side of the hips is doing something different, it's important to still try to maintain an even ground through both sit bones.

FUN FACT

The Ashtanga tradition of yoga practice has you holding each asana for five breaths; whereas, in Iyengar-style practice, you hold postures for much, much longer. Each tradition has valid points for why they believe their style of practice is better. I think it depends on the body you're in and what would benefit it most at any given time.

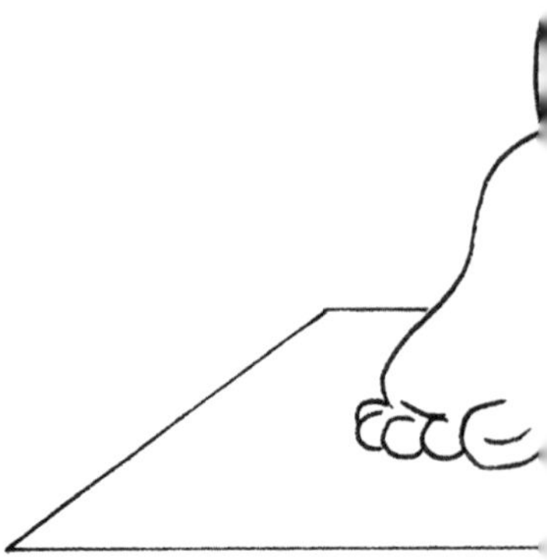

COLORING TIP

The latissimus dorsi muscle originates along a huge swath, including the iliac crest and thick connective tissue of the lower back and spine, the lower six thoracic vertebrae, and the lower ribs. Color this area a lighter shade than the actual muscle bellies to show how big the origin site of this muscle really is.

ANTERIOR DELTOID
LATISSIMUS DORSI
TERES MAJOR
PECTORALIS MAJOR
SUBSCAPULARIS

JOINTS OF THE PELVIS

Most folks don't realize that your pelvis is composed of more than just your acetabulofemoral joint (most commonly refer to as the hip joint). This is where the leg attaches to the torso. The sacroiliac joint (most commonly referred to as the SI joint) attaches the pelvis to the axial skeleton. The pubic symphysis, the least movable joint of the pelvis, joins the pubic bones together and is the most anterior of the pelvic joints.

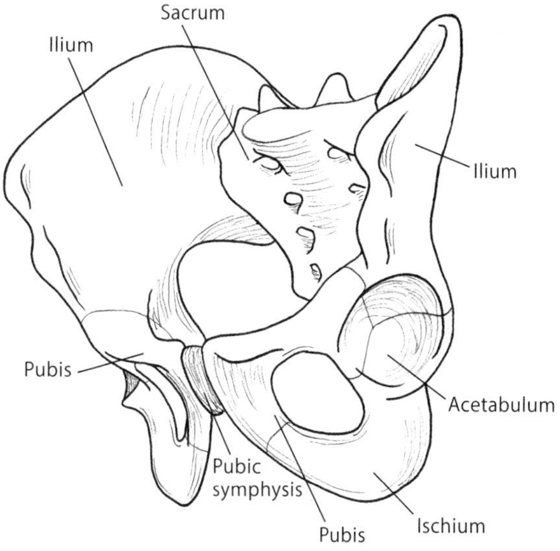

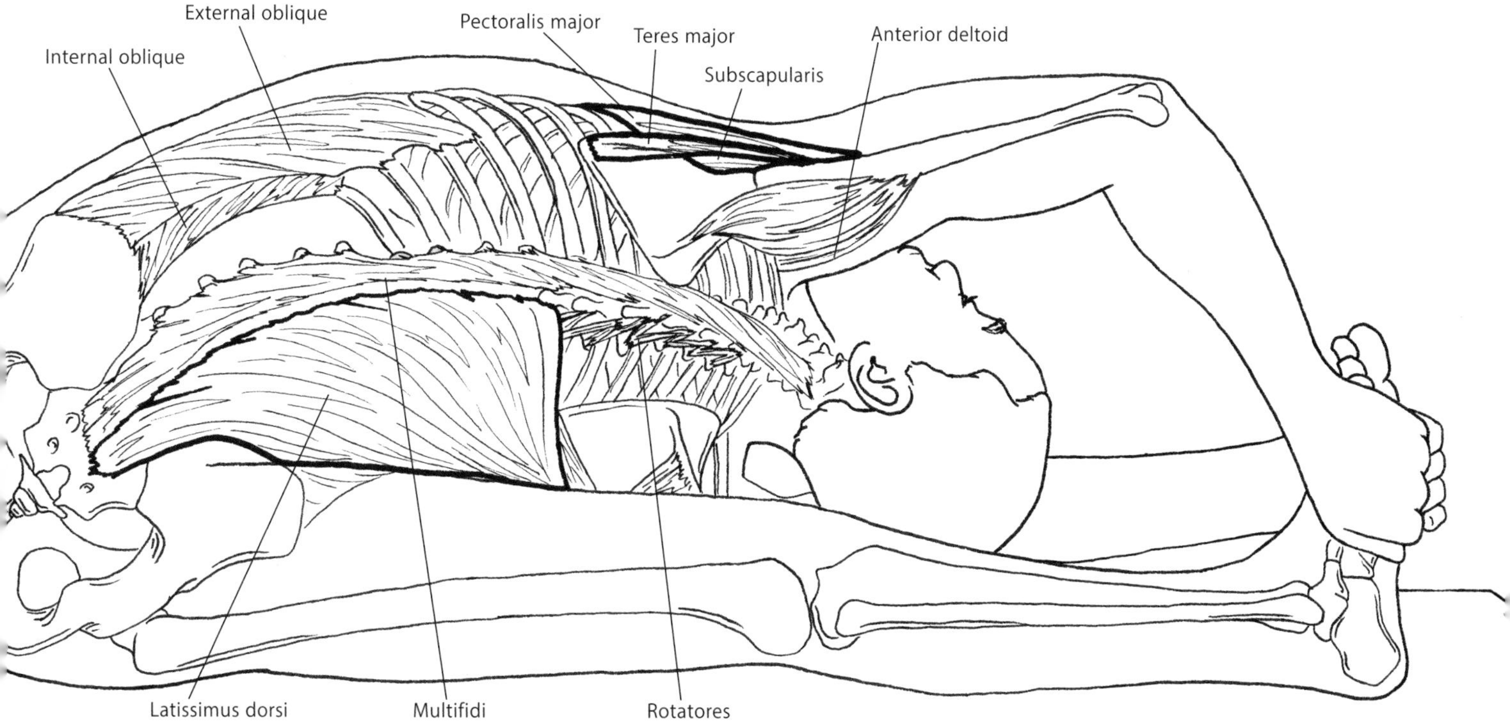

Navasana

nah-VAH-sah-nah

Boat

Navasana is a very core-centric posture. While some asanas may work just your lower or upper core, navasana wants it all. This is available to most everyone; it is just a matter of degree. Bending the knees makes it easier. Using your hands to hold behind the knees makes it easier. Don't avoid this asana; just modify as needed and keep doing it until you like it!

Seated on your mat, bring your knees toward your chest, flexing your hips. Retract and depress your scapula (bring your shoulder blades together and down), and lift your sternum (heart center). It is imperative that you stay up on your ischial tuberosities (sit bones) and resist allowing the spine to go into flexion and the hips to posteriorly tilt. (If you lose heart here, everyone will know, as you will roll backward on your mat!) Then, extend your legs as much as you can, pressing the balls of the feet forward as the toes spread wide and pull back. The biggest challenge here is resisting gravity.

LOWER BODY

Your psoas and iliacus muscles are concentrically contracted to hold the hips in flexion and keep both the legs and the upper body elevated. They are not working alone; the rectus femoris, sartorius, gluteus minimus, and tensor fasciae latae (TFL) are also fully engaged. In the beginning, you may feel this mainly in the front of the thighs, but as your core strengthens and your quadriceps get stronger, this will get easier. Promise.

As you try to extend the knees and hold them in extension, all four of your quadriceps muscles will concentrically contract and hold like crazy. Some practitioners' legs will get a little shaky here. Everyone's legs will get shaky here if you hold it long enough.

UPPER BODY

Your rhomboids and trapezius muscles will contract to retract the scapula. The serratus anterior muscles depress or draw the scapula down. You want to feel like the scapulae are propping up your heart and lungs. The chest should feel lifted.

The traditional arm positioning here is to reach the arms straight out in front of you with your elbows fully extended, palms facing in. The biceps brachii will be working to keep the shoulders in flexion, and the triceps brachii will be working to keep the elbows fully extended. Just when you thought this asana was all core!

Practice Tip

Engaging your zygomaticus muscle here will make **navasana** and every other asana easier. (The zygomaticus is also known as your smiling muscle. It is a muscle in your face that draws the mouth upward and outward.)

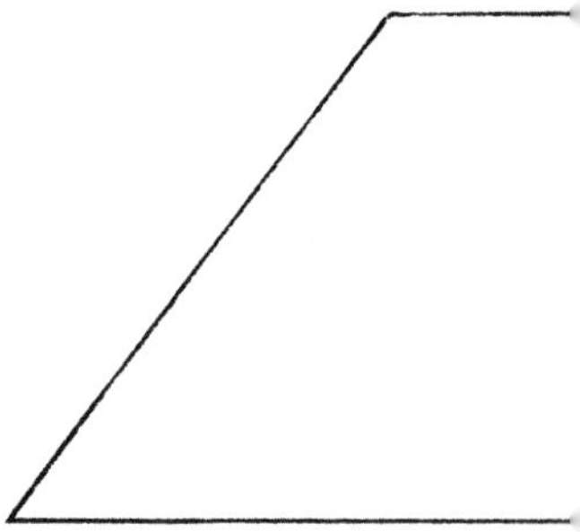

ILIACUS
RECTUS FEMORIS
SARTORIUS
GLUTEUS MINIMUS
TENSOR FASCIAE LATAE (TFL)

COLORING TIP

When you color the biceps brachii muscle on the right arm, note that the muscle originates from two heads at the shoulder. Use a sharp pencil and when you see the fork in the road, take it. Your left arm has two heads on the biceps muscle as well; you just can't see it from this view.

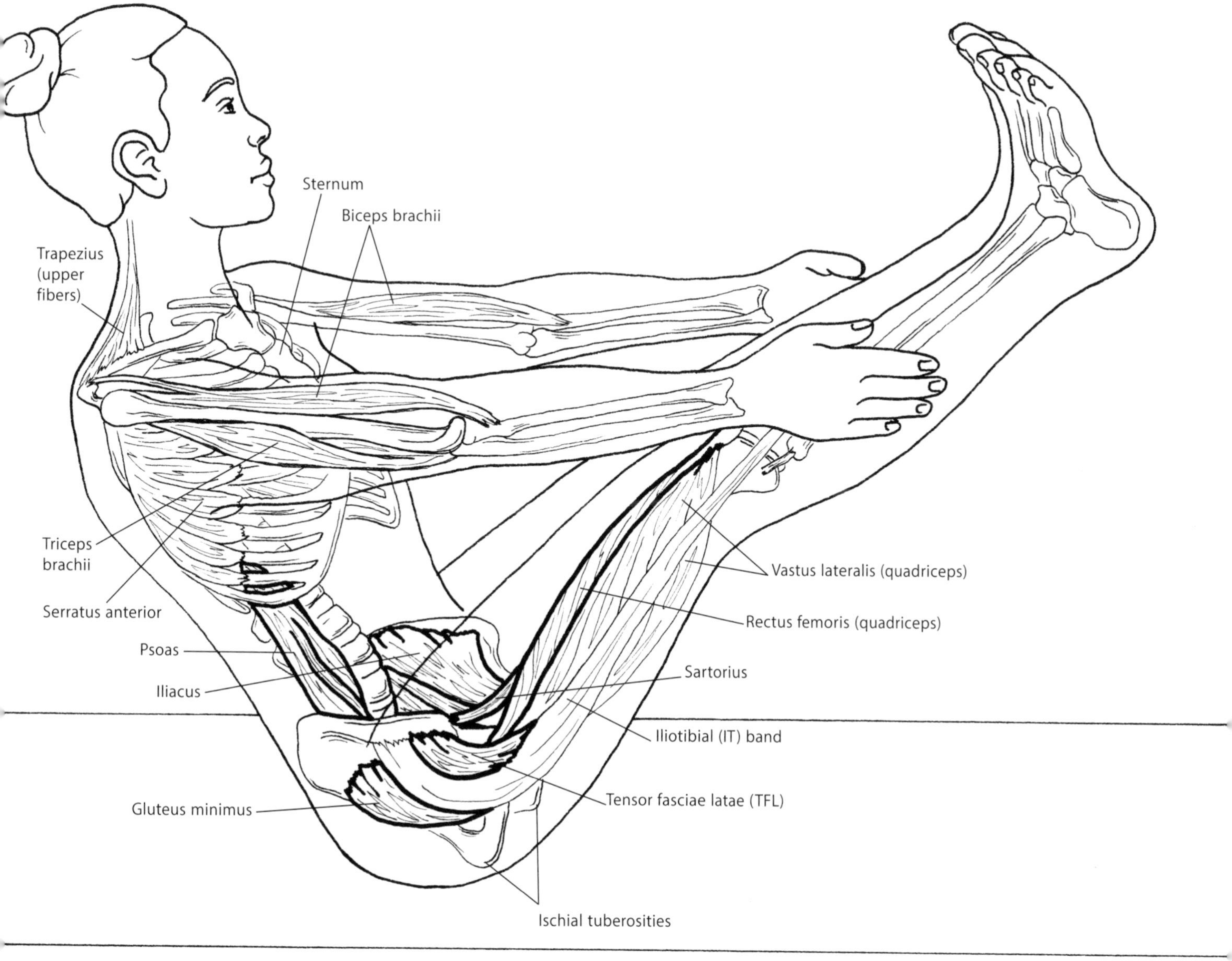

Krounchasana

kruhn-CHAH-sah-nah

Heron

Krounchasana is an advanced asana, and there are a lot of other foundational postures that should be at a level of competency before making this a part of your practice. It is akin to **triang mukha eka pada paschimottanasana**, except instead of pulling your upper body toward the straight leg, you're pulling the leg toward the upper body. And you're moving against gravity, adding to the challenge. Krounchasana will stretch your hamstrings, but what needs more of your attention here is the strength necessary in the spinal muscles to keep the pelvis neutral and the spine from being pulled into flexion (i.e., rounding).

Sitting on your mat, bend one leg back in **ardha virasana** (half hero), deeply internally rotating the hip. If you need to sit up on a block to keep the knee happy, you should. Once you've settled your seat, reach for your other foot and extend the knee as much as possible. Use a strap to pick up the slack, if needed. This hip is in pure hip flexion, as deep as you can get it without affecting the spine. Keep your sit bones evenly grounded, even as they are not doing exactly the same thing. Then stretch those hamstrings and find that edge.

LOWER BODY

You have to be careful with the bent leg in **krounchasana**. The medial hamstrings—the semimembranosus and semitendinosus—along with the gracilis—the one adductor muscle that crosses the knee—and the sartorius—the longest muscle you have—can all act to rotate the knee. These muscles also engage to internally rotate the hip. This is where you need to be careful. You want deep internal rotation in the hip, but very, very little rotation in the knee. The semitendinosus, gracilis, and sartorius all insert at the same point on the tibia. This is called the pes anserinus, which lies right above your medial collateral ligament (MCL). Any tension in these muscles' tendinous attachments on the lower leg should be avoided. Everything is truly connected, and you want to keep everything connected! This foundation should feel solid so the pose gets to those hamstrings.

UPPER BODY

Your erector spinae muscles are working hard with some help from the quadratus lumborum muscles and other deeper muscles along the posterior spine to keep the spine from being pulled toward flexion. They also help to keep the pelvis from being pulled into posterior tilt. The spinalis, longissimus, and Iliocostalis muscles make up the erector spinae group of muscles and will all be working here to maintain correct alignment from the pelvis all the way up to the neck.

Practice Tip

There are many asanas that ask for the hips to do asymmetrical ranges of motion but still stay even. It is too easy to fall into bad habits of letting the hips get misaligned because we think we are getting deeper in the pose or it just feels easier. Don't fall for it. Stay vigilant.

SEMIMEMBRANOSUS
SEMITENDINOSUS
GRACILIS
SARTORIUS
PES ANSERINUS

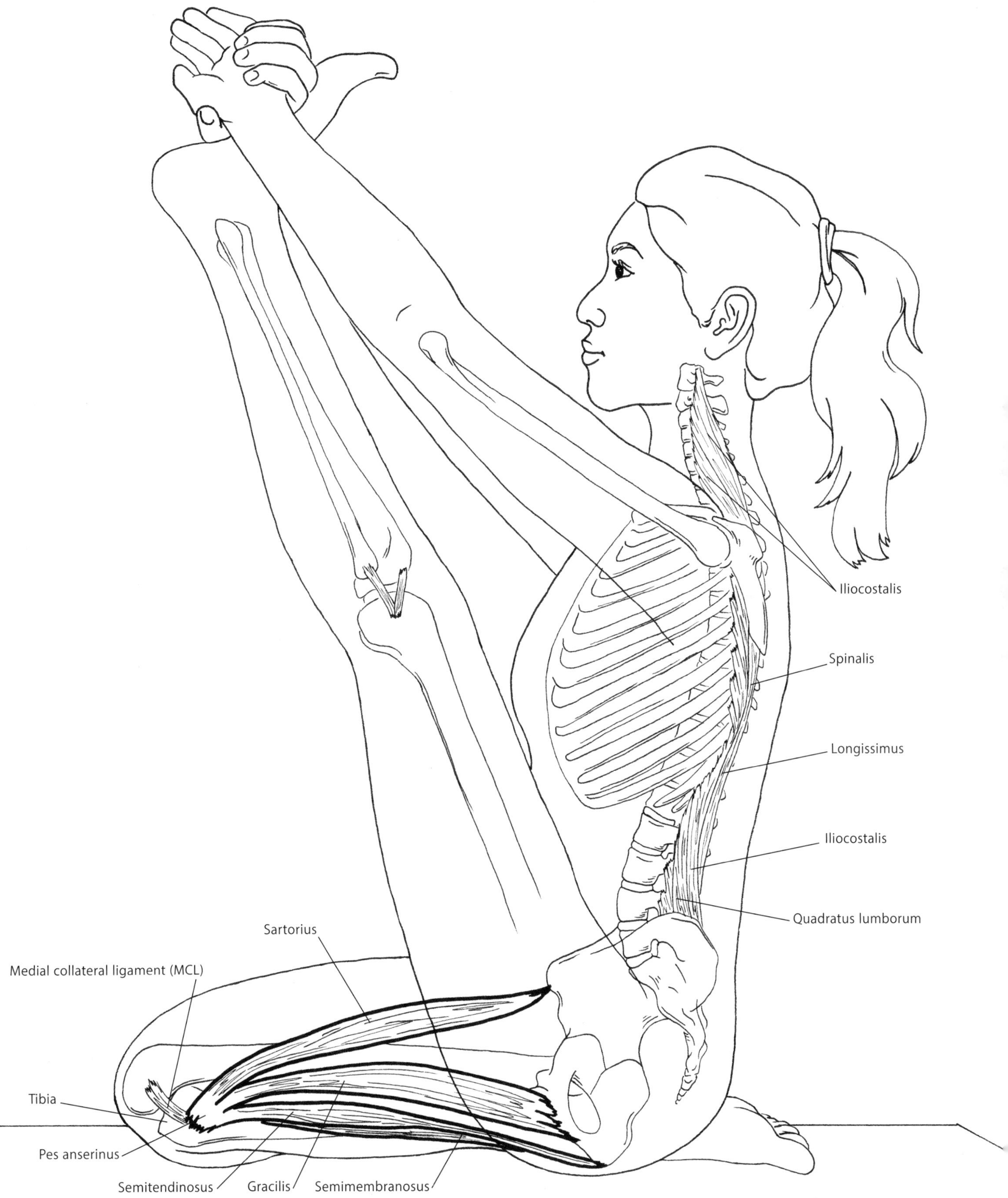
Iliocostalis
Spinalis
Longissimus
Iliocostalis
Quadratus lumborum
Sartorius
Medial collateral ligament (MCL)
Tibia
Pes anserinus
Semitendinosus
Gracilis
Semimembranosus

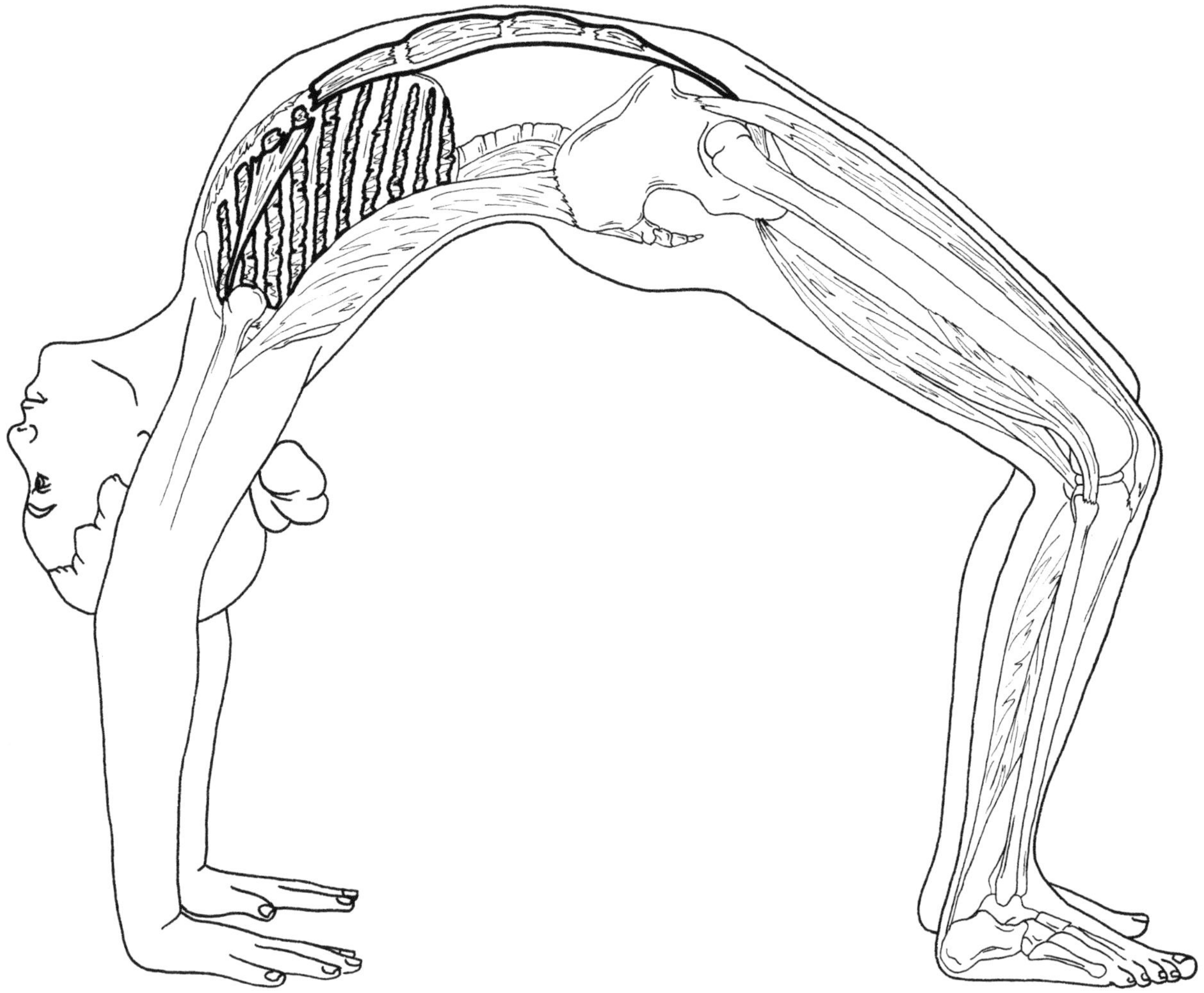

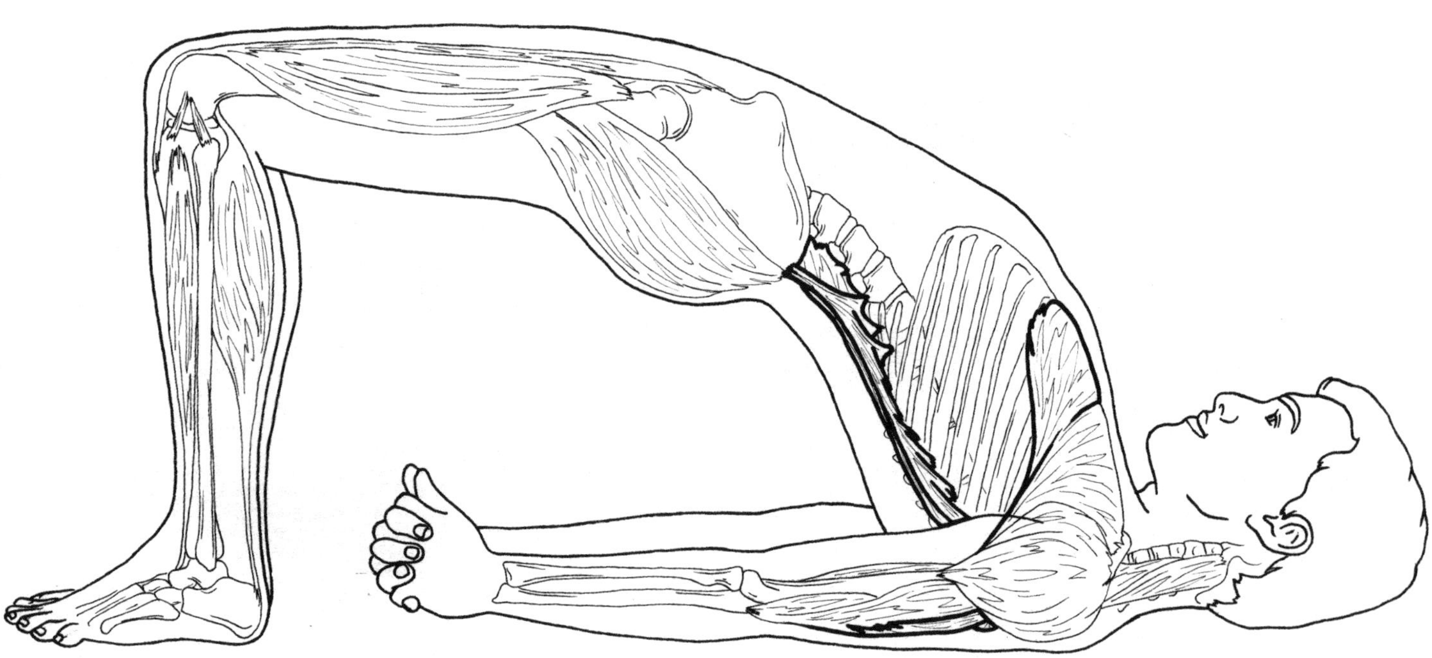

PART 4

Backbends

Practicing asanas that emphasize spinal extension are part and parcel of a well-rounded yoga asana practice. There are some folks in this world who are natural backbenders and others who will find these asanas some of the most challenging. Thankfully, there are some foundational backbends that most anyone can do. So there is always a place to start. The asanas requiring very deep spinal extension may never be fully achieved by some, maybe most, but with the proper use of props and appropriate modifications, most are available to some degree.

FUN FACT

Backbending asanas encourage the opening of the anahata (heart) chakra, the seat of love, anger, trust, and doubt, which sit behind the sternum. These emotions may unexpectedly show themselves in the midst of a backbend. Yoga is definitely working on the emotional level, and sometimes the physicality of a posture can unlock these emotions.

When you practice backbends, it is not just that the muscles along the posterior body have to work; the muscles along the anterior body have to stretch as well. You are moving through the sagittal plane in virtually every backbend that you practice. For cranky backs, backbending postures can be a lifesaver. All postures asking for spinal extension, which all backbends are calling for, will strengthen your back muscles, and this is good for a healthy back. For all the core junkies out there, this will give those "stomach-crunching" muscles some well-deserved room to breathe.

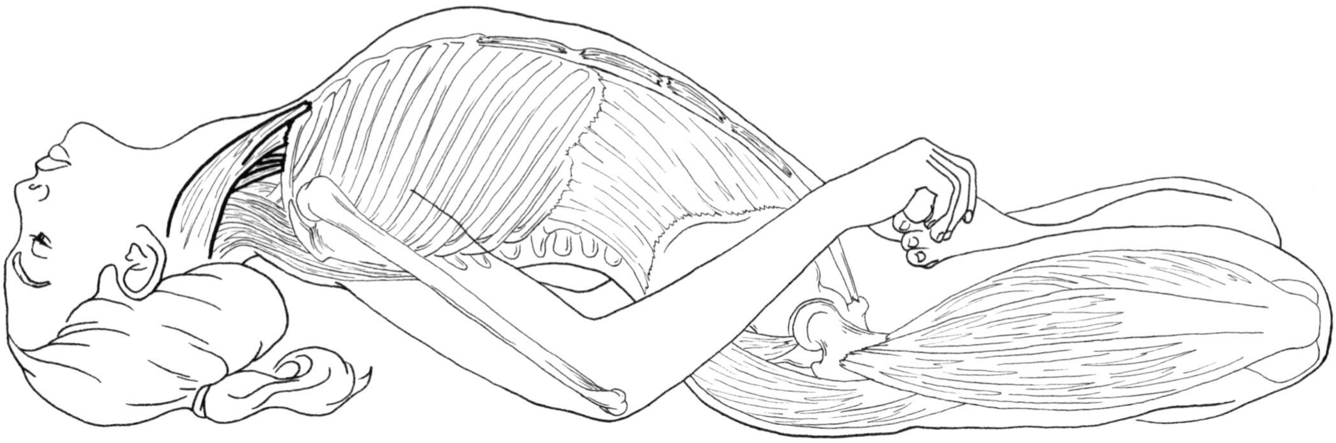

Salabhasana

sah-lah-BAH-sah-nah

Locust

Salabhasana is a fundamental and foundational backbending asana. It will inform and prepare the body for the more challenging backbends to come. This asana essentially asks all of your back muscles to contract and lift the upper and lower body, in defiance of gravity. This asana should always be challenging. There really is no getting to the finish line or moving on and leaving it behind.

Starting in the prone position, bring your pelvis into posterior tilt and internally rotate your hips. With your center as your ground, lift the upper and lower body as high as you can, and bring the hips into extension as most of the spine moves into extension as well. It is imperative that you keep your lower back feeling strong as you hold the posture.

LOWER BODY

Keeping the hips in internal rotation and pelvis in posterior tilt is majorly important. You need to keep the space between the vertebrae down there as you lift into the backbend. You do not want to feel any compression. If you keep crunching your back in this posture, you will pay a price, so tuck that tailbone!

What's obvious in **salabhasana** is the extension in the hips. The gluteus maximus along with the biceps femoris, semimembranosus, and semitendinosus (the hamstrings) are all concentrically contracting to extend at the hips and keep the legs lifted. The upper fibers of all three hamstring muscles must also work along with the gluteus maximus to maintain the posterior tilt of the pelvis. The other two gluteal muscles, gluteus medius and minimus, are your strongest internal rotators of the hips and should be engaging here to keep your sacroiliac (SI) joint from getting jammed up.

FUN FACT

Light on Yoga by B. K. S. Iyengar is considered the bible of yoga asana for many practitioners. Iyengar advises that one of the primary benefits of the practice of **salabhasana** is relief of flatulence. I guess this makes sense since your gluteal muscles are clenched so tight in this posture that nothing should be able to get out.

Practice Tip

Warm up by lifting opposite limbs first, in other words, lift the right arm and the left leg, and then switch. This will not only warm up the muscles for the full expression of the posture, but it will also warm up your brain and keep you paying attention.

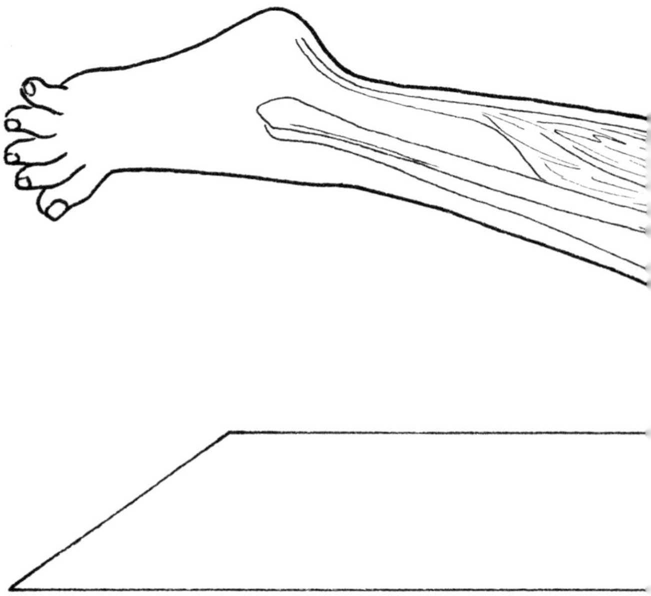

UPPER BODY

The lower fibers of the rectus abdominis muscles must be engaged along with the hamstrings and gluteus maximus muscles to maintain posterior pelvic tilt. The rectus abdominis acts to pull the pelvis by virtue of its attachment on the pubic bone. As you extend the spine, the rest of the rectus abdominis must lengthen. Good thing this is a big muscle as it has to do two things at once here.

All of your spinal erectors—spinalis, longissimus, and iliocostalis—are working hard to extend the spine and hold the backbend. They're getting a fair amount of help from the multifidi, rotatores, and latissimus dorsi muscles, among others.

There are many different arm variations practitioners can choose from, though certain traditions do have their own ideas. Keeping the shoulders in extension and arms extended is great for strengthening those arms. Whatever variation you choose, have fun with it!

COLORING TIP

The rectus abdominis muscle is commonly referred to as the "six pack." But we know there are actually ten muscle bellies (five on each side) that make up the muscle. Coloring each belly a different color will really make this clear.

BICEPS FEMORIS
SEMIMEMBRANOSUS
SEMITENDINOSUS
GLUTEUS MEDIUS
GLUTEUS MINIMUS
LATISSIMUS DORSI

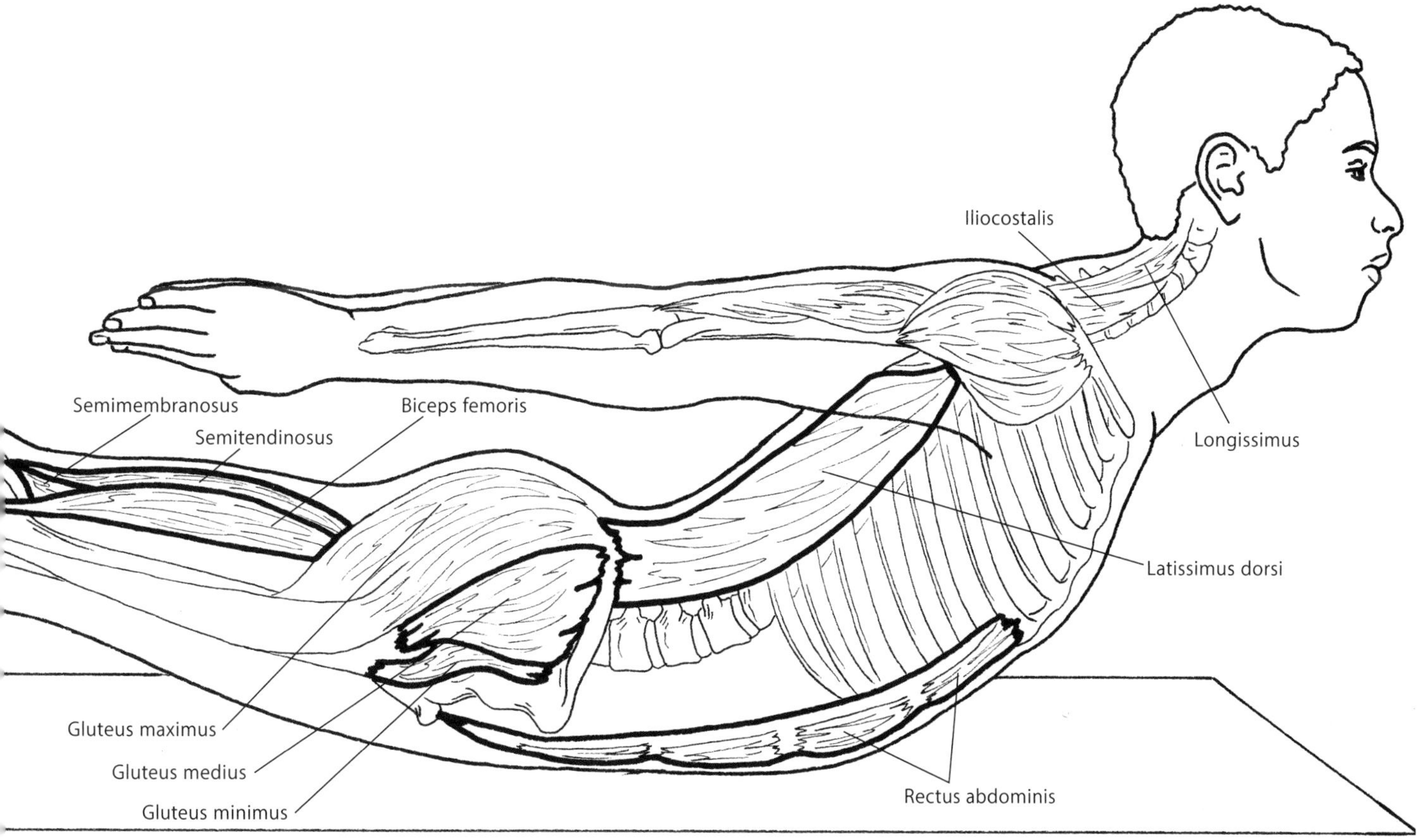

Setu Bandha Sarvangasana

SET-oo BAHN-dah sar-vahn-GAH-sah-nah

Bridge

Setu bandha sarvangasana is another fundamental and foundational backbend. You're still defying gravity as in **salabhasana**, but you have a lot more to ground here. With your feet pressing down and the scapula acting as a platform, along with the back of the head also remaining on the mat, you get a lot of surface area of the body to ground. Setu bandha sarvangasana will start to make your backbends feel strong and get them stronger.

Lying supine on your mat, bend your knees, taking care to keep your ankles and knees hip-distance apart with the ankles lined up under your knees and all ten toes pointing straight ahead. Take the time to set up your foundation. Before lifting the hips, it is a good idea to walk your shoulder blades together and down your back (i.e., retract and depress the scapula to help lengthen the neck). You should posteriorly tilt the hips before you lift off as well. Everything on the mat should ground as you lift the pelvis to the sky and breathe.

LOWER BODY

All your hip flexor muscles will get a good stretch here as the hips are held in extension. Since gravity is working against you, you really have to work for this stretch! All four quadriceps muscles will lengthen by virtue of keeping the knees bent. You will really be working your gluteus maximus to keep the pelvis lifted; just be sure not to overwork it.

UPPER BODY

As you engage the back muscles to bring the spine into extension, maintain the space between your T12 and L1 vertebrae. For most folks, this is where the angle of the backbend is most acute. This is why you maintain that posterior tilt. All of the spinal erectors—spinalis, longissimus, and iliocostalis—with a strong assist from the quadratus lumborum, will be concentrically contracted to maintain the asana and keep the bridge from collapsing.

The shoulders are in extension, external rotation, and adduction. The strongest muscles that will extend the shoulders here are the latissimus dorsi and teres major muscles. The strongest muscles that adduct the shoulders include the long head of the triceps along with the latissimus and teres major muscles. Your big back muscles are all really working here. If you're unable to keep the arms down on the mat, all these muscles have to work even harder.

The weight of the body will hold the shoulders in external rotation. That is why it is so important to set this up first. External rotation at the shoulder will work the posterior deltoid. As you bring your spine into extension and lift the pelvis off the mat, this creates shoulder extension, so the posterior deltoid will be pulling double duty. Keep your shoulders feeling good, and don't ask for more than they can give.

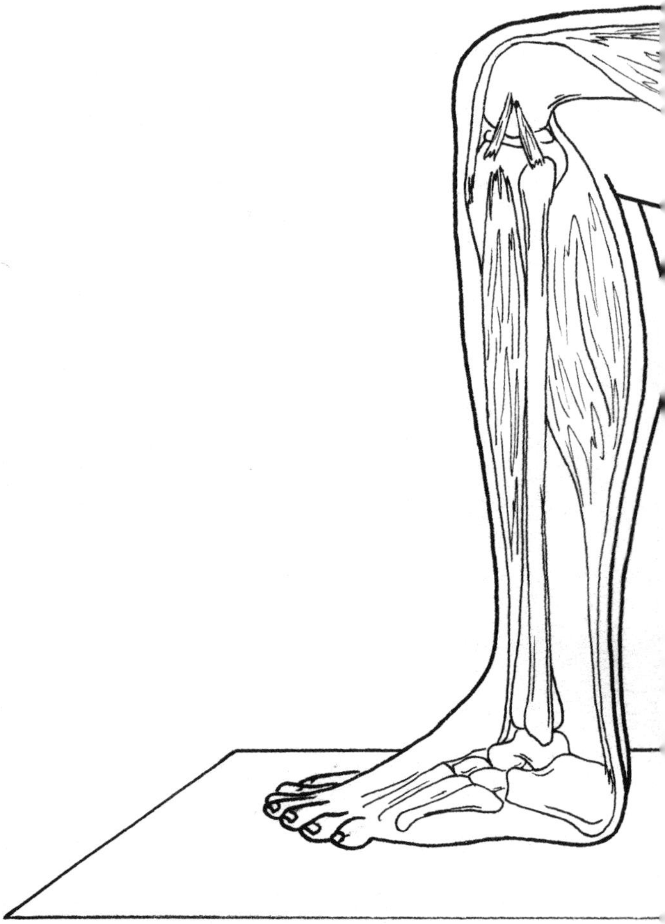

FUN FACT

Setu bandha sarvangasana is symbolic of the bridge constructed by Rama's army to rescue his princess Sita, who was being held by the demon Ravana in Lanka (modern day Sri Lanka). Recently archeologists have discovered what they believe to be remnants of a bridge on the sea floor in the same location described in the "myth."

Practice Tip

Placing a block under the sacrum will allow you to maintain **setu bandha sarvangasana** rather effortlessly, and rather than "working" the posture, you can enjoy the juicy stretch in all those hip flexor muscles.

PECTORALIS MAJOR

TERES MAJOR

TRICEPS BRACHII (LONG HEAD)

LONGISSIMUS

ILIOCOSTALIS

QUADRATUS LUMBORUM

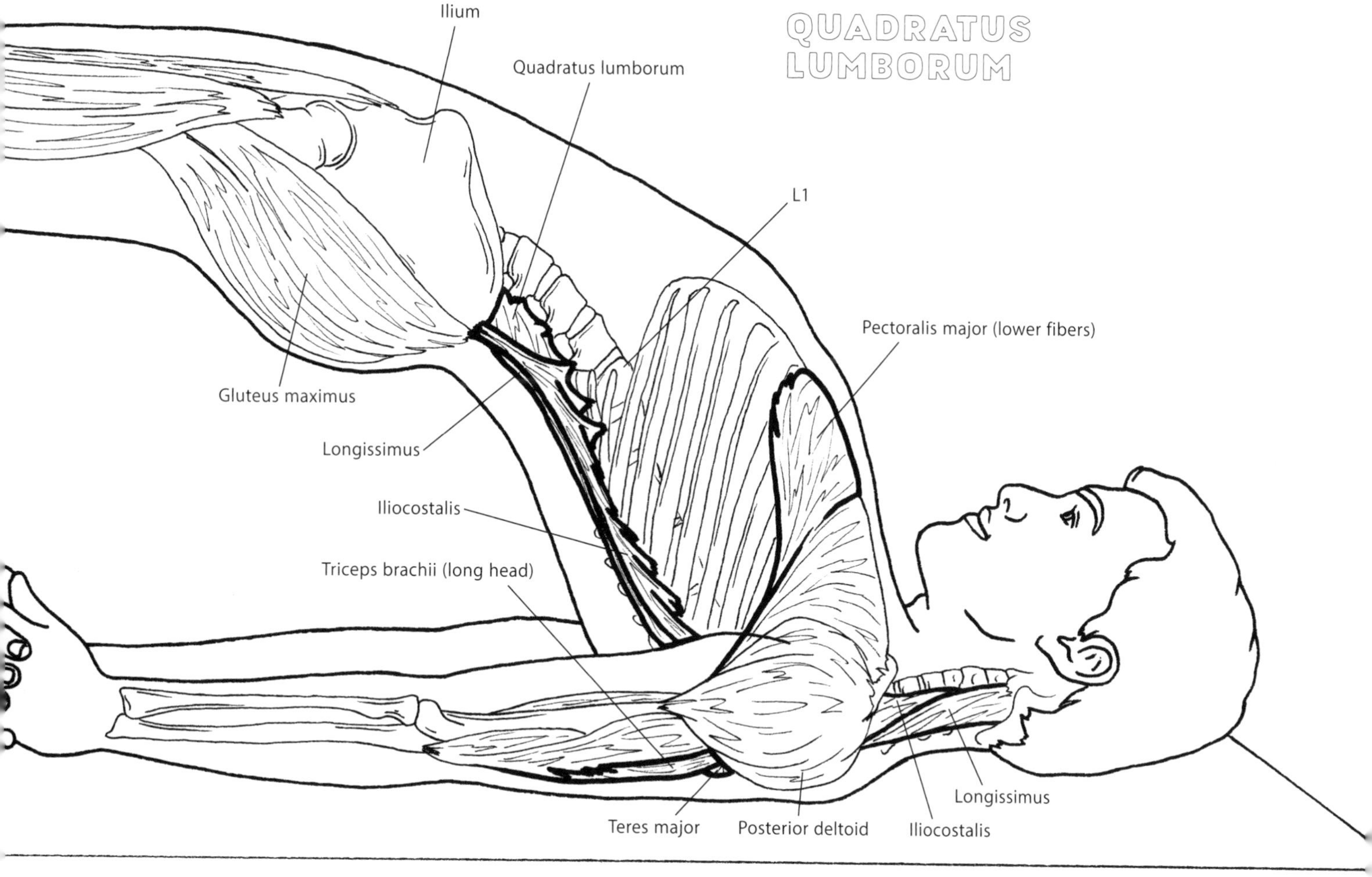

Urdhva Dhanurasana

URD-vah dah-nur-AH-sah-nah

Upward Bow

Urdhva dhanurasana is known in the West as the "full" backbend. There are some yoga asana traditions that refer to this posture as **chakrasana**, or "wheel." Whatever you call it, it is a challenging asana. Most practitioners just think of this posture as bringing the spine into deep extension. While that's true, it also requires deep flexion and external rotation in the shoulders in addition to deep internal rotation and extension in the hips. It is not all about just bending your spine backward. As you improve in this posture, it will open the door to even more challenging asanas.

Most practitioners will approach this posture lying supine on the mat. As the backbends deepen, you may be able to practice this from standing and dropping back. But you have to start somewhere, so start flat on your back with knees fully flexed, feet hip-distance apart, all ten toes pointing forward. Flex your shoulders and elbows to bring your hands under your shoulders, keeping elbows no wider than your shoulders and pointing straight up, fingers pointing toward your toes. Before pressing up, you should internally rotate your hips and externally rotate your shoulders. This will help keep space in the joints as the shoulders flex and the hips extend.

Most muscles along the posterior body are working here. We are going to focus on what has to stretch in the anterior body to allow this to happen.

Practice Tip

Always take time after backbends, particularly a deep back bend like **urdhva dhanurasana** to "counterpose." Take your spine into rotation with a gentle twist and/or a gentle forward bend and allow the spine to rotate and flex. Always bring back the balance.

LOWER BODY

As you press up, the hips go into deep extension. This will ask all your hip flexors to lengthen, a lot. Primarily the psoas, iliacus, and rectus femoris muscles will have to give the hips the room to extend.

UPPER BODY

The full span of the rectus abdominis will lengthen as the spine extends, stretching the anterior torso. The intercostal muscles will also have to give a little stretch here as well. This is why it may be more challenging to breathe in this asana as the intercostal muscles are primarily respiratory muscles and usually are just accommodating the lungs.

The deep flexion in the shoulders will stretch out those big pectoralis major and latissimus dorsi muscles and will also give the deeper pectoralis minor muscles some length as well.

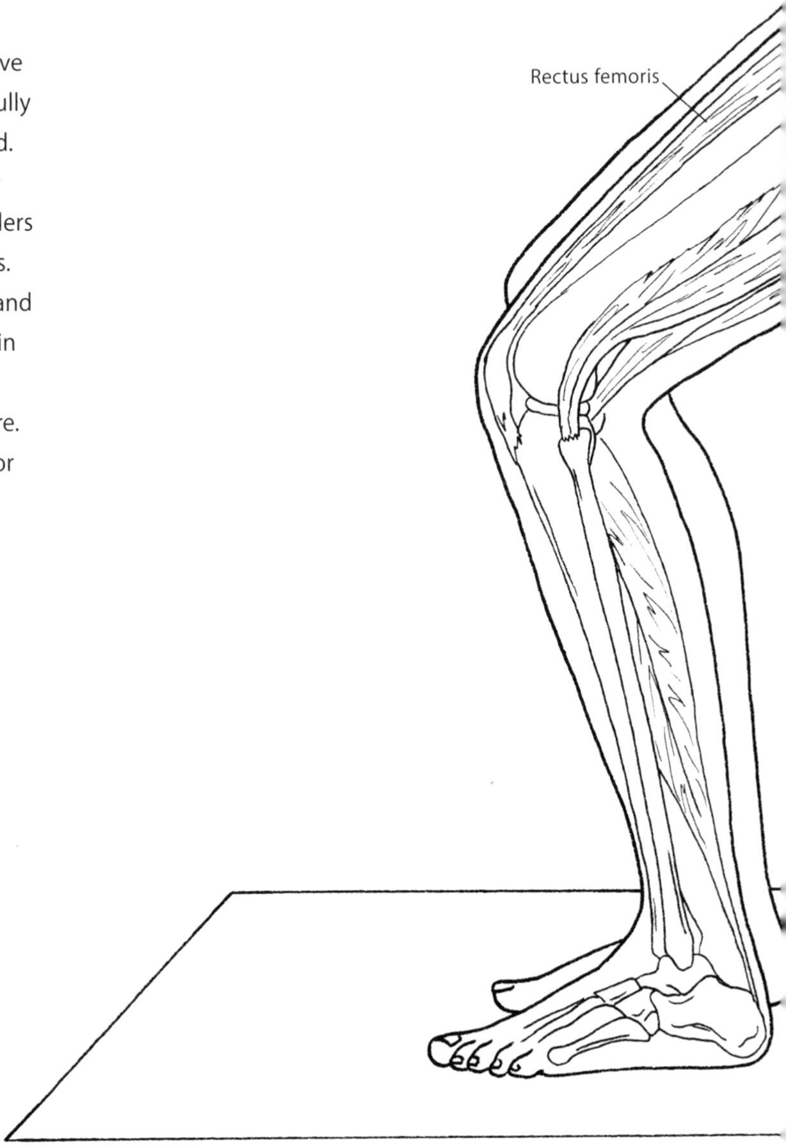

RECTUS ABDOMINIS
INTERCOSTAL MUSCLES
PECTORALIS MINOR

FUN FACT

This asana symbolizes Arjuna's famous shot with a bow and arrow. Arjuna shot an arrow through the eye of a metal fish revolving on the top of a pole in the middle of a fountain. As if that wasn't hard enough, he did it by looking at the target in the reflection of the water as he raised his bow upward.

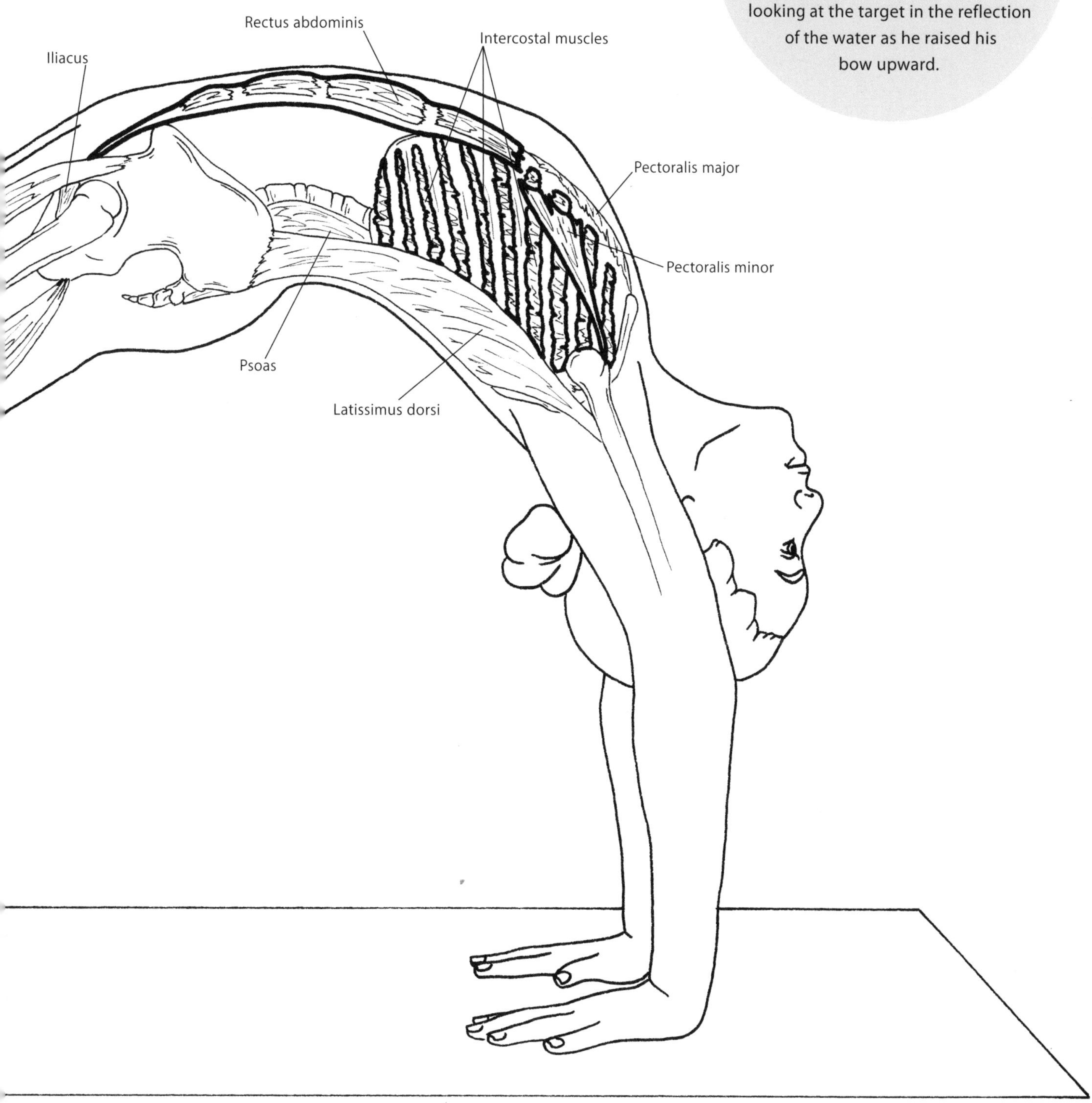

Kapotasana

kah-poh-TAH-sah-nah

Pigeon

As the back gets bendier, the muscles along the anterior body really start to lengthen, and the posterior muscles strengthen, **kapotasana** may become within reach, literally. Kapotasana wants deeper spinal extension and more open hip flexors and quadriceps muscles.

Set up this asana by kneeling on the mat, hips lined up over the knees, upper body tall. Before moving into spinal extension, establish the pelvis in posterior tilt and hips in internal rotation. Keep this alignment as you bring the spine into deep extension. The shoulders are externally rotated as the arms reach back in deep shoulder flexion, elbows flexed. Ideally, the forearms make it all the way down to the mat, with the palms resting on the heels and your head resting on the soles of your feet.

LOWER BODY

The psoas, iliacus, rectus femoris (strongest of the quadriceps), and sartorius muscles are the biggest, strongest hip flexors and will all have to lengthen here to provide for the deep hip extension. Because the knees are flexed, the other three quadriceps muscles—vastus lateralis, vastus medialis, and vastus intermedius—will also have to lengthen, vastly.

To maintain internal rotation in the hips, a bunch of big muscles get involved. The adductor muscle group, tensor fasciae latae (TFL), and the anterior fibers of both the gluteus medius and minimus are all called to action to rotate the femur bone medially. The medial hamstrings also assist in internal rotation, but have to pull "triple duty" as they are also assisting, along with the biceps femoris, to maintain posterior pelvic tilt and knee flexion.

UPPER BODY

To maintain posterior pelvic tilt, the rectus abdominis muscles pull the pubic bone anteriorly from its origin site on the pubic crest. At the same time, they must lengthen to allow for spinal extension. There is no way around this. Keep your back happy and don't let your ego write a check that your spine can't cash.

Practice Tip

Most everyone can start to approach this asana by setting up with their back facing a wall and reaching the hands up and over the head, making contact with the wall. The closer your feet are to the wall, the easier it will be. As you improve, you will walk your hands down the wall closer and closer to the floor. It's a journey!

FUN FACT

Legend has it that master teacher Krishnamacharya stood on his student Pattabhi Jois as he held this asana and gave a 20-minute lecture on yoga.

PSOAS

ILIACUS

RECTUS FEMORIS

SARTORIUS

TENSOR FASCIAE LATAE (TFL)

RECTUS ABDOMINIS

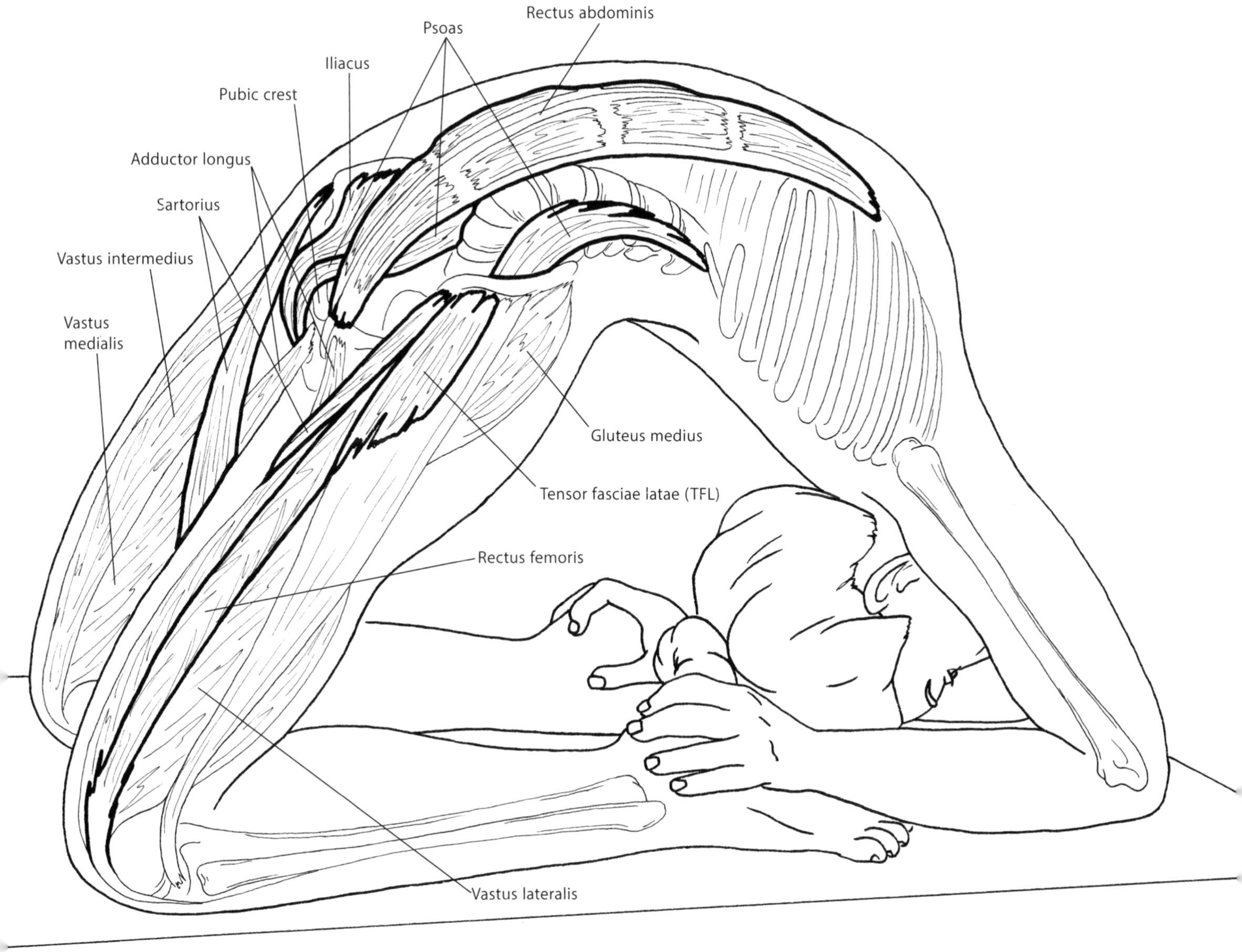

Matsyasana

mots-sy-AH-sah-nah

Fish

Matsyasana is the standard counterpose for **salamba sarvangasana**, the shoulder stand. It makes sense as it brings the cervical spine to deep extension, countering the deep flexion of the cervicals in sarvangasana. Ideally, the rest of the spine is neutral in sarvangasana, but for most of us mere mortals, we do end up with some flexion. The deep spinal extension in matsyasana is a welcome relief from that as well.

Start seated on the mat. If you're not able to get your legs in full **padmasana**, start with the legs fully extended. Extend your spine as you lean back, using your forearms to ground. Place the crown of your head on the mat. If you're unable to get the head all the way down, bring your elbows closer to your hips until you can. Then, try to take hold of your feet if you have your legs in padmasana; otherwise, keep the forearms down. Most students will first learn this asana with the legs extended, but that doesn't look much like a fish; try to find your tail!

LOWER BODY

What's going on here depends on which variation of **matsyasana** you're practicing. If you're able to practice with a lotus, you will mostly feel the gluteus maximus muscles working hard trying to keep the knees down and on the mat.

UPPER BODY

We're going to focus on the neck muscles that really work and stretch here. The muscles along the back of the neck and posterior cervical spine will all have to engage to pull the cervical spine into deep extension and work to keep the neck stable. The strongest muscles you have back there are the upper fibers of the trapezius muscles, the levator scapula muscles, the splenius capitis, and the splenius cervicis muscles. The strength of these muscles must be agreeable to the length of the muscles along the anterior cervical spine and front of the neck. The biggest are the sternocleidomastoid (SCM), anterior scalene, longus capitis, and longus colli muscles. Be mindful of the weight you're taking in your head. With the head on the mat, you will be holding the cervical spine in place; make sure it's a place you want to be.

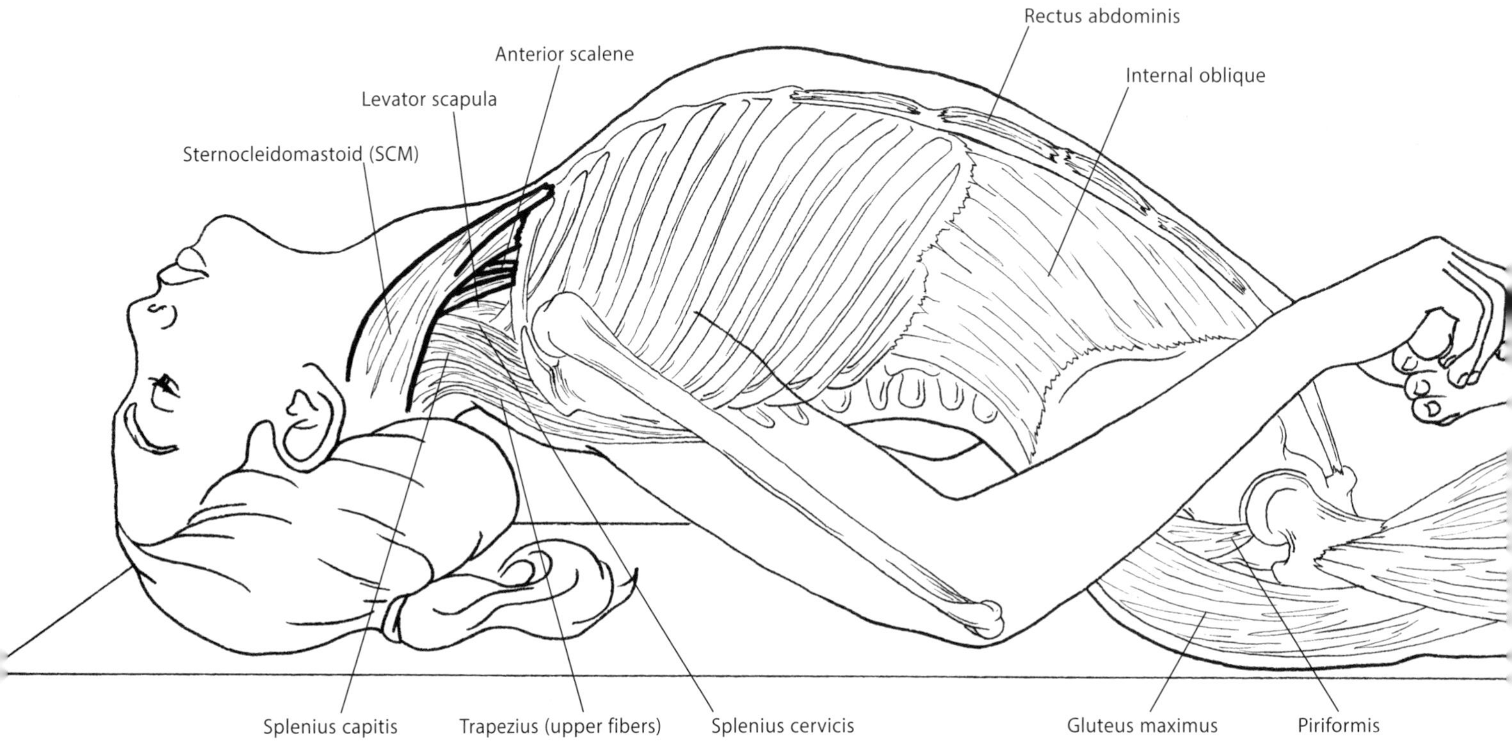

Posterior View of Neck and Upper Back

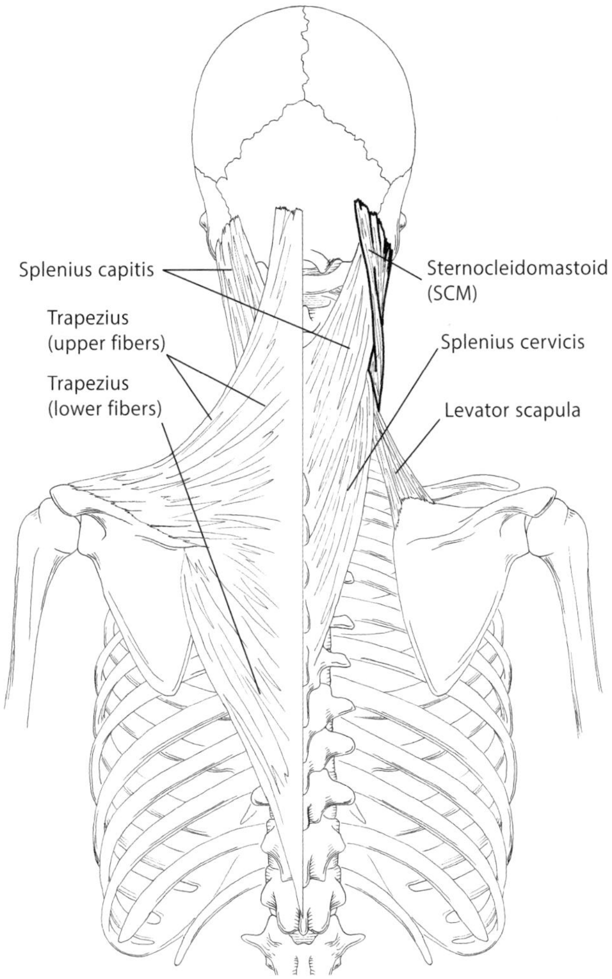

Anterior View of Neck

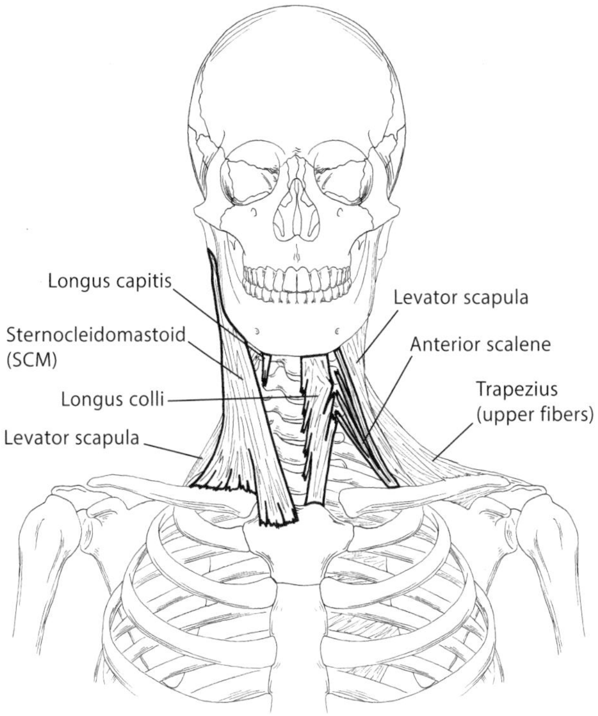

FUN FACT

Matsya is an avatar of Vishnu. Vishnu was called to Earth to save it from a great flood, and so he incarnated on Earth as a fish. He befriended Manu and advised him to gather all the plants and animals to place on a boat that he would send before the flood to save the flora and fauna. All life was saved and returned to land once the waters subsided. Sound familiar?

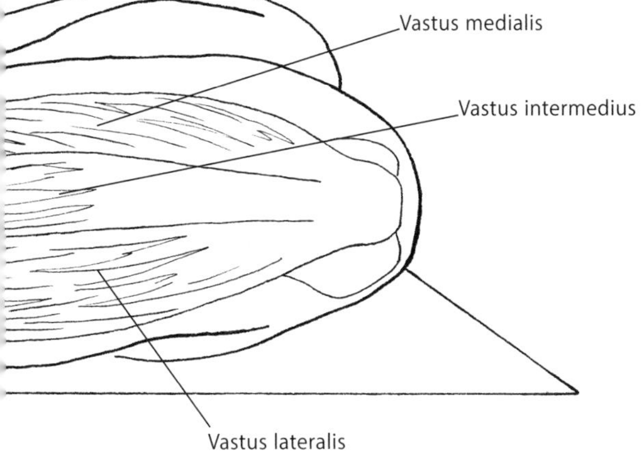

STERNOCLEIDOMASTOID (SCM)

ANTERIOR SCALENE

LONGUS CAPITIS

LONGUS COLLI

Glossary

A

Abduction
Moving a limb away from the midline.

Acetabulofemoral joint
The connection of the femur (upper leg bone) to the pelvis.

Adduction
Moving a limb toward the midline.

Anjali mudra
Holding palms together in front of the heart center. Also known as "prayer position."

Anterior (ventral)
Toward the front of the body.

Anterior cruciate ligament (ACL)
A ligament of the knee.

Anterior pelvic tilt
The pelvis tilts forward, pulling the sit bones back.

Asana
Sanskrit term meaning "posture" or "seat."

Atlantoaxial joint
The connection of the C1 vertebra to the C2 vertebra.

B

Ball-and-socket joint
A type of joint characterized by the rounded surface of one bone articulating around a depression in another bone and allowing for the greatest range of motion between bones.

Bilateral
Both sides of the body working together.

C

Center of gravity
The balancing point of the body in relation to the force of gravity.

Cervical spine
The seven vertebrae that form the neck.

Chakra
Sanskrit term meaning "wheel." Usually refers to the energy vortices in the body.

Coccyx
The vertebrae that form the tailbone.

Concentric contraction
Muscle fibers shorten.

Coronal plane
See frontal plane.

D

Deep
Farther away from the skin.

Distal
Located away from the center of the body in relation to another structure.

Dorsal
See posterior.

Dorsal flexion
Stretches sole of foot; heel pulls away from the knee and the toes pull in toward the lower leg.

Downward rotation of scapula
Scapula pulls inferiorly and anteriorly.

Drishti
Sanskrit term for "gazing point."

E

Eccentric contraction
Muscle fibers lengthen while still exerting strength.

Eversion
Turning the calcaneus (heel) bone medially.

Extension
The angle of a joint is increased.

External rotation
See lateral rotation.

F

Flexion
The angle of a joint is decreased.

Frontal (or coronal) plane
Divides the body into front and back (anterior and posterior) sections.

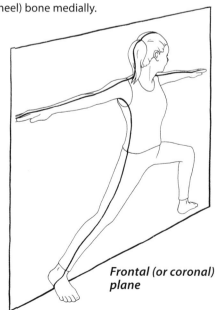

Frontal (or coronal) plane

G

Glenohumeral joint
The joint that connects the humerus (upper arm) to the scapula (shoulder blade).

Ground(ing)
Making an energetic connection to the earth.

H

Hamstrings
Three muscles that compose the posterior area of the upper leg.

Heart center
The energetic heart located just behind the sternum in the seat of the heart chakra.

Hinge joint
A joint that can only flex or extend.

Horizontal adduction of shoulder
Arm is parallel to the floor and moving medially.

I

Inferior
Toward the bottom of the body.

Insertion site
The attachment of a tendon to a lighter bone.

Internal rotation
See medial rotation.

K

Kyphosis
Exaggeration of the curve of the thoracic spine.

L

Lateral
Toward the side of the body.

Lateral collateral ligament (LCL)
A ligament of the knee.

Lateral flexion
Side bend of the spine.

Lateral rotation
A joint moves toward the side of the body through the transverse plane.

Ligament
The connective tissue that connects bone to bone.

Lordosis
Exaggeration of the curve of the lumbar spine.

Lumbar spine
The five vertebrae that make up the lower back.

M

Medial
Closer to the middle of the body.

Medial collateral ligament (MCL)
A ligament of the knee.

Medial rotation
A joint moves toward the center of the body through the transverse plane.

Meniscus
The connective tissue that cushions a joint.

N

Namaste
A Sanskrit greeting with many translations. My favorite: "I bow to the light within you from the light within me." Often spoken with a slight bow and the palms in prayer position in front of the heart.

Neutral
Correct alignment of bones and joints that creates uniform and even spacing between the bones.

O

Origin site
The attachment of tendon to heavier bone.

P

Plantar flexion
Toes point, stretching the top of the foot.

Posterior (dorsal)
Toward the back of the body.

Posterior cruciate ligament (PCL)
A ligament of the knee.

Posterior pelvic tilt
The pelvis tilts back as the sit bones are pulled forward, tucking the pelvis.

Prime mover
The strongest muscle involved in a particular movement.

Pronation
From the Western anatomical position, the lower arm rotates so palms face back, or the soles of the feet turn away from each other.

Prone
Lying facedown.

Proximal
Located toward the center of the body in relation to another structure.

Q

Quadriceps
A group of four muscles along the anterior upper leg.

R

Reciprocal inhibition
A neuromuscular response in the body that relaxes opposing muscles during muscular contraction.

Retraction
Scapulae pull closer together.

Rotation
Spinal twist.

S

Sacroiliac (SI) joint
Joins the sacrum to the ilium.

Sagittal plane
Divides the body into right and left sides.

Sit bones
Common term in yoga for the ischial tuberosities.

Spinous process
The part of the vertebral body that protrudes posteriorly.

Suboccipital muscles
A group of four deep muscles located just below the occiput in the posterior neck.

Superficial
Closer to the skin.

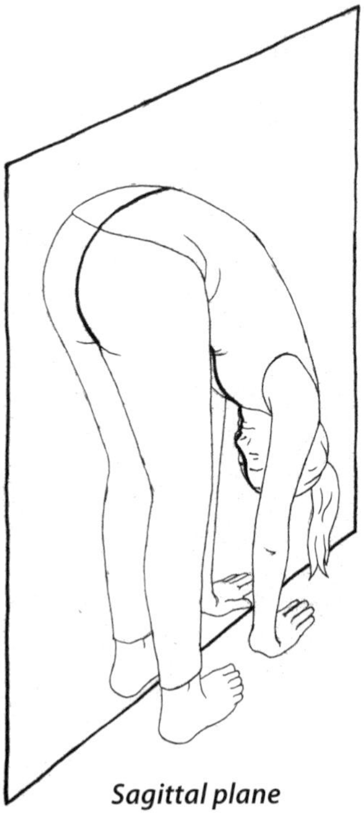

Sagittal plane

Superior
Closer to the head.

Supination
Turns palm to face forward or up, or turns the soles of the feet in.

Supine
Lying face up.

Synergist
A muscle that helps the prime mover perform an action.

T

Tendon
Attaches muscles to bones.

Thoracic spine
The twelve vertebrae that make up the upper back.

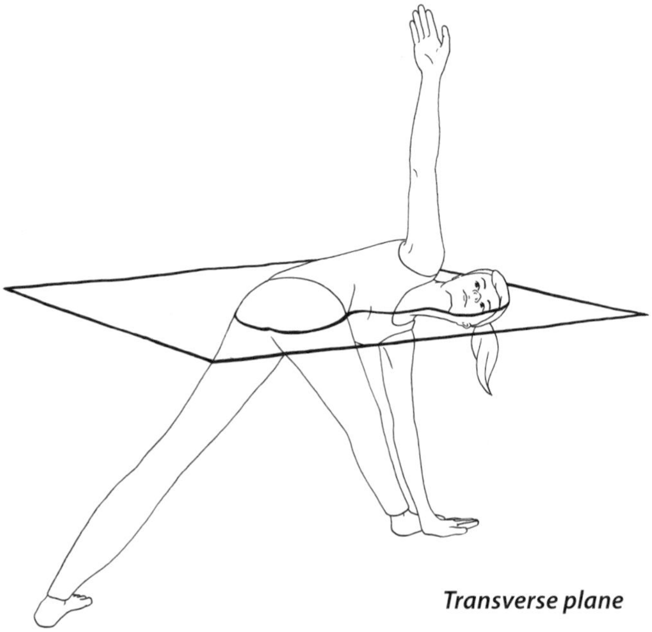

Transverse plane

Transverse plane
Divides the body into upper and lower portions.

Transverse process
The part of the vertebral body that protrudes laterally.

Tuberosity
A larger bump on a bone.

U

Unilateral
Occurring on one side of the body.

Index

A

adductor brevis 34–35, 68–69
adductor longus 34–35, 68–69
adductor magnus 34–35, 68–69
adductors 34–35, 68–69, 100–101
  adductor brevis 34–35, 68–69
  adductor longus 34–35, 68–69
  adductor magnus 34–35, 68–69
  gracilis 34–35, 68–69, 100–101
  pectineus 34–35, 68–69
adho mukha svanasana 20
adho mukha vrksasana 56
Anjaneya 14
anjaneyasana 14
anterior cruciate ligament (ACL) 42–43
ardha baddha padma paschimottanasana 74
ardha matsyendrasana 80
ardha padmasana 74, 84
ardha virasana 76, 84, 96, 100
arm balances 48–59
ashtangasana 16
Ashtavakra 49
astavakrasana 48

B

backbends 102–113
back muscles 113
baddhakonasana 70
bakasana 54
balancing poses 38–63
  arm balances 48–59
  on one leg 40–47
Bharadvaja 84
Bharadvaja's twist 84
bharadvajasana 84
bhujangasana 18
biceps brachii 14–15, 16–17, 26–27, 54–55
biceps femoris 12–13, 20–21, 22–23, 28–29, 66–67, 104–105
boat 98
bound-angle posture 70
brachialis 52–53, 54–55, 58–59
brachioradialis 54–55, 56–57, 58–59
bridge 106

C

calcaneus 10–11, 40–41
cervical spine 10–11, 34–35
chair 30
chakrasana 108
chaturanga 16
clavicle 10–11
cobra 18
coracobrachialis 14–15, 32–33
crow 54
cuneiform 40–41

D

Daksha 32, 34
deep 6 81
deltoid 14–15, 16–17, 18–19, 20–21, 24–25, 28–29, 34–35, 44–45, 58–59, 82–83, 94–95, 96–97
  anterior 14–15, 16–17, 34–35, 82–83, 96–97
  middle 24–25, 34–35, 94–95
  posterior 18–19, 20–21, 24–25, 28–29, 44–45, 58–59, 86–87, 94–95
downward-facing dog 20
downward-facing tree 56

E

eagle 42
easy seated posture 88
eight-bends posture 48
eight-limbs posture 16
eka pada bakasana 54
erector spinae 16–17
extended side angle 26
extended triangle 24
extensor carpi radialis brevis 22–23, 48–49
extensor carpi radialis longus 22–23, 48–49
extensor carpi ulnaris 22–23, 48–49
extensor digiti minimi 54–55
extensor digitorum 22–23, 48–49
extensor digitorum longus 30–31, 48–49, 78–79
extensor hallucis longus 30–31, 78–79
extensor indicis 54–55
extensor muscles 23
extensor pollicis brevis 54–55
extensor pollicis longus 54–55
external oblique 14–15, 18–19, 30–31, 40–41, 86–87

F

feather of the peacock 58
fibula 90–91
fish 112
flexor carpi radialis 50–51, 84–85
flexor carpi ulnaris 50–51, 84–85
foot bones 77
foot-hand posture 22
forward bends, seated 66–79

G

Garuda 42
garudasana 42
gastrocnemius 12–13, 20–21, 22–23, 66–67
gate (Ashtanga) 96
gate (Iyengar) 94
gluteus maximus 14–15, 18–19, 22–23, 30–31, 36–37, 44–45, 50–51, 54–55, 70–71, 80–81
gluteus medius 36–37, 70–71, 74–75, 90–91, 104–105
gluteus minimus 36–37, 70–71, 74–75, 76–77, 90–91, 98–99, 104–105
gracilis 34–35, 68–69, 100–101

H

half-bound lotus forward bend 74
half hero 76, 84, 96, 100
half lord of the fishes 80
half lotus 74, 84
hamstrings 30–31
  biceps femoris 12–13, 20–21, 22–23, 28–29, 66–67, 104–105
  semimembranosus 12–13, 20–21, 24–25, 28–29, 36–37, 66–67, 100–101, 104–105
  semitendinosus 12–13, 20–21, 22–23, 24–25, 28–29, 36–37, 66–67, 100–101, 104–105
Hanuman 30, 92
Hatha Yoga Pradipika 66
head-to-knee posture 72
hero 92
heron 100

I

iliacus 14–15, 18–19, 44–45, 46–47, 52–53, 88–89, 98–99, 110–111
iliocostalis 16–17
iliotibial (IT) band 14–15, 80–81
infraspinatus 18–19, 28–29, 50–51, 58–59, 78–79, 86–87
intense stretch posture 12
intercostal muscles 108–109
internal oblique 46–47, 52–53, 86–87
inversions 60–63
Iyengar, B. K. S. 4, 104

J

janu sirsasana 72

K

kapotasana 110
King Daksha 32, 34
king dancer 44
King of All Birds 42
knee stabilizers 72
Krishnamacharya 111
krounchasana 100
kukkutasana 52

L

Lakshmi 58
lateral collateral ligament (LCL) 42–43
latissimus dorsi 58–59, 82–83, 96–97, 104–105
levator scapula 36–37, 60–61
ligamentum nuchae 60–61
Light on Yoga 104
locust 104
longissimus 16–17, 94–95
longus capitis 62–63, 112–113
longus colli 62–63, 112–113
lotus 90
low lunge 14
lumbar spine 10–11

M

mandible 10–11
Manu 113
Marichi's pose A 78
Marichi's pose C 82
marichyasana A 78
marichyasana C 82
Matsya 113
matsyasana 112
medial collateral ligament (MCL) 42–43, 92–93
medial meniscus 90–91, 92–93,
metatarsals 40–41
mountain 10
multifidi 18–19, 36–37, 84–85

N

natarajasana 44
navasana 98
neck muscles 61, 62, 113
noose 86

O

obliquus capitis inferior 62–63
obliquus capitis superior 62–63
one-legged crow 54

P

padahastasana 22
padmasana 90
palmaris longus 50–51, 84–85
parighasana (Ashtanga) 96
parighasana (Iyengar) 94
parivrtta trikonasana 36
parsva bakasana 50
parsvottanasana 28
pasasana 86
paschimottanasana 66
Patanjali 40
patella 10–11
pectineus 34–35, 68–69
pectoralis major 14–15, 16–17, 30–31, 44–45, 58–59, 82–83, 96–97, 106–107
pectoralis minor 108–109
pelvis 81, 97
peroneal brevis 26–27, 42–43
peroneal longus 26–27, 42–43
pes anserinus 100–101
pigeon 110
pincha mayurasana 58
piriformis 24–25, 26–27, 34–35, 80–81
plantaris 12–13
popliteus 30–31
posterior cruciate ligament (PCL) 42–43
pronator quadratus 56–57
pronator teres 56–57
psoas 14–15, 18–19, 24–25, 44–45, 46–47, 52–53, 70–71, 88–89, 110–111
pyramid 28

Q

quadratus lumborum 72–73
quadriceps
  rectus femoris 26–27, 32–33, 44–45, 46–47, 74–75, 76–77, 92–93, 98–99, 110–111
  vastus intermedius 32–33, 92–93
  vastus lateralis 32–33, 74–75, 92–93
  vastus medialis 32–33, 74–75, 92–93

R

Ram 107
Rama 92
Ravana 30, 107
rectus abdominis 14–15, 18–19, 32–33, 40–41, 46–47, 52–53, 108–109, 110–111
rectus capitis anterior 62–63
rectus capitis posterior major 62–63
rectus capitis posterior minor 62–63
rectus femoris 26–27, 32–33, 44–45, 46–47, 74–75, 76–77, 92–93, 98–99, 110–111
revolved triangle 36
rhomboid major 60–61
rhomboid minor 60–61
rooster 52
rotator cuff muscles 79
rotatores 18–19, 36–37, 84–85

S

salabhasana 104
salamba sarvangasana 60
sartorius 14–15, 46–47, 76–77, 98–99, 100–101, 110–111
Sati 32, 34, 47
scalenes 60–61, 82–83, 112–113
  anterior 60–61, 112–113
  middle 60–61
scorpion 58
seated asanas 64–101
seated forward bends 66-79
seated twists 80–87
semimembranosus 12–13, 20–21, 24–25, 28–29, 36–37, 66–67, 100–101, 104–105
semispinalis capitis 18–19
semitendinosus 12–13, 20–21, 22–23, 24–25, 28–29, 36–37, 66–67, 100–101, 104–105
serratus anterior 56–57
setu bandha sarvangasana 106
Shiva 32, 34, 47, 84
shoulders 61
side crow 50
sirsasana B 62
Sita 107
soleus 12–13, 20–21, 22–23, 66–67
spinal erectors 17
spinalis 16–17, 94–95
spine 10–11, 34–35
  cervical 10–11, 34–35
  lumbar 10–11
  thoracic 10–11
splenius cervicis 80–81
standing asanas 8–37
sternocleidomastoid (SCM) 80–81, 82–83, 112–113
subclavius 68–69
suboccipital muscles 62
subscapularis 82–83, 96–97
sukhasana 88
sun salute 8–21
supported all-limbs posture 60
supraspinatus 24–25, 26–27
surya namaskar 8–21

T

tadasana 10
talus 40–41
tensor fasciae latae (TFL) 70–71, 76–77, 98–99, 90–91, 110–111
teres major 58–59, 96–97, 106–107
teres minor 18–19, 28–29, 50–51, 58–59, 78–79, 86–87
thoracic spine 10–11
three-limb-facing one-leg forward bend 76
tibialis anterior 30–31, 32–33, 48–49, 72–73
tibialis posterior 72–73
transverse abdominis 88–89, 94–95
transversospinalis muscles 17
trapezius 82–83
tree 40
triang mukha eka pada paschimottanasana 76
triceps brachii 44–45, 58–59, 60–61, 106–107
tripod headstand 62
twists, seated 80–87

U

upavishta konasana 68
upward bow 108
urdhva dhanurasana 108
utkatasana 30
uttanasana 12
utthita hasta tadasana 46
utthita parsvakonasana 26
utthita trikonasana 24

V

vastus intermedius 32–33, 92–93
vastus lateralis 32–33, 74–75, 92–93
vastus medialis 32–33, 74–75, 92–93
Virabhadra 32, 34, 47
virabhadrasana I 32
virabhadrasana II 34
virabhadrasana III 46
virasana 92
Vishnu 42, 113
vrishchikasana 58
vrksasana 40

W

warrior I 32
warrior II 34
warrior III 46
Warriors 32, 34
wheel 108
wide-angle seated forward bend 68

Y

Yoga Sutras 40

Pose Index

Sanskrit

adho mukha svanasana 20
adho mukha vrksasana 56
anjaneyasana 14
ardha baddha padma paschimottanasana 74
ardha matsyendrasana 80
ashtangasana 16
astavakrasana 48
baddhakonasana 70
bharadvajasana 84
bhujangasana 18
eka pada bakasana 54
garudasana 42
janu sirsasana 72
kapotasana 110
krounchasana 100
kukkutasana 52
marichyasana A 78
marichyasana C 82
matsyasana 112
natarajasana 44
navasana 98
padahastasana 22
padmasana 90
parighasana (Ashtanga) 96
parighasana (Iyengar) 94
parivrtta trikonasana 36
parsva bakasana 50
parsvottanasana 28
pasasana 86
paschimottanasana 66
pincha mayurasana 58
salabhasana 104
salamba sarvangasana 60
setu bandha sarvangasana 106
sirsasana B 62
sukhasana 88
tadasana 10
triang mukha eka pada paschimottanasana 76
upavishta konasana 68
urdhva dhanurasana 108
utkatasana 30
uttanasana 12
utthita parsvakonasana 26
utthita trikonasana 24
virabhadrasana I 32
virabhadrasana II 34
virabhadrasana III 46
virasana 92
vrksasana 40

English

Bharadvaja's twist 84
boat 98
bound-angle posture 70
bridge 106
chair 30
cobra 18
downward-facing dog 20
downward-facing tree 56
eagle 42
easy seated posture 88
eight-bends posture 48
eight-limbs posture 16
extended side angle 26
extended triangle 24
feather of the peacock 58
fish 112
foot-hand posture 22
gate (Ashtanga) 96
gate (Iyengar) 94
half lord of the fishes 80
half-bound lotus forward bend 74
head-to-knee posture 72
hero 92
heron 100
intense stretch posture 12
king dancer 44
locust 104
lotus 90
low lunge 14
Marichi's pose A 78
Marichi's pose C 82
mountain 10
noose 86
one-legged crow 54
pigeon 110
pyramid 28
revolved triangle 36
rooster 52
seated forward bend 66
side crow 50
supported all-limbs posture 60
three-limb-facing one-leg forward bend 76
tree 40
tripod headstand 62
upward bow 108
warrior I 32
warrior II 34
warrior III 46
wide-angle seated forward bend 68

About the Author

Kelly Solloway is a born-and-raised Jersey girl. She has been practicing yoga since 2001 and teaching since 2003. In 2007, in an effort to escape from the rat race and finally reach the cheese, she decided to quit her day job to go to massage school with the hopes of earning a living as a yoga teacher and massage therapist. It was in massage school that she discovered her love for anatomy. She soon realized that once you get a better understanding of how the body is put together and moves around, the asana practice becomes that much deeper and more profound. And at the same time very visceral and real. She currently teaches public and private yoga classes at Yoga Synthesis, run by Raji Thron, her beloved teacher, in Ramsey, New Jersey, and teaches anatomy in teacher-training programs. She also runs her own Gentle Restorative Teacher Trainings, workshops, and classes and continues to share her love of yoga and anatomy in the northern New Jersey area.

Kelly holds a bachelor's degree in sociology. She is a registered 500 E-RYT yoga teacher and is a licensed practicing massage therapist. She is the author of *The Yoga Anatomy Coloring Book*.

About the Illustrator

Samantha Stutzman is an artist and medical illustrator based in Grand Rapids, Michigan. She studied human anatomy at Michigan State's College of Human Medicine and graduated from Kendall College of Art and Design as the Medical Illustration Excellence Award recipient. Samantha completed her post-college internship with Thieme Medical Publishers in New York City, and then went on to create her company, Blue Leaf Illustrations LLC. Samantha is skilled with oil, graphite, colored pencil, charcoal, ink, and digital illustration. She illustrated *The Yoga Anatomy Coloring Book*.

Flash Cards

The following pages contain 48 flash cards. In them, you will find most of the asanas and anatomy covered in this book. I hope that you will use these cards to test your knowledge of the names of the asanas and the highlighted anatomy. Don't worry if you don't remember everything, especially the first time around; we just covered a huge amount of information.

The flash card pages are perforated. Carefully tear out each page and separate it into four cards. On the front of each card is a yoga asana with the anatomy labeled with letters. It will test you on both the English and Sanskrit names of the asanas and your ability to name the anatomy. The answers are right on the back, so it's easy to check yourself. This is a great way to solidify your knowledge, beyond reading and coloring.

In addition, you may use the flash cards to sequence the postures to create a yoga practice either for yourself or for your classes.

These cards are easy to travel with. You can keep these cards with you for a convenient way to study or plan yoga practices at any time! I hope you find them useful as you continue to expand your knowledge of the anatomy of yoga!

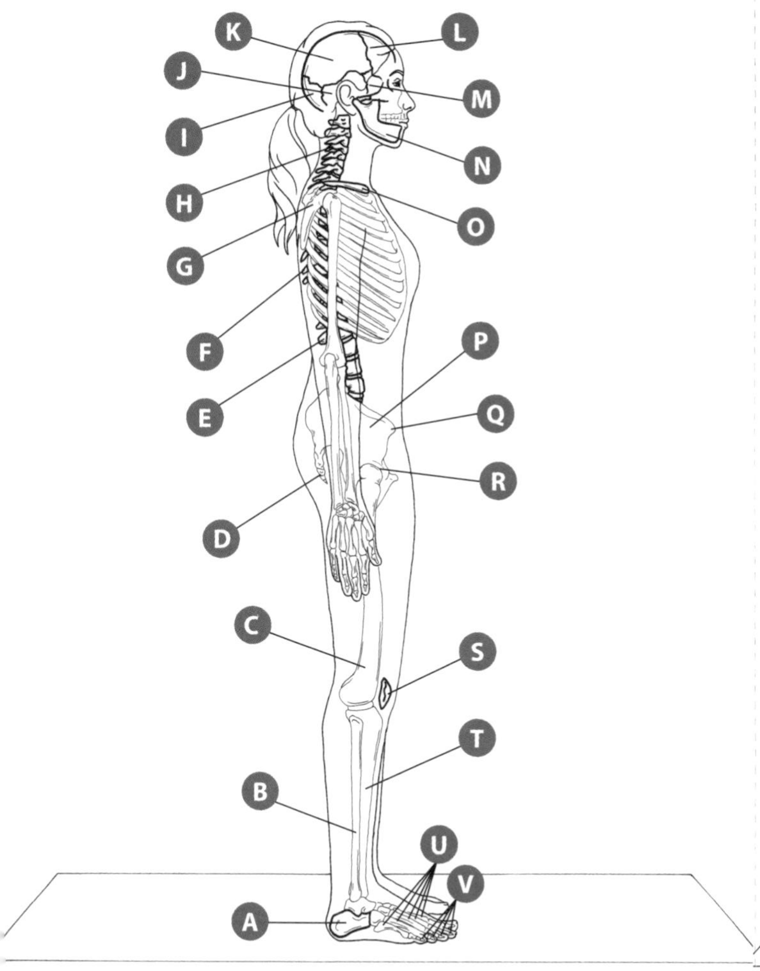
K
L
J
M
I
N
H
O
G
F
P
E
Q
R
D
C
S
T
B
U
V
A

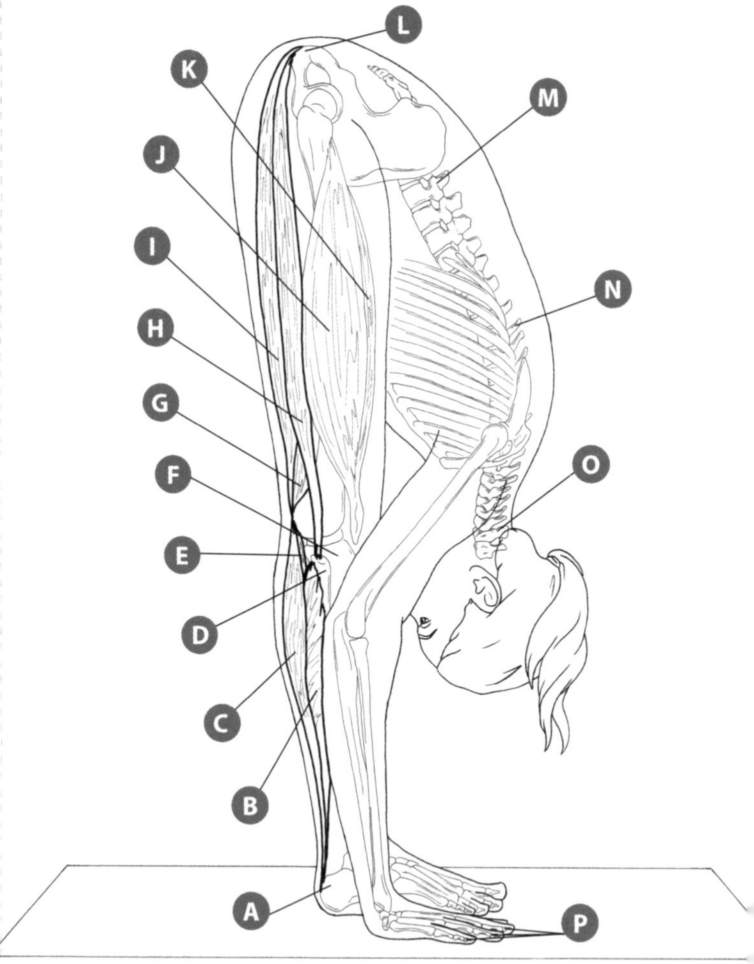
L
K
M
J
I
N
H
G
O
F
E
D
C
B
A
P

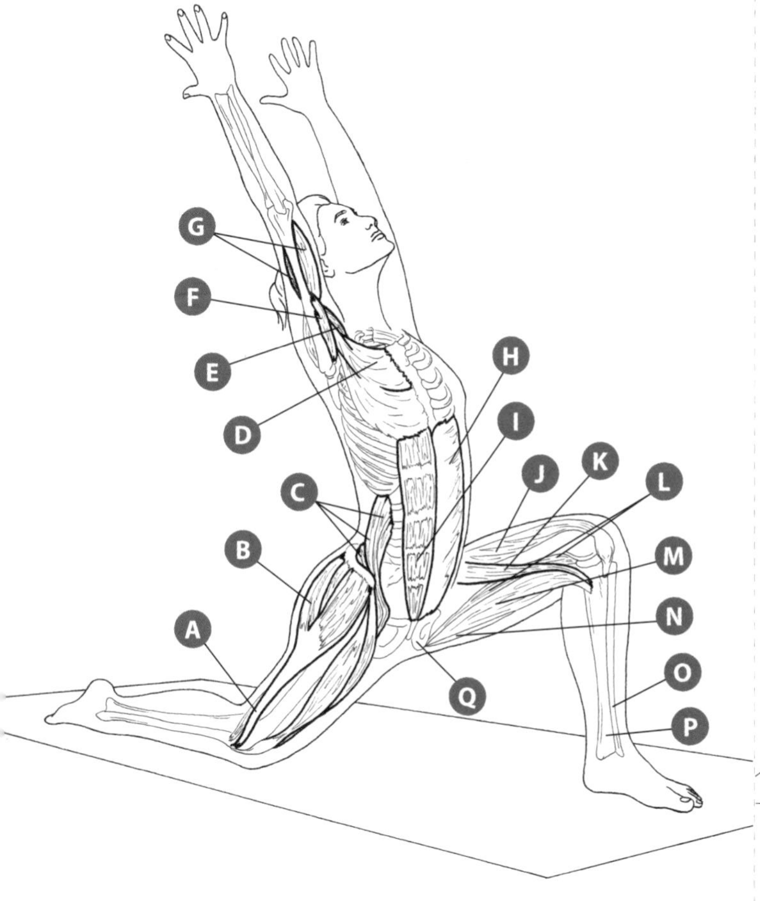
G
F
E
D
H
I
C
J
K
L
B
M
A
N
Q
O
P

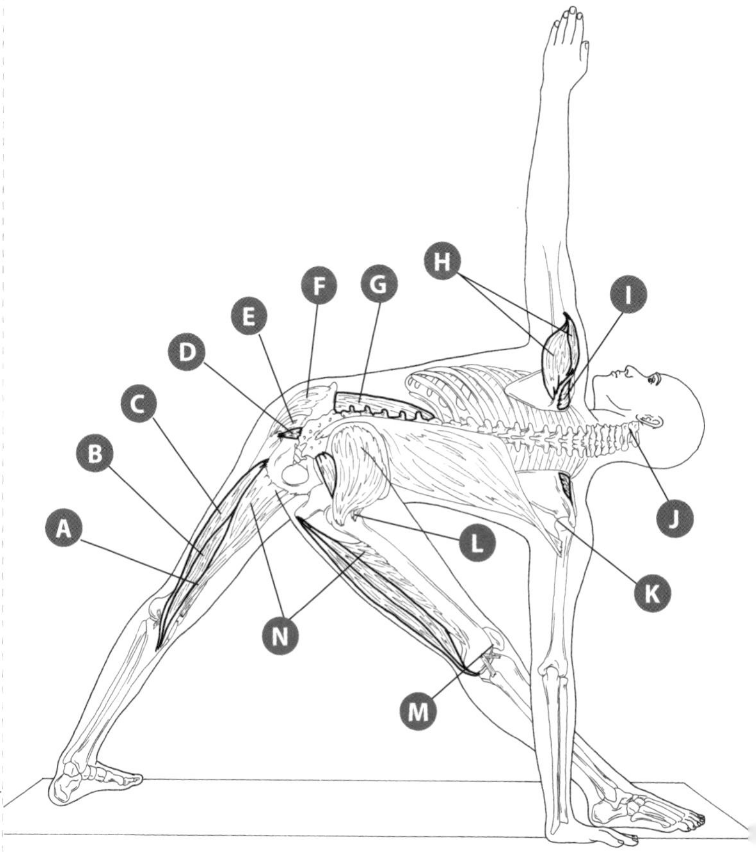
H
F
G
I
E
D
C
B
A
J
L
K
N
M

Uttanasana

Intense Stretch Posture

A.... Calcaneus
B.... Soleus
C.... Gastrocnemius
D.... Fibula
E.... Plantaris
F.... Tibia
G.... Semimembranosus
H.... Biceps femoris
I .... Semitendinosus
J .... Vastus lateralis
K.... Rectus femoris
L.... Ischial tuberosity
M ... Lumbar spine
N.... Thoracic spine
O.... Cervical spine
P.... Phalanges

Tadasana

Mountain

A.... Calcaneus
B.... Fibula
C.... Femur
D.... Coccyx
E.... Lumbar spine
F.... Thoracic spine
G.... Scapula
H.... Cervical spine
I .... Occipital bone
J .... Temporal bone
K.... Parietal bone
L.... Frontal bone
M ... Sphenoid bone
N.... Mandible
O.... Clavicle
P.... Ilium
Q.... Anterior superior iliac spine (ASIS)
R.... Acetabulofemoral (hip) joint
S.... Patella
T.... Tibia
U.... Metatarsals
V.... Phalanges

Utthita Trikonasana

Extended Triangle

A.... Gracilis
B.... Semimembranosus
C.... Semitendinosus
D.... Piriformis
E.... Gluteus minimus
F.... Gluteus medius
G.... Psoas
H.... Deltoid
I .... Supraspinatus
J .... Atlantoaxial joint
K.... Glenohumeral joint
L.... Iliacus
M ... Patella
N.... Adductor magnus

Anjaneyasana

Low Lunge

A.... Iliotibial (IT) band
B.... Gluteus maximus
C.... Iliopsoas
D.... Pectoralis major (upper fibers)
E.... Anterior deltoid
F.... Coracobrachialis
G.... Biceps brachii
H.... External oblique
I .... Rectus abdominis
J .... Rectus femoris
K.... Sartorius
L.... Biceps femoris
M ... Semimembranosus
N.... Semitendinosus
O.... Fibula
P.... Tibia
Q.... Pelvis

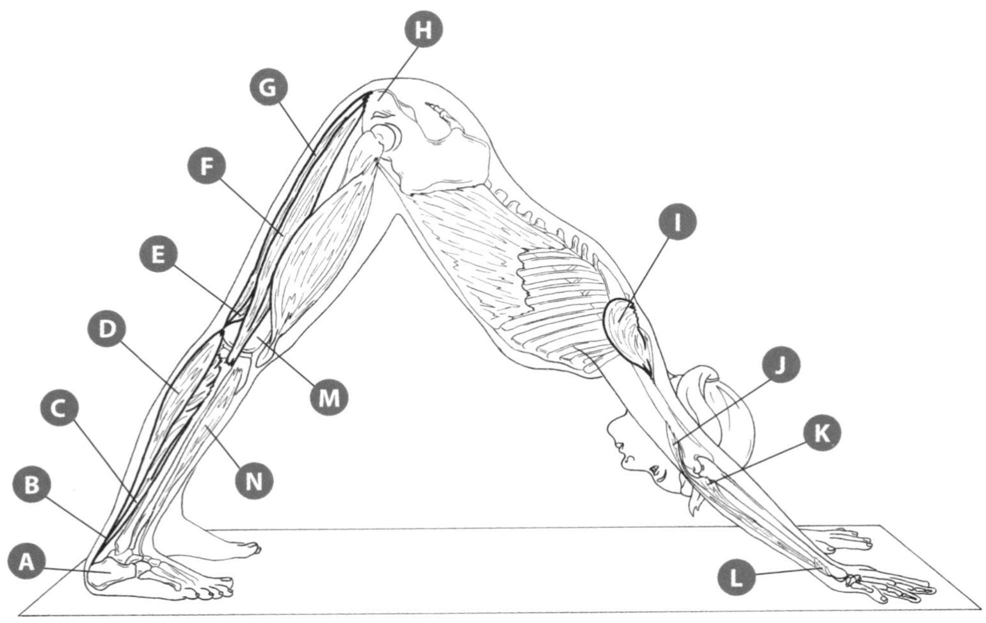
A
B
C
D
E
F
G
H
I
J
K
L
M
N

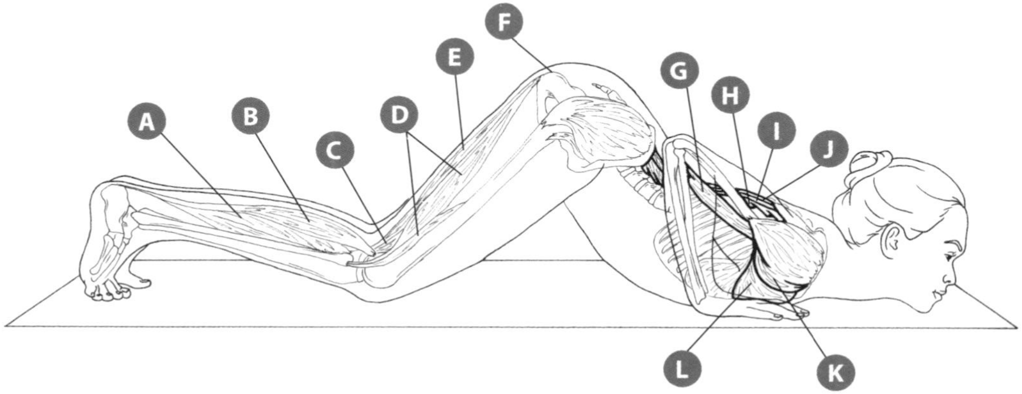
A
B
C
D
E
F
G
H
I
J
K
L

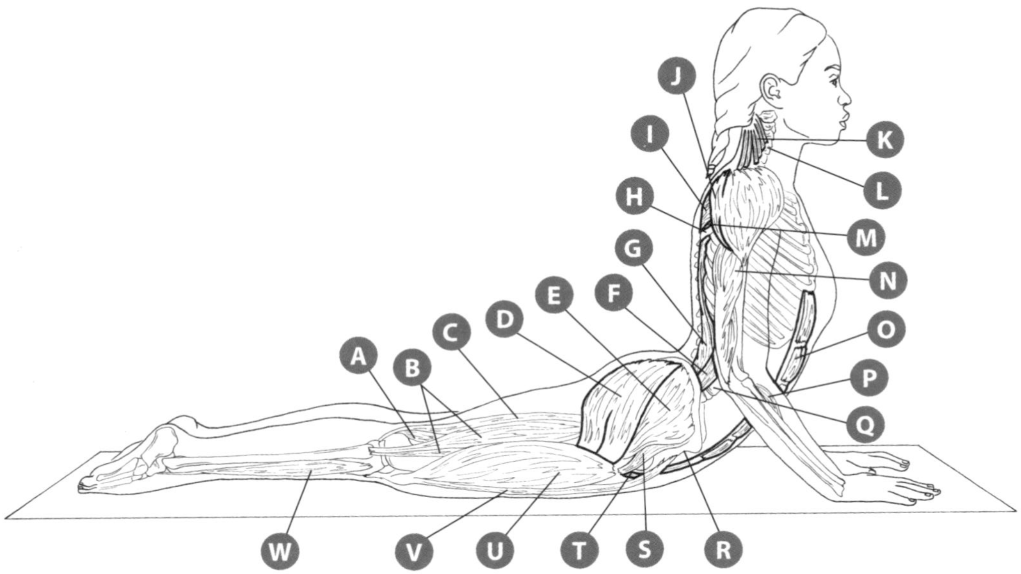
A
B
C
D
E
F
G
H
I
J
K
L
M
N
O
P
Q
R
S
T
U
V
W

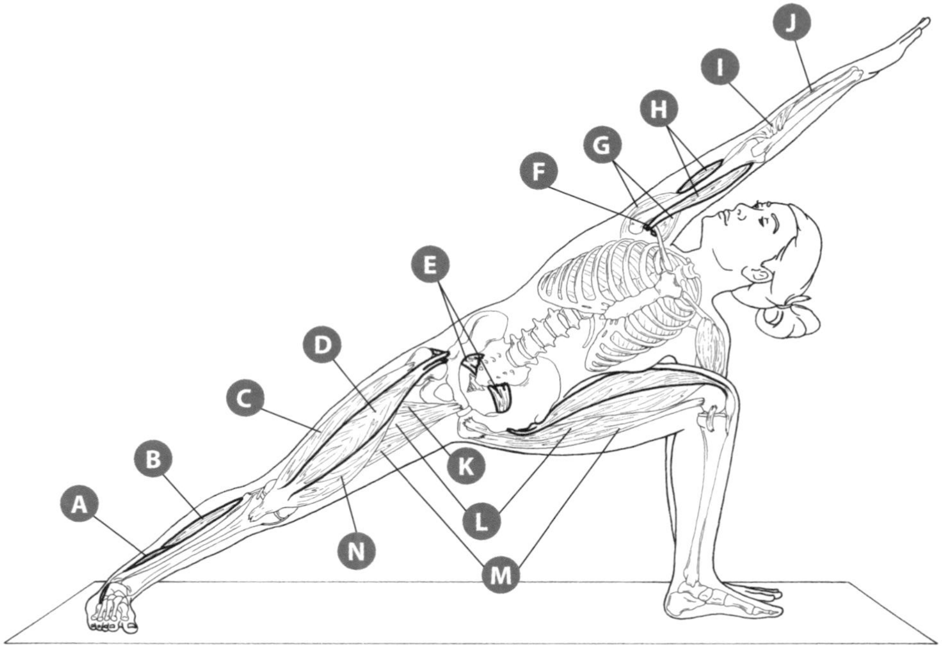
A
B
C
D
E
F
G
H
I
J
K
L
M
N

Adho Mukha Svanasana
Downward-Facing Dog

A. . . . Calcaneus
B. . . . Achilles tendon
C. . . . Soleus
D. . . . Gastrocnemius
E. . . . Semimembranosus
F. . . . Biceps femoris
G. . . . Semitendinosus
H. . . . Ischial tuberosity
I . . . . Posterior deltoid
J . . . . Brachioradialis
K. . . . Pronator teres
L . . . . Pronator quadratus
M . . . Femur
N. . . . Tibialis anterior

Bhujangasana
Cobra

A. . . . Semimembranosus
B. . . . Biceps femoris
C. . . . Semitendinosus
D. . . . Gluteus maximus
E. . . . Gluteus medius
F. . . . Psoas
G. . . . Multifidi
H. . . . Scapula
I . . . . Infraspinatus
J . . . . Posterior deltoid
K. . . . Semispinalis capitis
L . . . . Cervical spine
M . . . Teres minor
N. . . . Triceps brachii
O. . . . Rectus abdominis
P. . . . Pronator teres
Q. . . . Lumbar spine
R. . . . Spine of the ilium
S. . . . Gluteus minimus
T. . . . Iliacus
U. . . . Vastus lateralis
V. . . . Rectus femoris
W . . . Tibialis anterior

Ashtangasana
Eight-Limbs Posture

A . . . . Soleus
B . . . . Gastrocnemius
C . . . . Semimembranosus
D . . . . Biceps femoris
E . . . . Semitendinosus
F . . . . Ischial tuberosity
G . . . . Biceps brachii
H . . . . Iliocostalis
I. . . . . Longissimus
J. . . . . Spinalis
K . . . . Anterior deltoid
L . . . . Pectoralis major (upper fibers)

Utthita Parsvakonasana
Extended Side Angle

A. . . . Peroneal brevis
B. . . . Peroneal longus
C. . . . Vastus lateralis
D. . . . Rectus femoris
E. . . . Piriformis
F. . . . Supraspinatus
G. . . . Deltoid
H. . . . Biceps brachii
I . . . . Supinator
J . . . . Brachioradialis
K. . . . Adductor brevis
L . . . . Adductor longus
M . . . Adductor magnus
N. . . . Vastus medialis

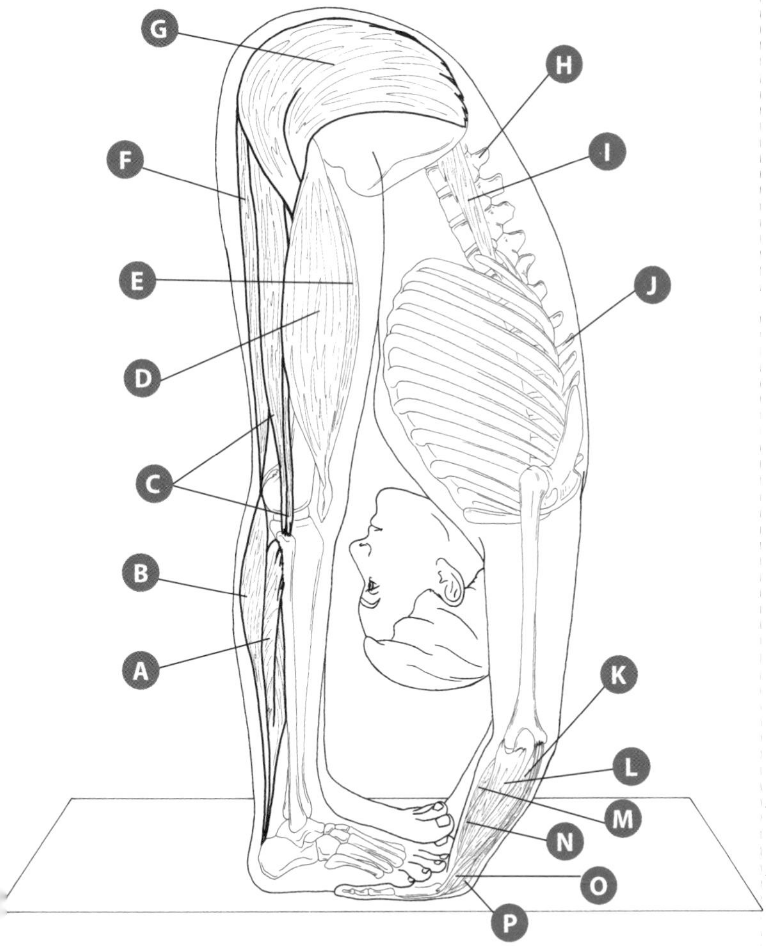
G
H
F
I
E
J
D
C
B
A
K
L
M
N
O
P

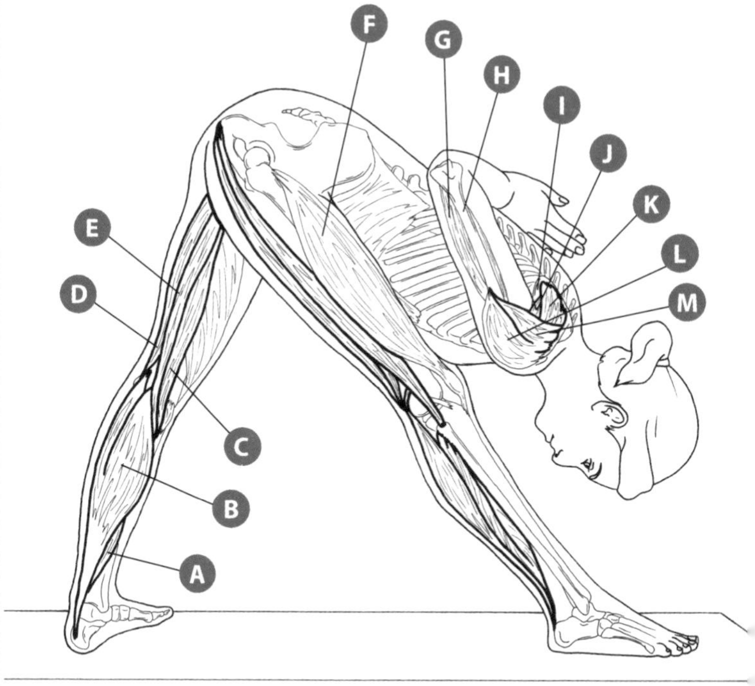
F
G
H
I
J
K
E
L
D
M
C
B
A

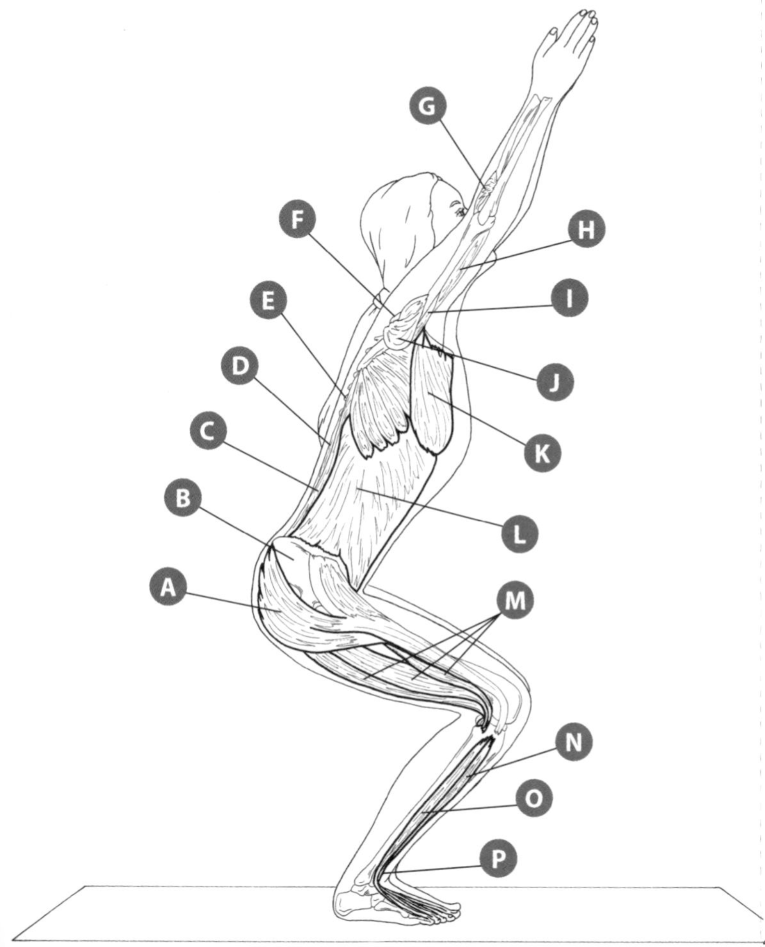
G
F
H
E
I
D
J
C
K
B
L
A
M
N
O
P

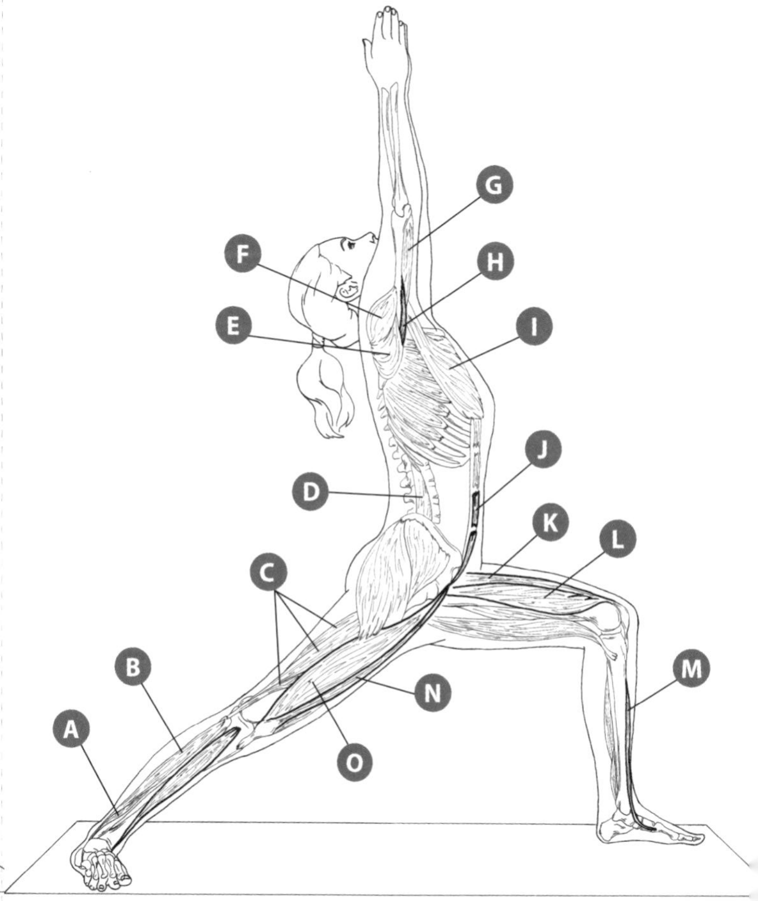
G
F
H
E
I
J
D
K
L
C
B
N
M
A
O

Parsvottanasana
Pyramid

A .... Soleus

B .... Gastrocnemius

C .... Semimembranosus

D .... Biceps femoris

E .... Semitendinosus

F .... Vastus lateralis

G .... Biceps brachii

H .... Humerus

I .... Scapula

J .... Teres minor

K .... Infraspinatus

L .... Middle deltoid

M .... Posterior deltoid

Padahastasana
Foot-Hand Posture

A.... Soleus

B.... Gastrocnemius

C.... Biceps femoris

D.... Vastus lateralis

E.... Rectus femoris

F.... Semitendinosus

G.... Gluteus maximus

H.... Lumbar spine

I .... Psoas

J .... Thoracic spine

K.... Extensor carpi ulnaris

L .... Flexor carpi ulnaris

M ... Palmaris longus

N.... Flexor digitorum superficialis

O.... Extensor digiti minimi

P.... Extensor digitorum

Virabhadrasana I
Warrior I

A.... Peroneal brevis

B.... Peroneal longus

C.... Hamstrings

D.... Psoas

E.... Posterior deltoid

F.... Middle deltoid

G.... Biceps brachii

H.... Coracobrachialis

I .... Pectoralis major

J .... Rectus abdominis

K.... Vastus intermedius

L .... Vastus medialis

M ... Tibialis anterior

N.... Rectus femoris

O.... Vastus lateralis

Utkatasana
Chair

A.... Gluteus maximus

B.... Pelvis

C.... Iliocostalis

D.... Longissimus thoracis

E.... Thoracic spine

F.... Serratus posterior superior

G.... Supinator

H.... Biceps brachii

I .... Coracobrachialis

J .... Posterior deltoid

K.... Pectoralis major

L .... External oblique

M ... Hamstrings

N.... Tibialis anterior

O.... Extensor digitorum longus

P.... Extensor hallucis longus

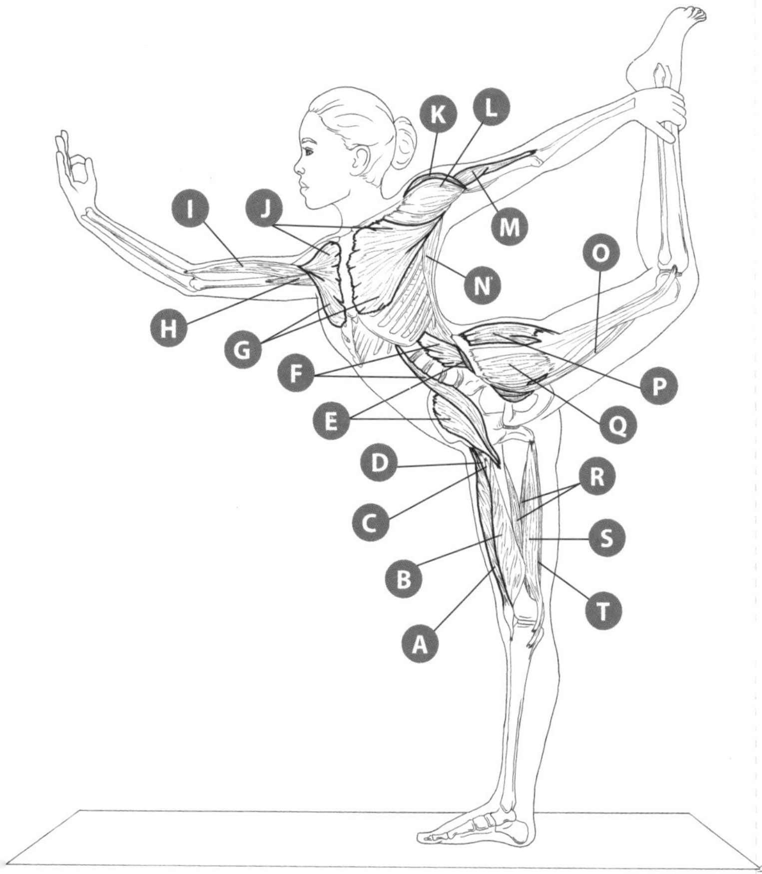
A
B
C
D
E
F
G
H
I
J
K
L
M
N
O
P
Q
R
S
T

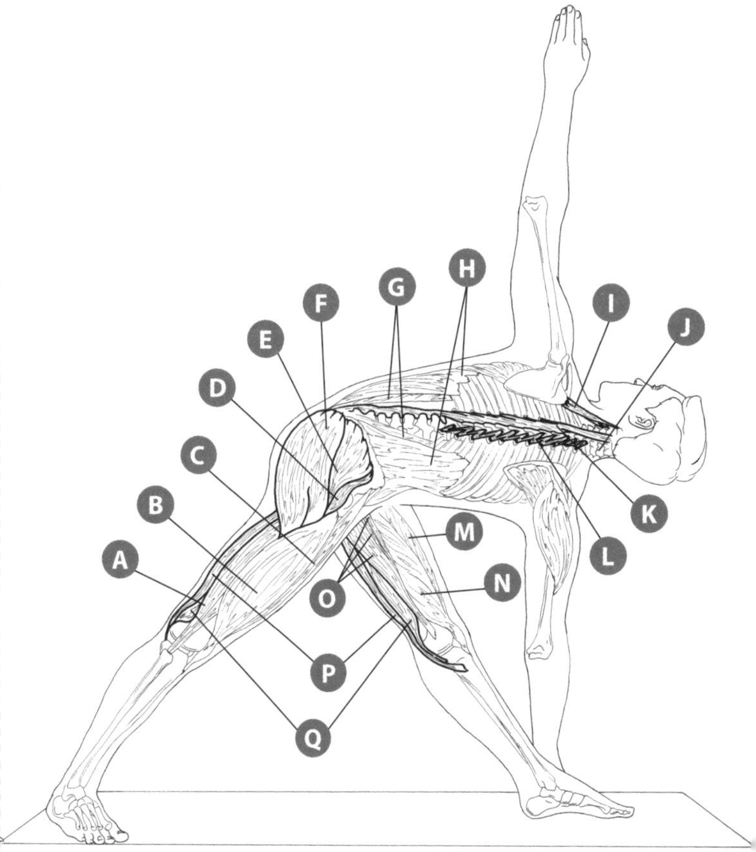
A
B
C
D
E
F
G
H
I
J
K
L
M
N
O
P
Q

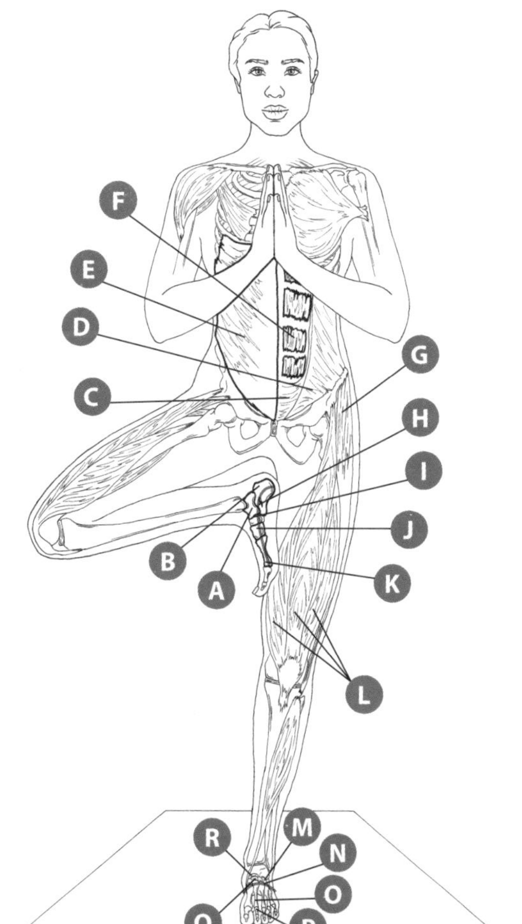
A
B
C
D
E
F
G
H
I
J
K
L
M
N
O
P
Q
R

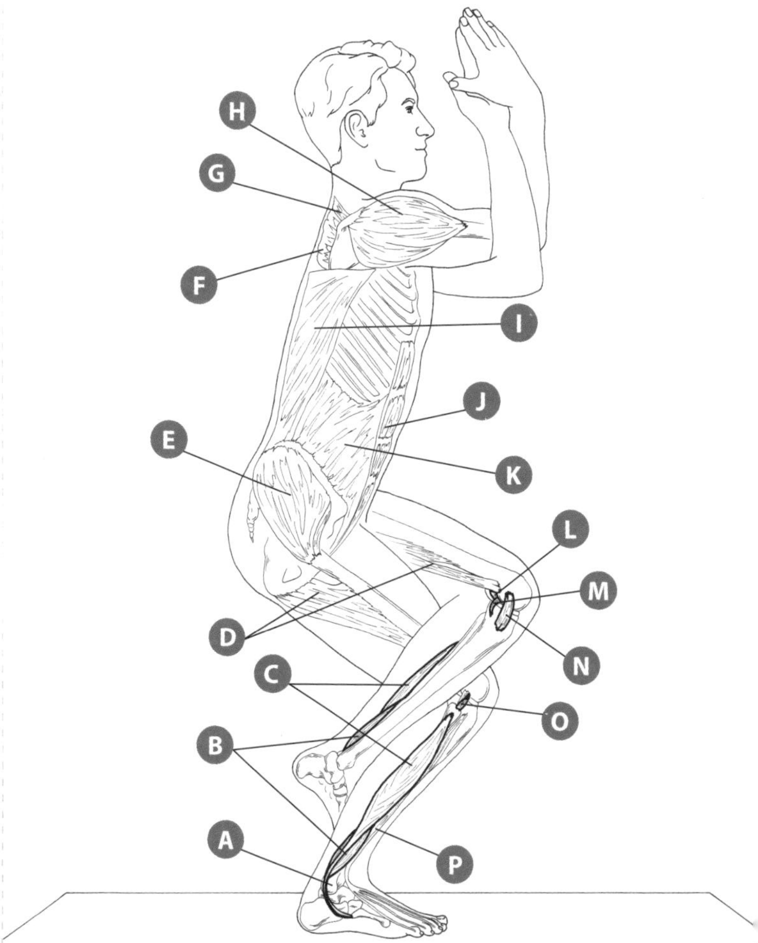
A
B
C
D
E
F
G
H
I
J
K
L
M
N
O
P

Parivrtta Trikonasana
Revolved Triangle

A . . . . Biceps femoris
B . . . . Vastus lateralis
C . . . . Rectus femoris
D . . . . Gluteus minimus
E . . . . Gluteus medius
F . . . . Gluteus maximus
G . . . . Internal obliques
H . . . . External obliques
I . . . . Levator scapula
J . . . . Cervical spine
K . . . . Multifidi
L . . . . Rotatores
M . . . Vastus intermedius
N . . . . Vastus medialis
O . . . . Adductors
P . . . . Semitendinosus
Q . . . . Semimembranosus

Natarajasana
King Dancer

A . . . . Rectus femoris
B . . . . Vastus medialis
C . . . . Vastus intermedius
D . . . . Vastus lateralis
E . . . . Iliacus
F . . . . Psoas
G . . . . Pectoralis major (lower fibers)
H . . . . Coracobrachialis
I . . . . Biceps brachii
J . . . . Pectoralis major (upper fibers)
K . . . . Posterior deltoid
L . . . . Middle deltoid
M . . . Triceps brachii
N . . . . Latissimus dorsi
O . . . . Sartorius
P . . . . Gluteus maximus
Q . . . . Tensor fasciae latae (TFL)
R . . . . Biceps femoris
S . . . . Semimembranosus
T . . . . Semitendinosus

Garudasana
Eagle

A . . . . Lateral malleolus
B . . . . Peroneal brevis
C . . . . Peroneal longus
D . . . . Adductor magnus
E . . . . Gluteus medius
F . . . . Rhomboid major
G . . . . Rhomboid minor
H . . . . Deltoid
I . . . . Latissimus dorsi
J . . . . Rectus abdominis
K . . . . Transverse abdominis
L . . . . Anterior cruciate ligament (ACL)
M . . . Posterior cruciate ligament (PCL)
N . . . . Medial collateral ligament (MCL)
O . . . . Lateral collateral ligament (LCL)
P . . . . Extensor digitorum longus

Vrksasana
Tree

A . . . . Talus
B . . . . Calcaneus
C . . . . Transverse abdominis
D . . . . Internal oblique
E . . . . External oblique
F . . . . Rectus abdominis
G . . . . Tensor fasciae latae (TFL)
H . . . . Longitudinal medial arch
I . . . . Navicular
J . . . . Cuneiform
K . . . . Metatarsals
L . . . . Quadriceps
M . . . Cuboid
N . . . . Transverse arch
O . . . . Metatarsals
P . . . . Phalanges
Q . . . . Cuneiforms
R . . . . Navicular

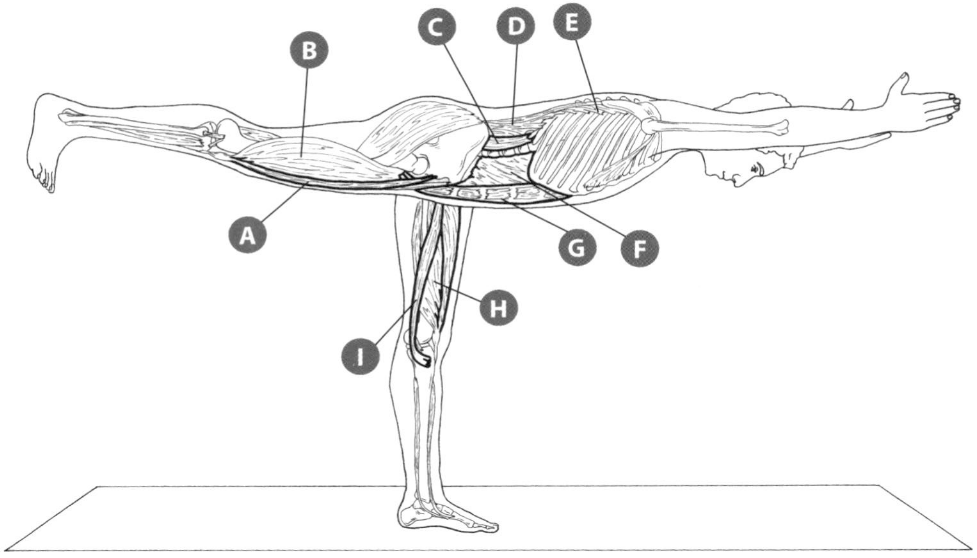
B
C
D
E
A
G
F
H
I

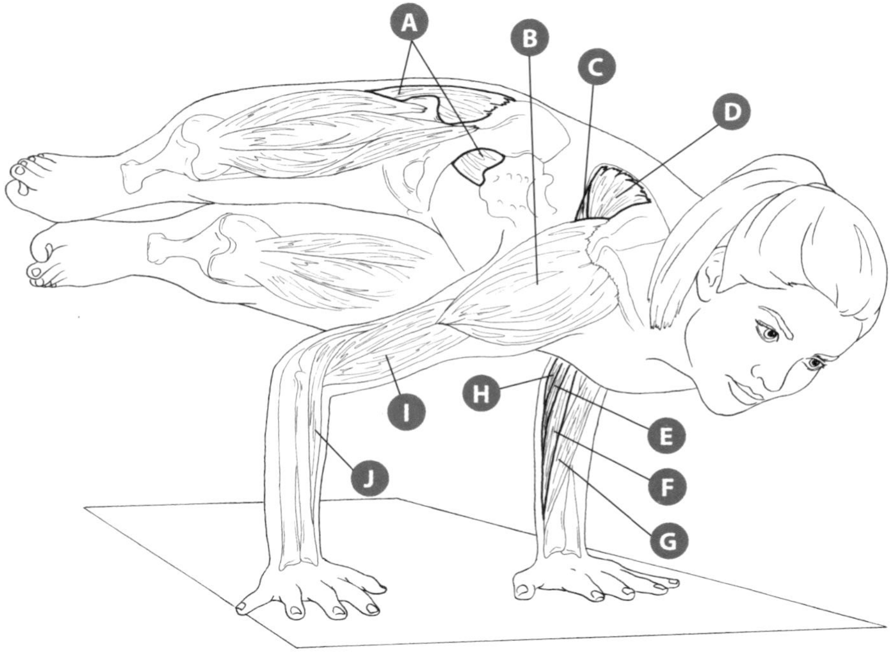
A
B
C
D
H
I
E
J
F
G

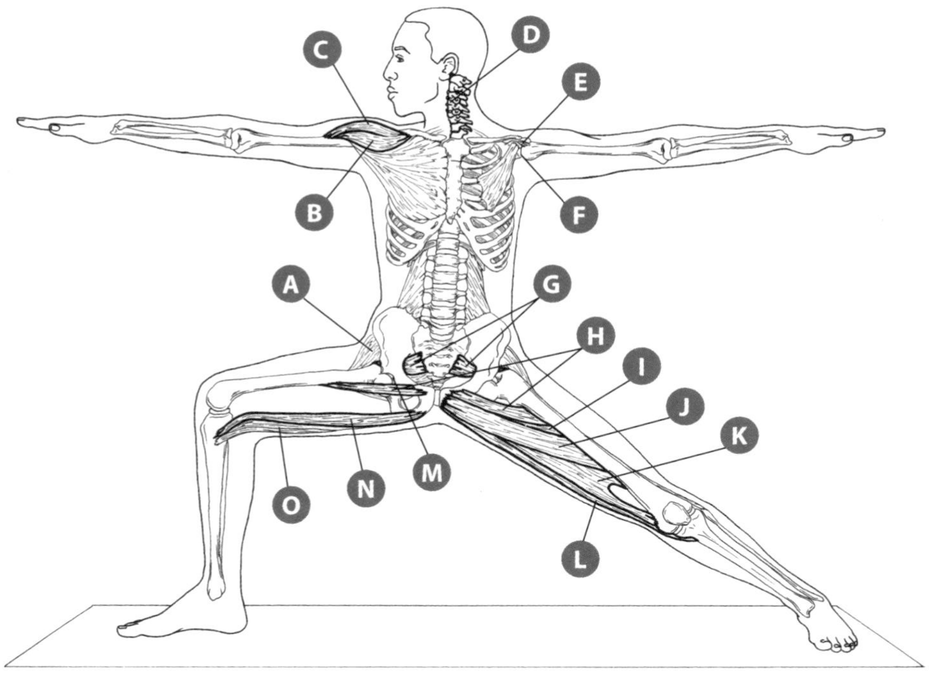
C
D
E
B
F
A
G
H
I
J
K
M
N
O
L

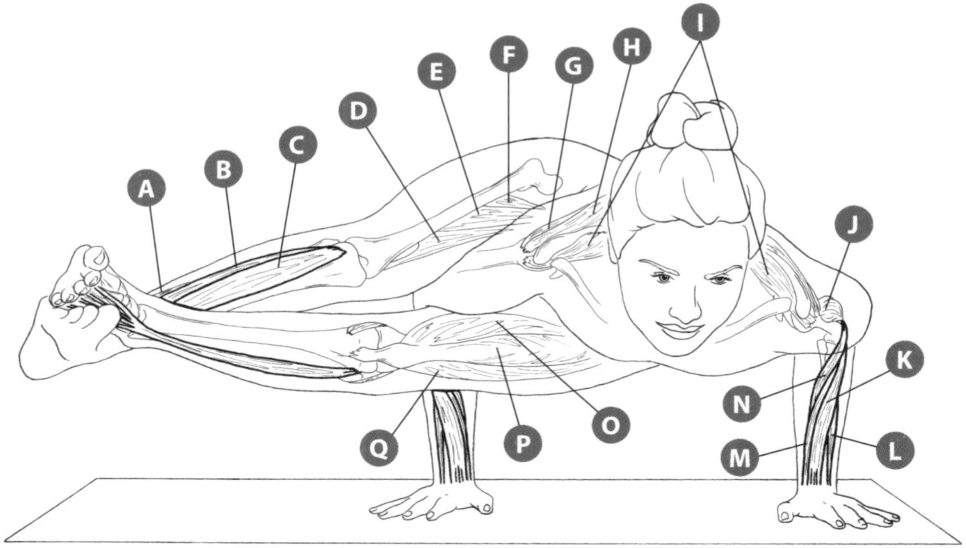
I
F
H
E
G
D
C
B
A
J
K
N
Q
P
O
L
M

Virabhadrasana III
Warrior III

A .... Rectus femoris

B .... Vastus lateralis

C .... Psoas

D .... Longissimus

E .... Iliocostalis

F .... Internal oblique

G .... Rectus abdominis

H .... Vastus medialis

I .... Sartorius

Virabhadrasana II
Warrior II

A.... Gluteus maximus

B.... Anterior deltoid

C.... Middle deltoid

D.... Cervical spine

E.... Supraspinatus

F.... Glenohumeral joint

G.... Piriformis

H.... Pectineus

I .... Adductor brevis

J .... Adductor longus

K.... Adductor magnus

L.... Gracilis

M ... Acetabulofemoral joint

N.... Semimembranosus

O.... Semitendinosus

Parsva Bakasana
Side Crow

A .... Gluteus maximus

B .... Deltoid

C .... Teres minor

D .... Infraspinatus

E .... Palmaris longus

F .... Flexor carpi radialis

G .... Brachioradialis

H .... Flexor carpi ulnaris

I .... Biceps brachii

J............. Brachialis

Astavakrasana
Eight-Bends Posture

A.... Peroneal brevis

B.... Extensor digitorum longus

C.... Tibialis anterior

D.... Adductor magnus

E.... Adductor longus

F.... Adductor brevis

G.... Teres minor

H.... Infraspinatus

I .... Supraspinatus

J .... Triceps brachii

K.... Extensor digitorum

L.... Extensor carpi ulnaris

M ... Extensor carpi radialis brevis

N.... Extensor carpi radialis longus

O.... Vastus medialis

P.... Rectus femoris

Q.... Vastus lateralis

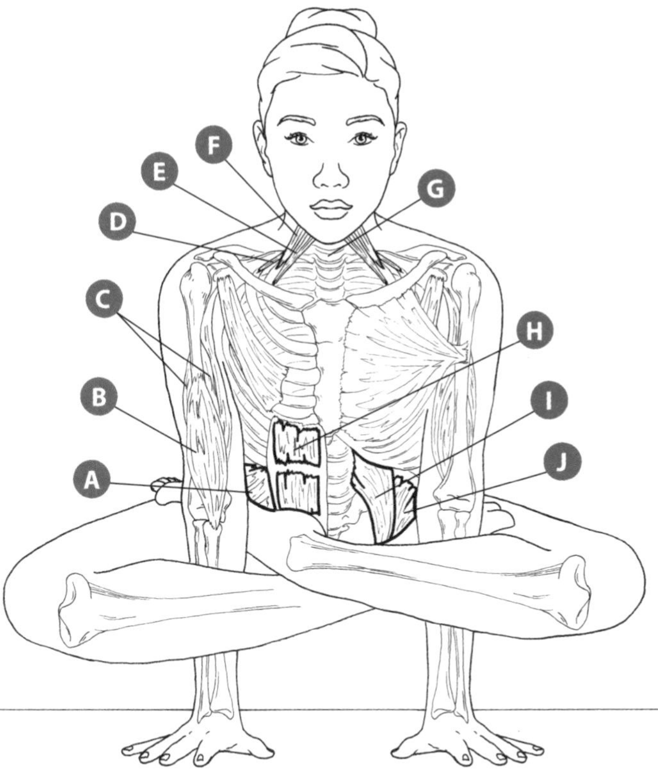
A
B
C
D
E
F
G
H
I
J

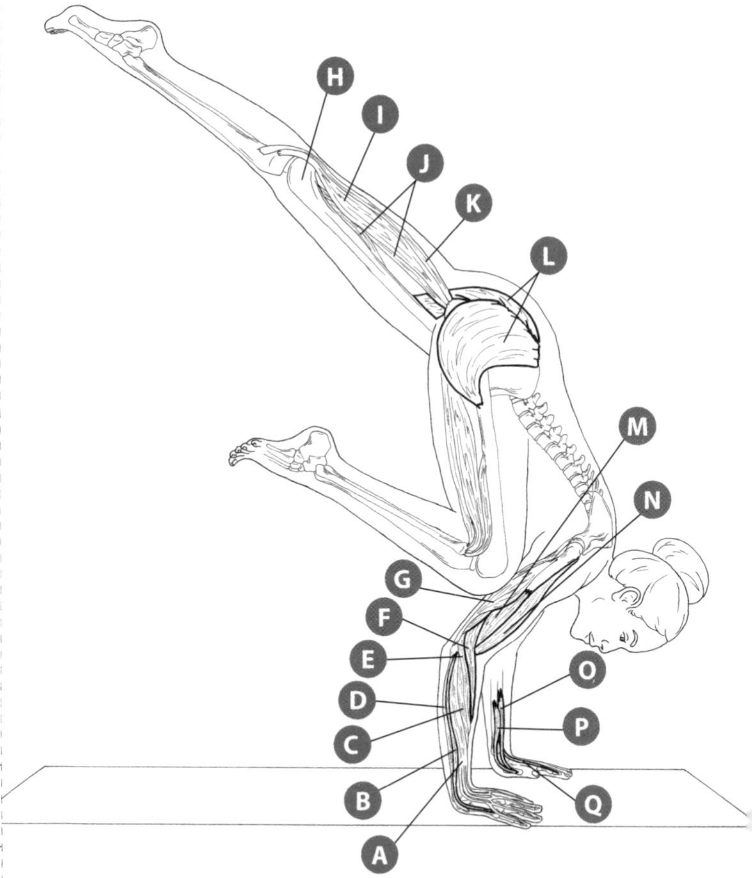
A
B
C
D
E
F
G
H
I
J
K
L
M
N
O
P
Q

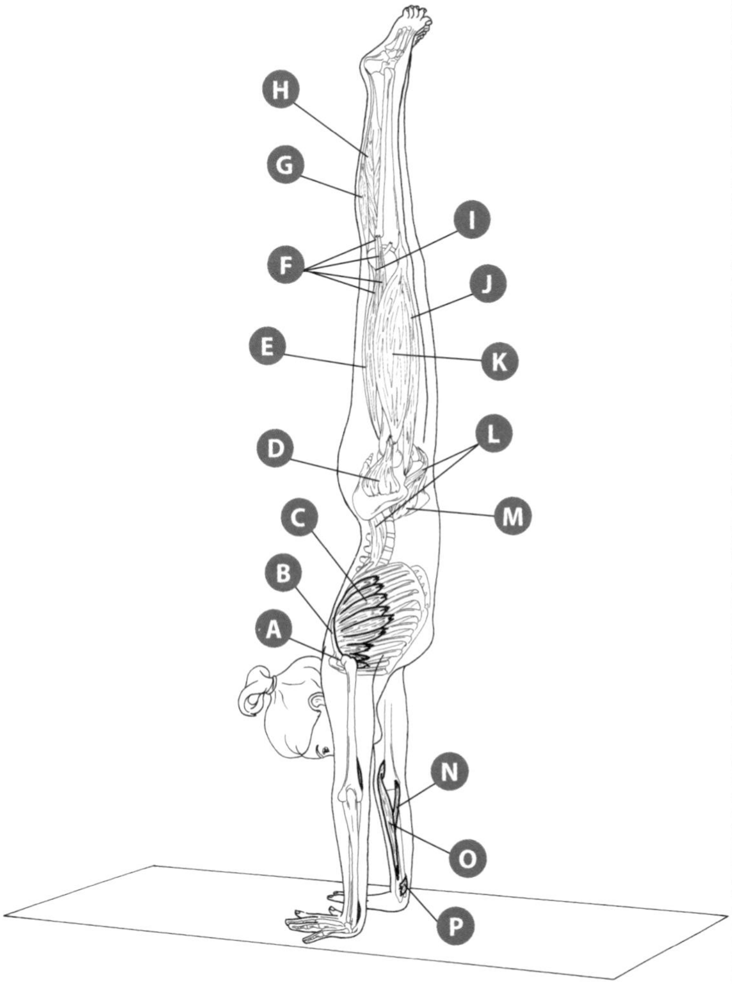
A
B
C
D
E
F
G
H
I
J
K
L
M
N
O
P

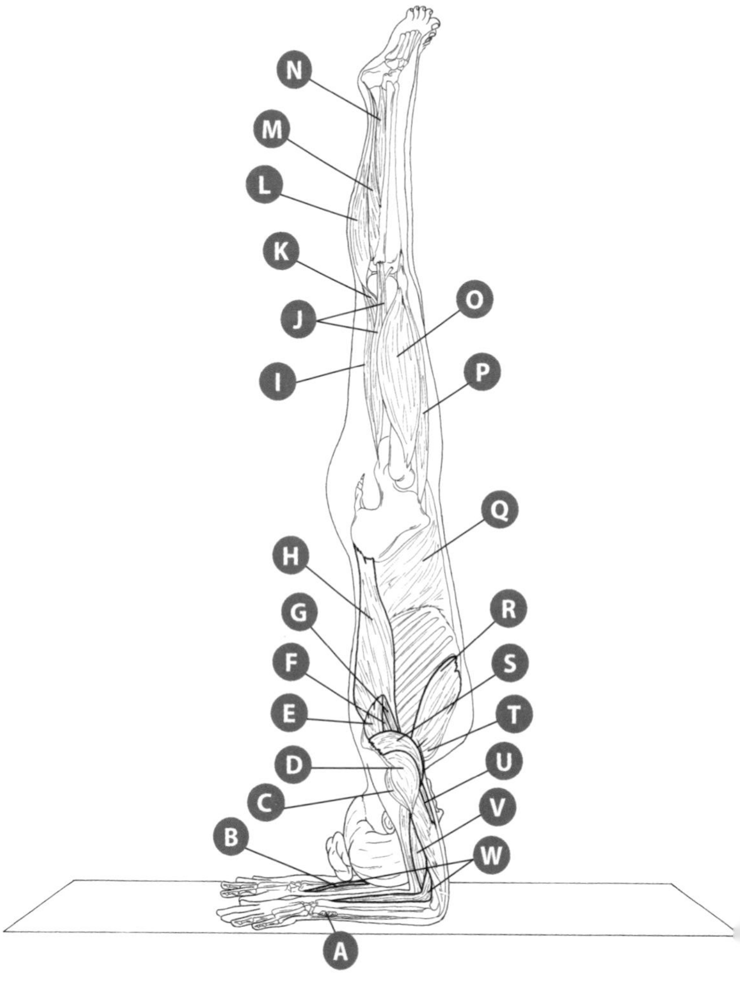
A
B
C
D
E
F
G
H
I
J
K
L
M
N
O
P
Q
R
S
T
U
V
W

Eka Pada Bakasana

One-Legged Crow

A. . . . Extensor digitorum

B. . . . Extensor carpi ulnaris

C. . . . Extensor carpi radialis brevis

D. . . . Extensor digiti minimi

E. . . . Extensor carpi radialis longus

F . . . . Brachioradialis

G. . . . Triceps brachii

H. . . . Femur

I . . . . Semimembranosus

J . . . . Biceps femoris

K. . . . Semitendinosus

L . . . . Gluteus maximus

M . . . Brachialis

N. . . . Biceps brachii

O. . . . Extensor pollicis longus

P . . . . Extensor pollicis brevis

Q. . . . Extensor indicis

Kukkutasana

Rooster

A . . . . Internal oblique

B . . . . Brachialis

C . . . . Triceps brachii

D . . . . Posterior scalene

E . . . . Anterior scalene

F . . . . Middle scalene

G . . . . Cervical spine

H . . . . Rectus abdominis

I. . . . . Psoas

J. . . . . Iliacus

Pincha Mayurasana

Feather of the Peacock

A. . . . Pronator quadratus

B. . . . Flexor carpi radialis

C. . . . Anterior deltoid

D. . . . Middle deltoid

E. . . . Infraspinatus

F . . . . Teres minor

G. . . . Teres major

H. . . . Latissimus dorsi

I . . . . Semitendinosus

J . . . . Biceps femoris

K. . . . Semimembranosus

L . . . . Gastrocnemius

M . . . Soleus

N. . . . Flexor hallucis longus

O. . . . Vastus lateralis

P. . . . Rectus femoris

Q. . . . Transverse abdominis

R. . . . Pectoralis major (lower fibers)

S. . . . Posterior deltoid

T. . . . Pectoralis major (upper fibers)

U. . . . Triceps brachii (long head)

V. . . . Brachialis

W . . . Brachioradialis

Adho Mukha Vrksasana

Downward-Facing Tree

A. . . . Glenohumeral joint

B. . . . Scapula

C. . . . Serratus anterior

D. . . . Gluteus minimus

E. . . . Semitendinosus

F. . . . Biceps femoris

G. . . . Gastrocnemius

H. . . . Soleus

I . . . . Semimembranosus

J . . . . Rectus femoris

K. . . . Vastus lateralis

L . . . . Psoas

M . . . Iliacus

N. . . . Pronator teres

O. . . . Brachioradialis

P. . . . Pronator quadratus

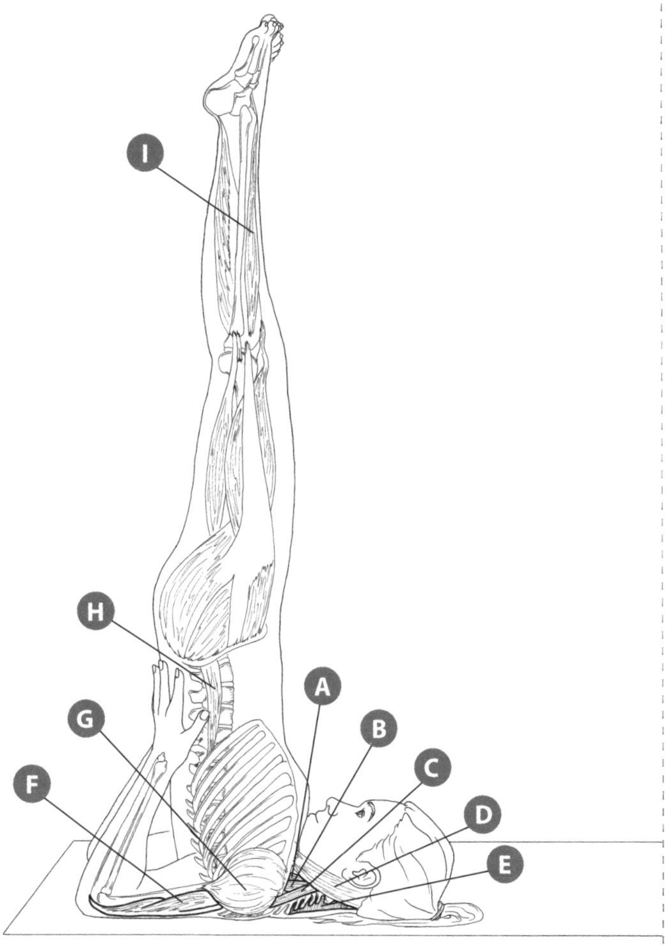
I
H
A
G
B
C
F
D
E

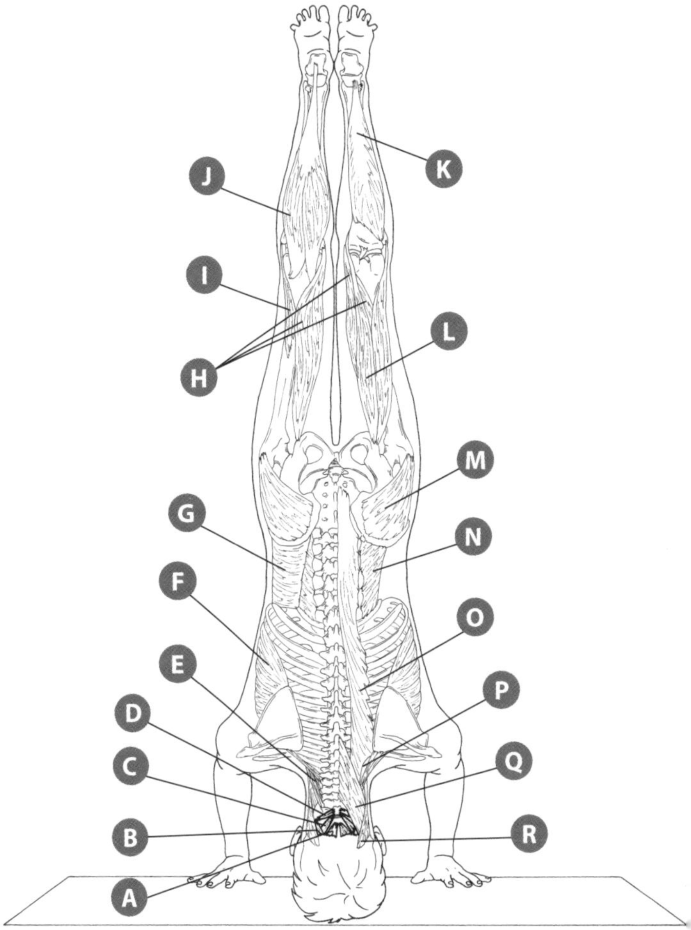
K
J
I
L
H
M
G
N
F
O
E
P
D
Q
C
B
R
A

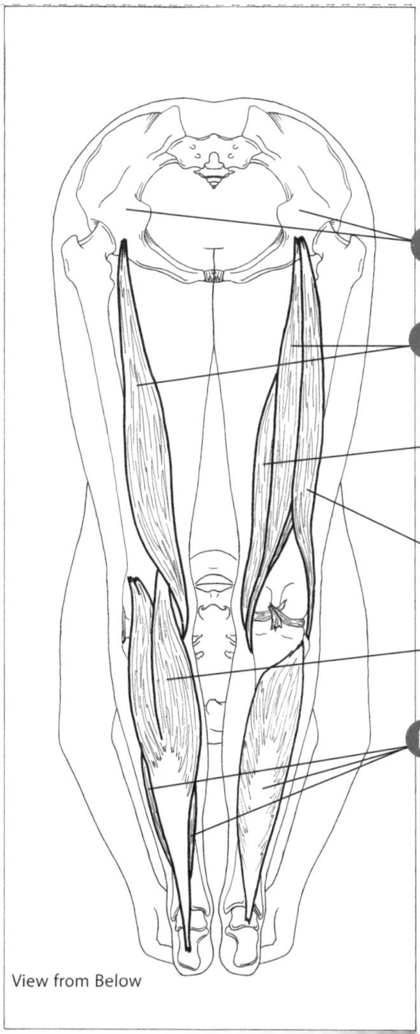
A
B
C
D
E
F
View from Below

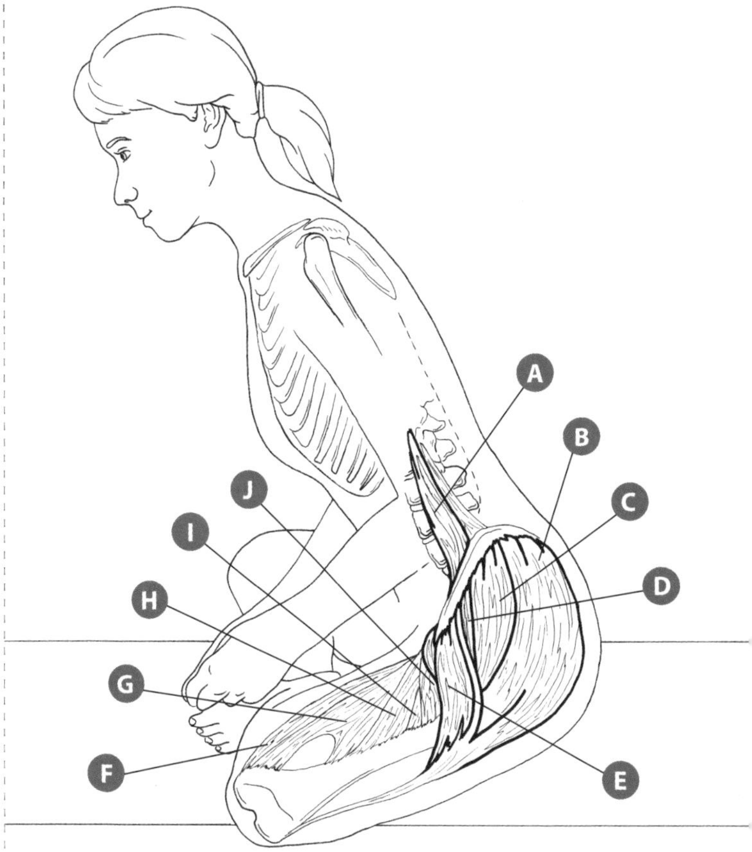
A
B
J
C
I
D
H
G
F
E

Sirsasana B
Tripod Headstand

A. . . . Rectus capitis posterior minor

B. . . . Obliquus capitis superior

C. . . . Rectus capitis posterior major

D. . . . Obliquus capitis inferior

E. . . . Scalenes

F. . . . Serratus anterior

G. . . . Transverse abdominis

H. . . . Semimembranosus

I . . . . Biceps femoris (short head)

J . . . . Gastrocnemius

K. . . . Soleus

L . . . . Semitendinosus

M . . . Gluteus medius

N. . . . Quadratus lumborum

O. . . . Longissimus capitis

P. . . . Levator scapula

Q. . . . Splenius capitis

R. . . . Sternocleidomastoid (SCM)

Salamba Sarvangasana
Supported All-Limbs Posture

A . . . . Anterior scalene

B . . . . Middle scalene

C . . . . Levator scapula

D . . . . Sternocleidomastoid

E . . . . Ligamentum nuchae

F . . . . Triceps brachii

G . . . . Deltoid

H . . . . Psoas

I . . . . Tibialis anterior

Baddhakonasana
Bound-Angle Posture

A . . . . Psoas

B . . . . Gluteus maximus

C . . . . Gluteus medius

D . . . . Gluteus minimus

E . . . . Tensor fasciae latae (TFL)

F . . . . Gracilis

G . . . . Adductor magnus

H . . . . Adductor longus

I . . . . Adductor brevis

J. . . . . Pectineus

Paschimottanasana
Seated Forward Bend

A . . . . Ischial tuberosities

B . . . . Semimembranosus

C . . . . Semitendinosus

D . . . . Biceps femoris

E . . . . Gastrocnemius

F . . . . Soleus

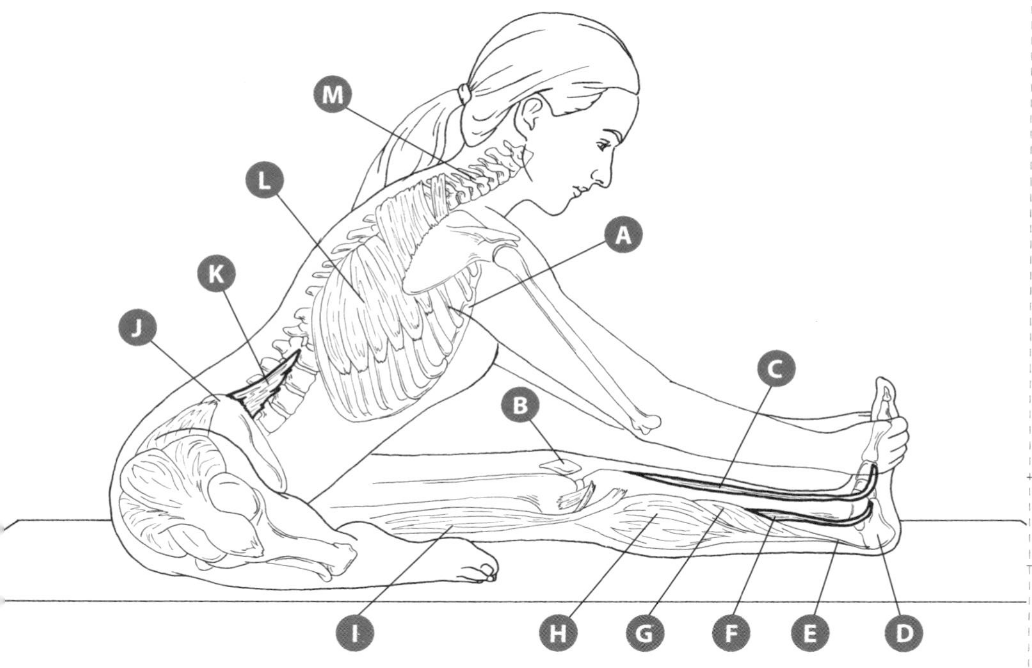
M
L
A
K
J
C
B
I
H
G
F
E
D

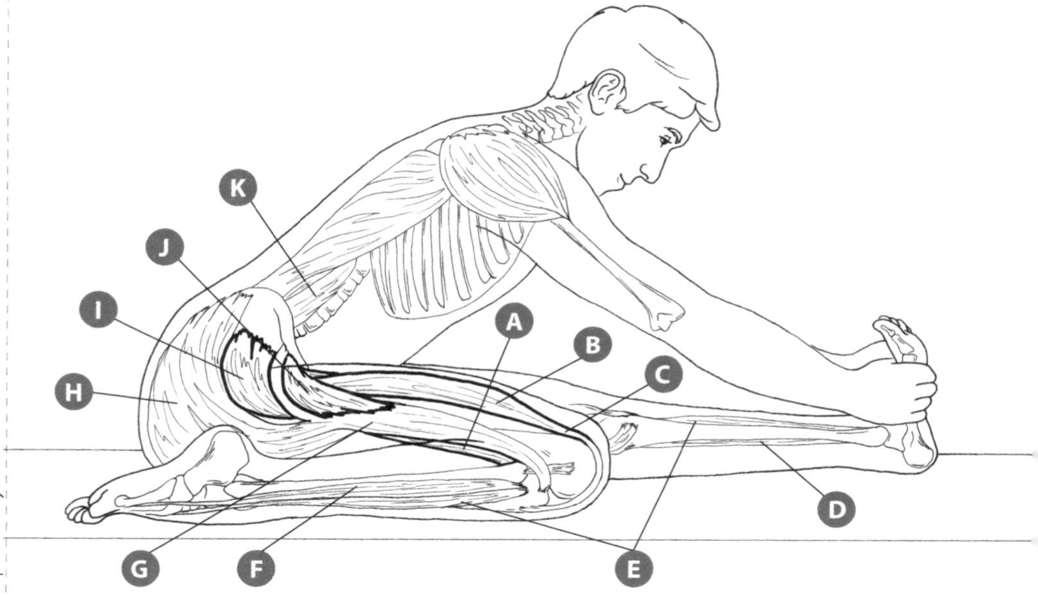
K
J
I
A
B
C
H
D
G
F
E

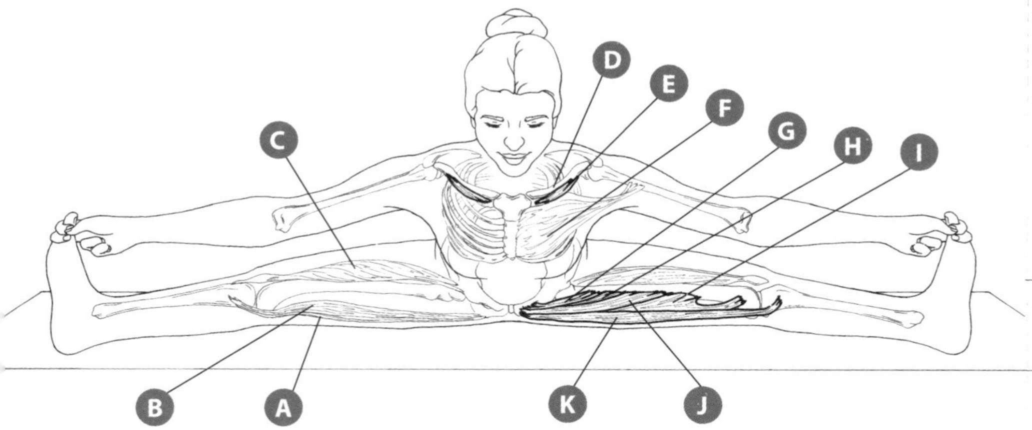
D
E
F
G
H
I
C
B
A
K
J

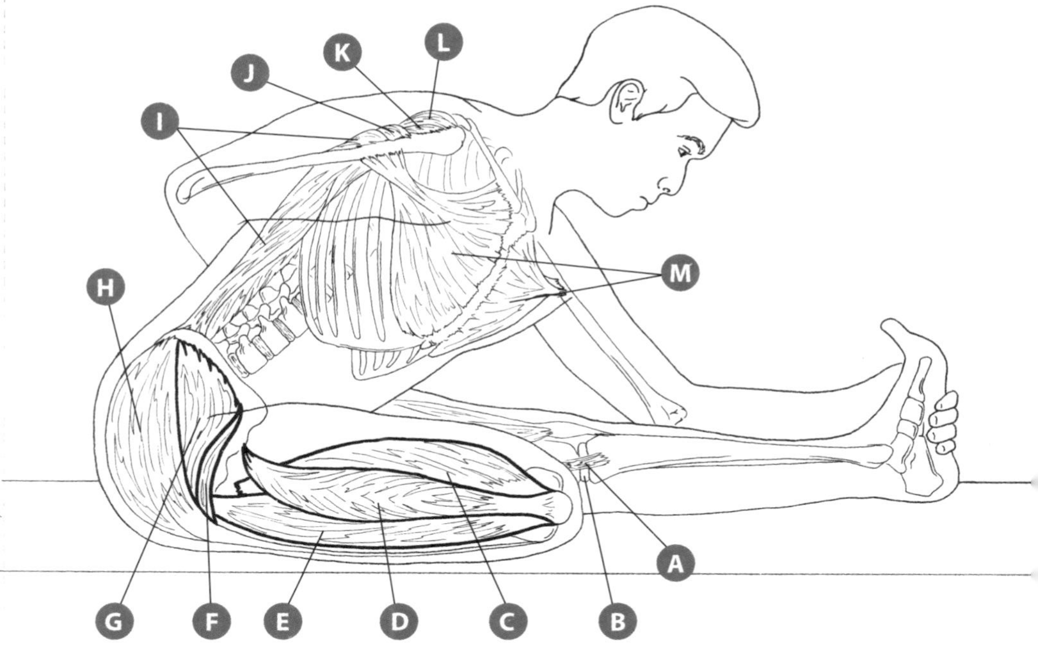
J
K
L
I
M
H
A
G
F
E
D
C
B

Janu Sirsasana
Head-to-Knee Posture

A .... Sternum

B .... Patella

C .... Tibialis anterior

D .... Calcaneus

E .... Achilles tendon

F .... Tibialis posterior

G .... Soleus

H .... Gastrocnemius

I .... Semitendinosus

J .... Iliac crest

K .... Quadratus lumborum

L .... Serratus anterior

M .... Cervical spine

Upavishta Konasana
Wide-Angle Seated Forward Bend

A .... Semitendinosus

B .... Semimembranosus

C .... Rectus femoris

D .... Clavicle

E .... Subclavius

F .... Pectoralis major

G .... Pectineus

H .... Adductor brevis

I .... Adductor magnus

J .... Adductor longus

K .... Gracilis

Triang Mukha Eka Pada Paschimottanasana
Three-Limb Facing One-Leg Forward Bend

A .... Sartorius

B .... Rectus femoris

C .... Quadriceps tendon

D .... Extensor hallucis longus

E .... Tibialis anterior

F .... Extensor digitorum longus

G .... Iliotibial (IT) band

H .... Gluteus maximus

I .... Gluteus minimus

J .... Tensor fasciae latae (TFL)

K .... Psoas

Ardha Baddha Padma Paschimottanasana
Half-Bound Lotus Forward Bend

A .... Medial collateral ligament (MCL)

B .... Medial meniscus

C .... Vastus medialis

D .... Rectus femoris

E .... Vastus lateralis

F .... Gluteus minimus

G .... Gluteus medius

H .... Gluteus maximus

I .... Latissimus dorsi

J .... Teres major

K .... Teres minor

L .... Infraspinatus

M .... Pectoralis major

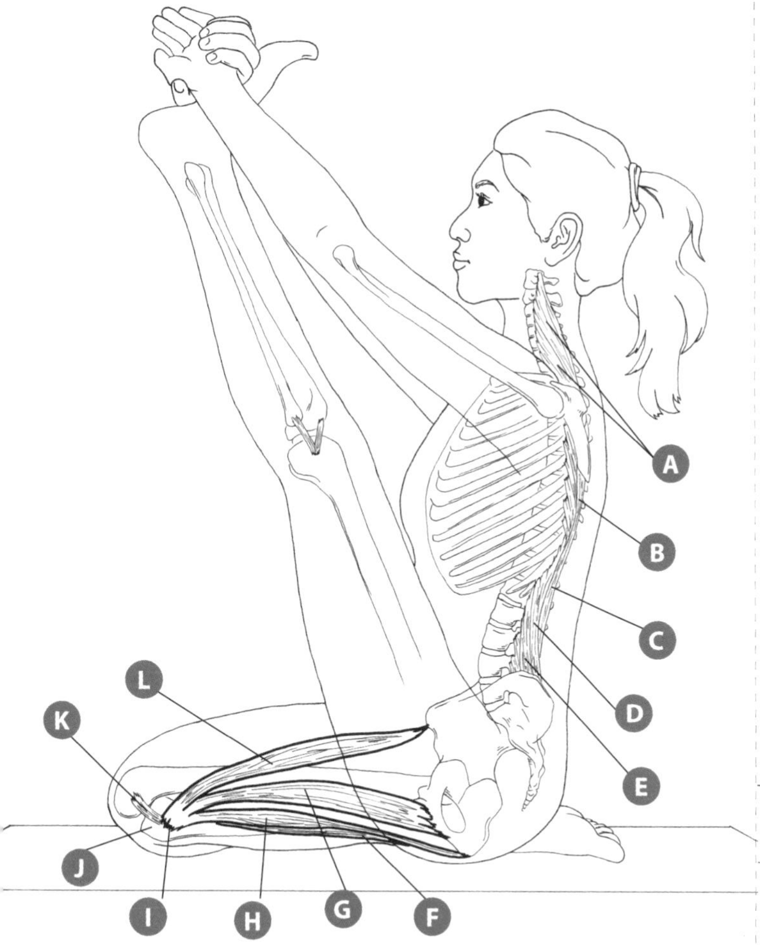
A
B
C
D
E
F
G
H
I
J
K
L

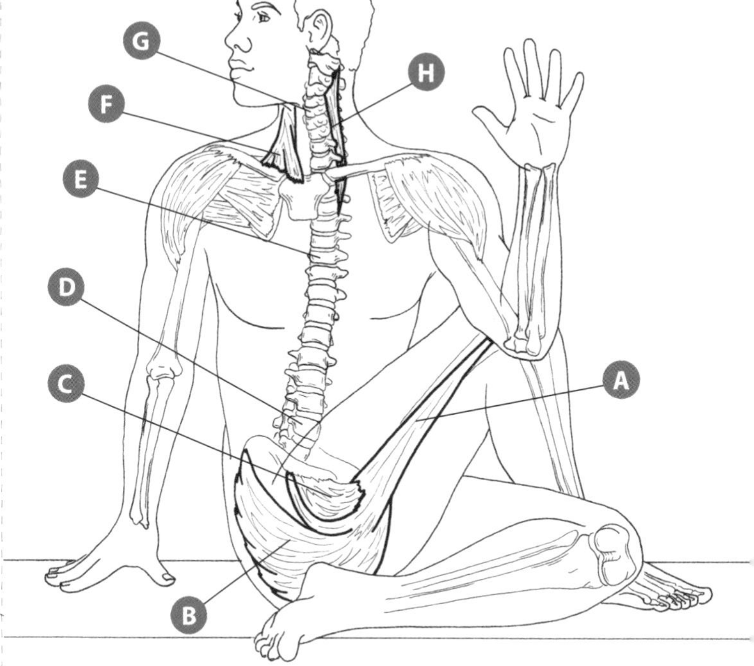
G
H
F
E
D
A
C
B

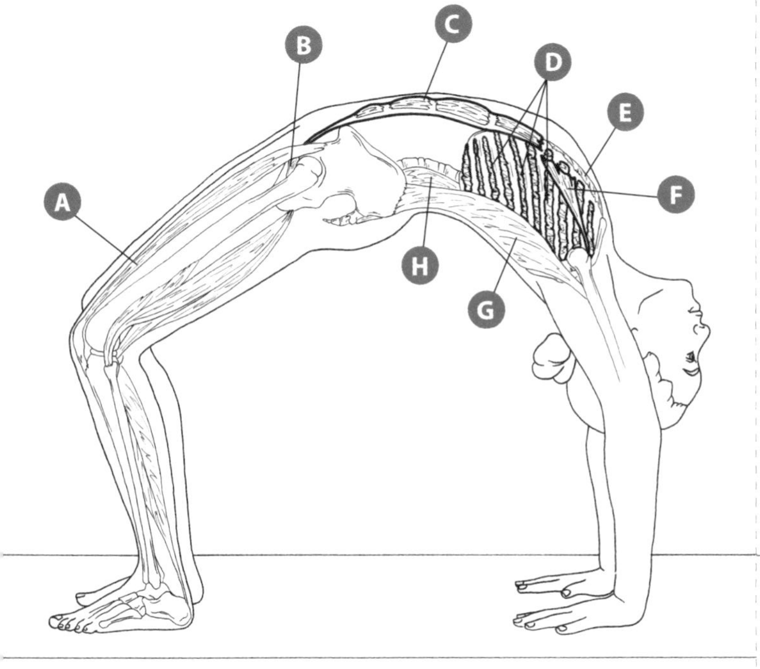
B
C
D
E
F
A
H
G

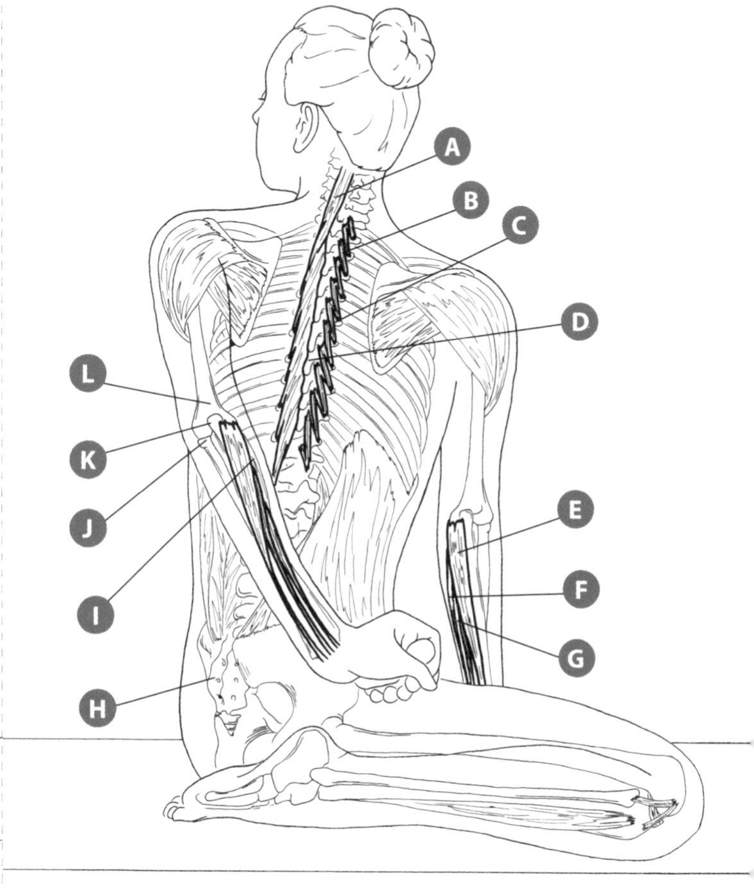
A
B
C
D
L
K
J
I
E
F
G
H

Ardha Matsyendrasana
Half Lord of the Fishes

A .... Iliotibial (IT) band
B .... Gluteus maximus
C .... Tensor fasciae latae (TFL)
D .... Lumbar spine
E .... Thoracic spine
F .... Sternocleidomastoid (SCM)
G .... Cervical spine
H .... Splenius cervicis

Krounchasana
Heron

A .... Iliocostalis
B .... Spinalis
C .... Longissimus
D .... Iliocostalis
E .... Quadratus lumborum
F .... Semimembranosus
G .... Gracilis
H .... Semitendinosus
I .... Pes anserinus
J .... Tibia
K .... Medial collateral ligament (MCL)
L .... Sartorius

The Yoga Anatomy Coloring Book: Pose by Pose

Bharadvajasana
Bharadvaja's Twist

A .... Multifidi
B .... Rotatores
C .... Transverse process
D .... Spinous process
E .... Flexor carpi radialis
F .... Flexor carpi ulnaris
G .... Palmaris longus
H .... Sacrum
I .... Pronator teres
J .... Radius
K .... Ulna
L .... Humerus

The Yoga Anatomy Coloring Book: Pose by Pose

Urdhva Dhanurasana
Upward Bow

A .... Rectus femoris
B .... Iliacus
C .... Rectus abdominis
D .... Intercostal muscles
E .... Pectoralis major
F .... Pectoralis minor
G .... Latissimus dorsi
H .... Psoas

The Yoga Anatomy Coloring Book: Pose by Pose

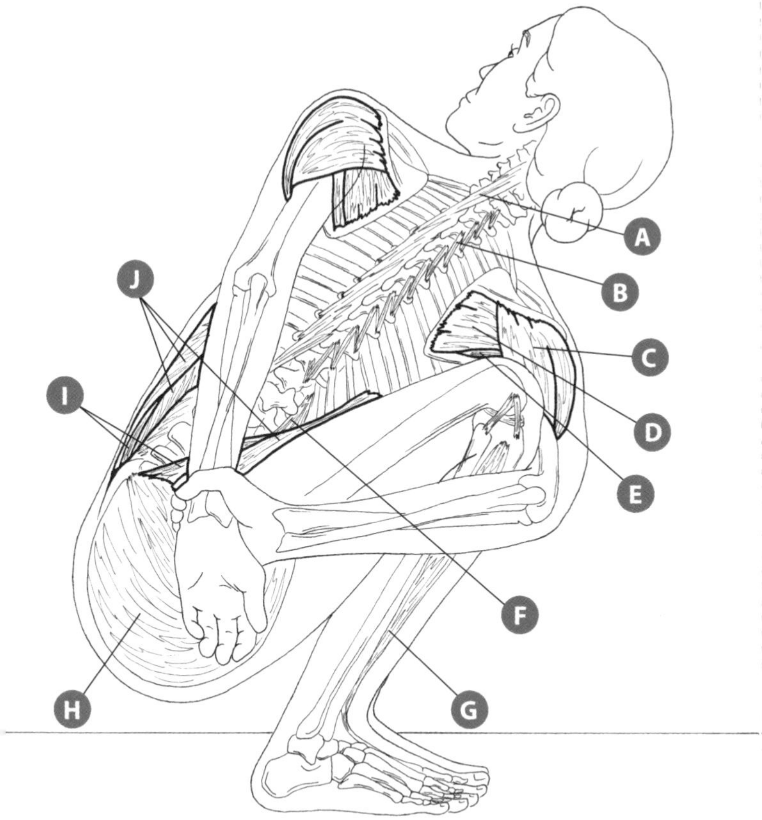
A
B
C
D
E
F
G
H
I
J

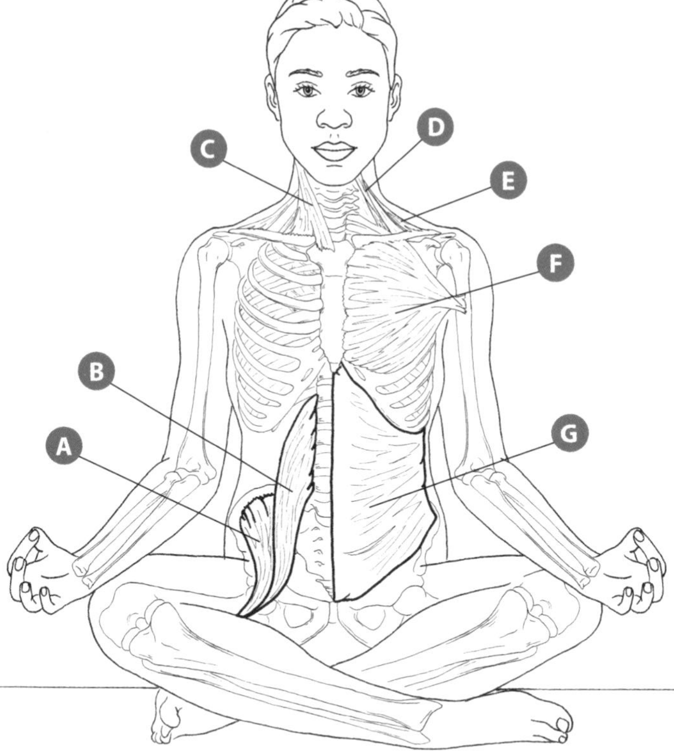
A
B
C
D
E
F
G

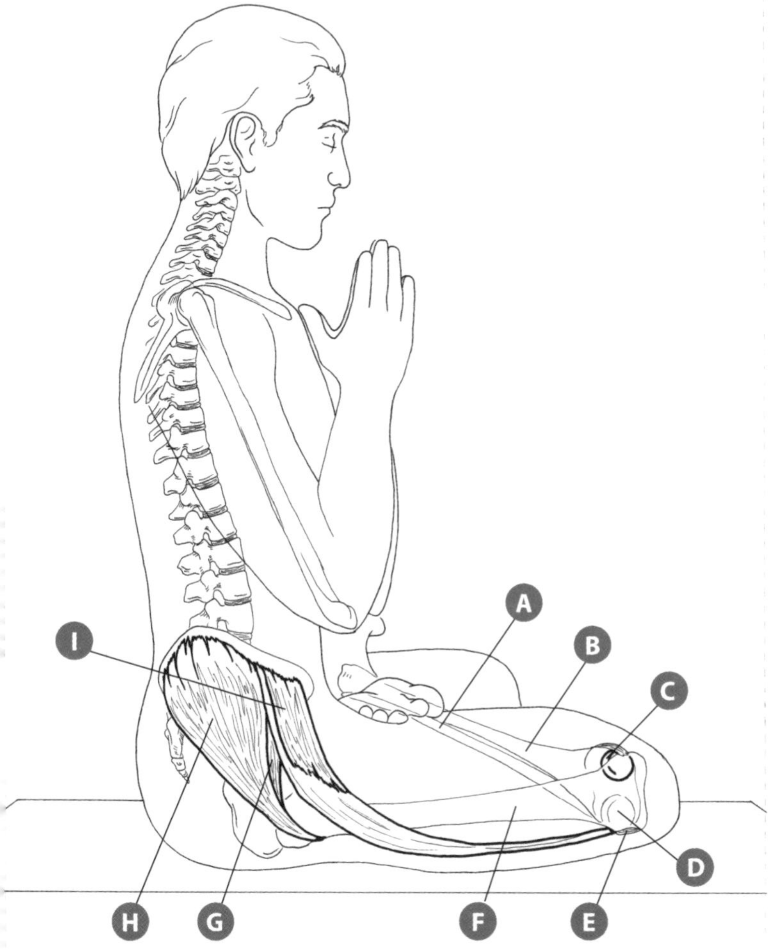
A
B
C
D
E
F
G
H
I

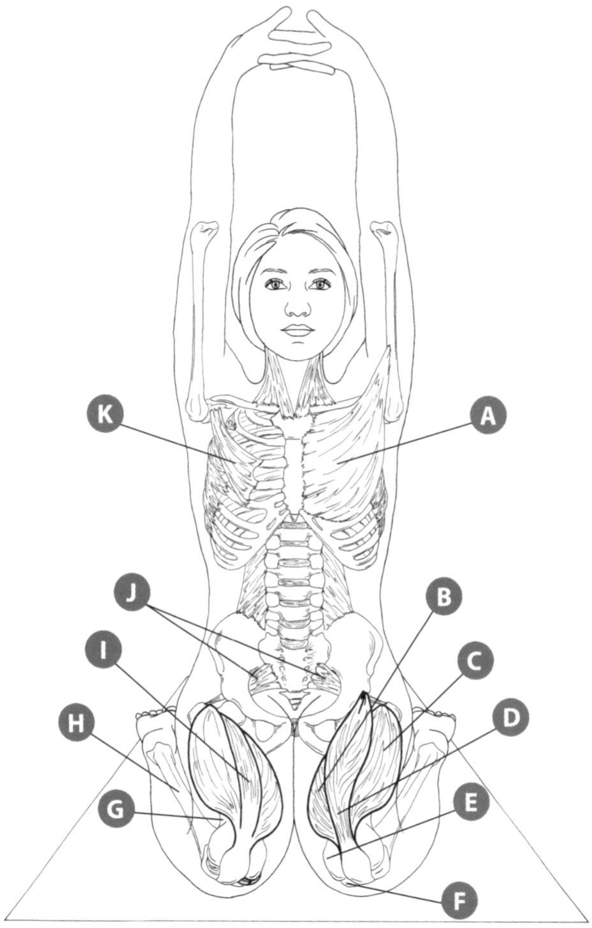
A
B
C
D
E
F
G
H
I
J
K

Sukhasana
Easy Seated Posture

A .... Iliacus

B .... Psoas

C .... Sternocleidomastoid (SCM)

D .... Levator scapula

E .... Trapezius

F .... Pectoralis major

G .... Transverse abdominis

Pasasana
Noose

A .... Multifidi

B .... Rotatores

C .... Posterior deltoid

D .... Infraspinatus

E .... Teres minor

F .... Psoas

G .... Tibialis anterior

H .... Gluteus maximus

I .... Internal obliques

J .... External obliques

Virasana
Hero

A .... Pectoralis major

B .... Vastus medialis

C .... Vastus lateralis

D .... Rectus femoris

E .... Medial condyle of the femur

F .... Medial condyle of the tibia

G .... Femur

H .... Tibia

I .... Vastus intermedius

J .... Piriformis

K .... Pectoralis minor

Padmasana
Lotus

A .... Fibula

B .... Tibia

C .... Medial meniscus

D .... Lateral condyle of the femur

E .... Lateral collateral ligament (LCL)

F .... Femur

G .... Gluteus minimus

H .... Gluteus medius

I .... Tensor fasciae latae (TFL)

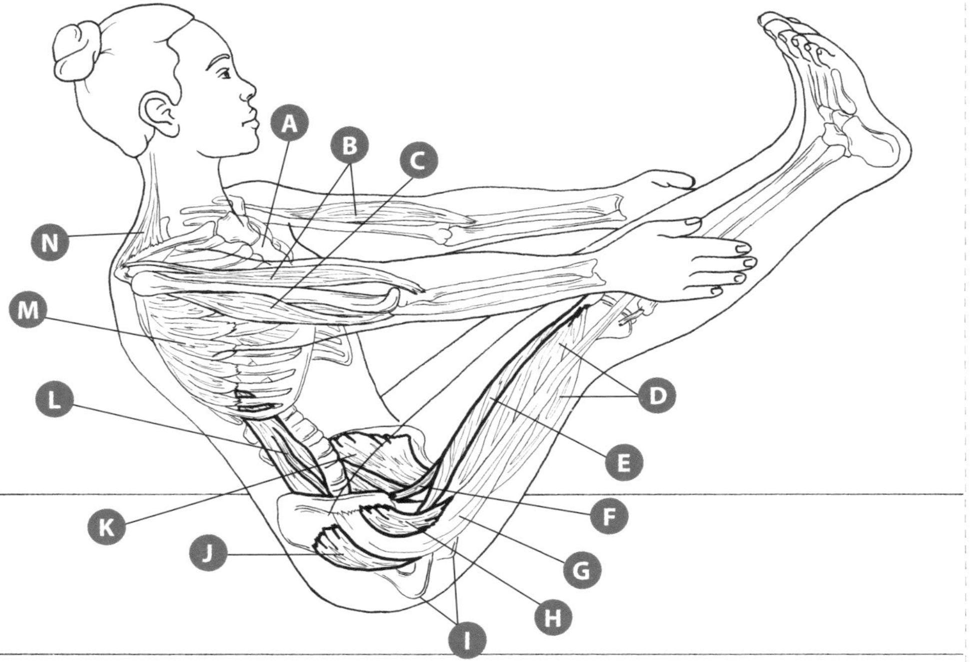
A
B
C
D
E
F
G
H
I
J
K
L
M
N

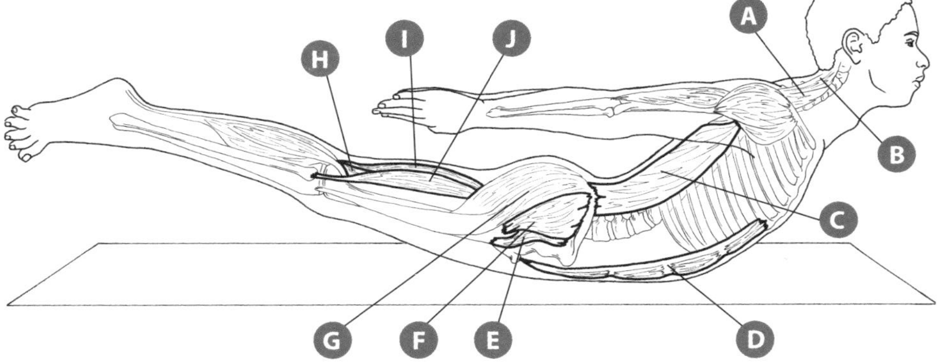
A
B
C
D
E
F
G
H
I
J

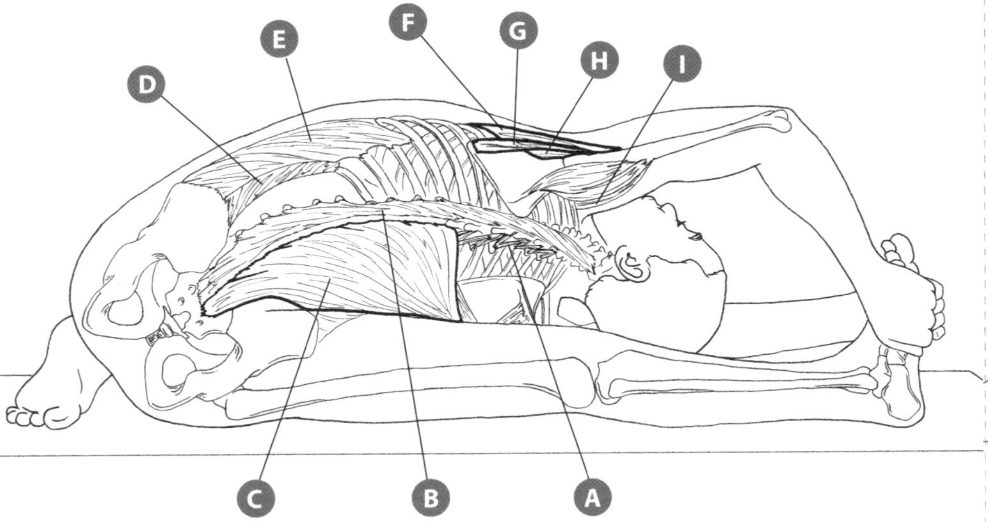
A
B
C
D
E
F
G
H
I

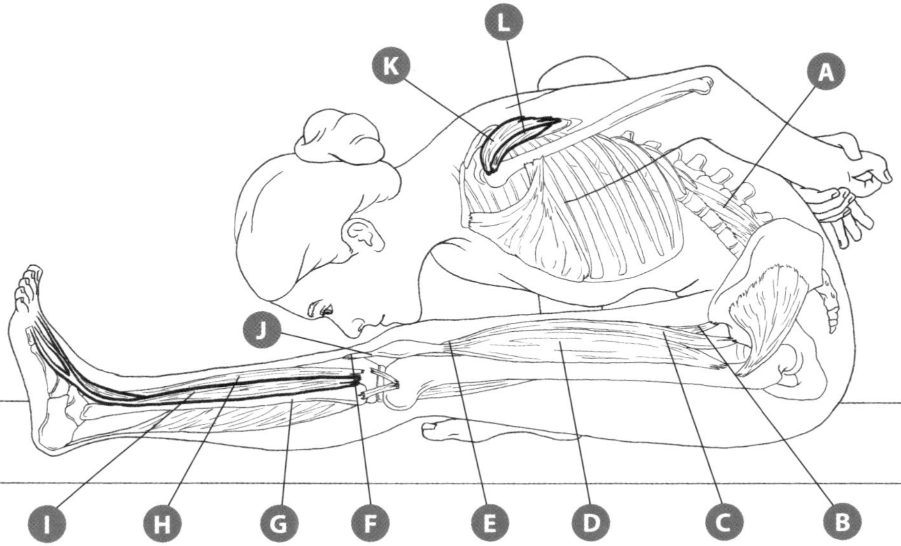
A
B
C
D
E
F
G
H
I
J
K
L

Navasana
Boat

A.... Sternum

B.... Biceps brachii

C.... Triceps brachii

D.... Vastus lateralis

E.... Rectus femoris

F.... Sartorius

G.... Iliotibial (IT) band

H.... Tensor fasciae latae (TFL)

I .... Ischial tuberosities

J .... Gluteus minimus

K.... Iliacus

L.... Psoas

M ... Serratus anterior

N.... Trapezius (upper fibers)

Parighasana (Ashtanga)
Gate

A .... Rotatores

B .... Multifidi

C .... Latissimus dorsi

D .... Internal oblique

E .... External oblique

F .... Pectoralis major

G............ Teres major

H............ Subscapularis

I............. Anterior deltoid

Salabhasana
Locust

A............ Iliocostalis

B .... Longissimus

C .... Latissimus dorsi

D............ Rectus abdominis

E .... Gluteus minimus

F .... Gluteus medius

G............ Gluteus maximus

H............ Semimembranosus

I............. Semitendinosus

J............. Biceps femoris

Marichyasana A
Marichi's Pose A

A............ Psoas

B .... Sartorius

C .... Rectus femoris

D............ Vastus intermedius

E .... Quadriceps tendon

F .... Tibial tuberosity

G............ Tibia

H............ Tibialis anterior

I............. Extensor digitorum longus

J............. Patella tendon

K .... Infraspinatus

L .... Teres minor

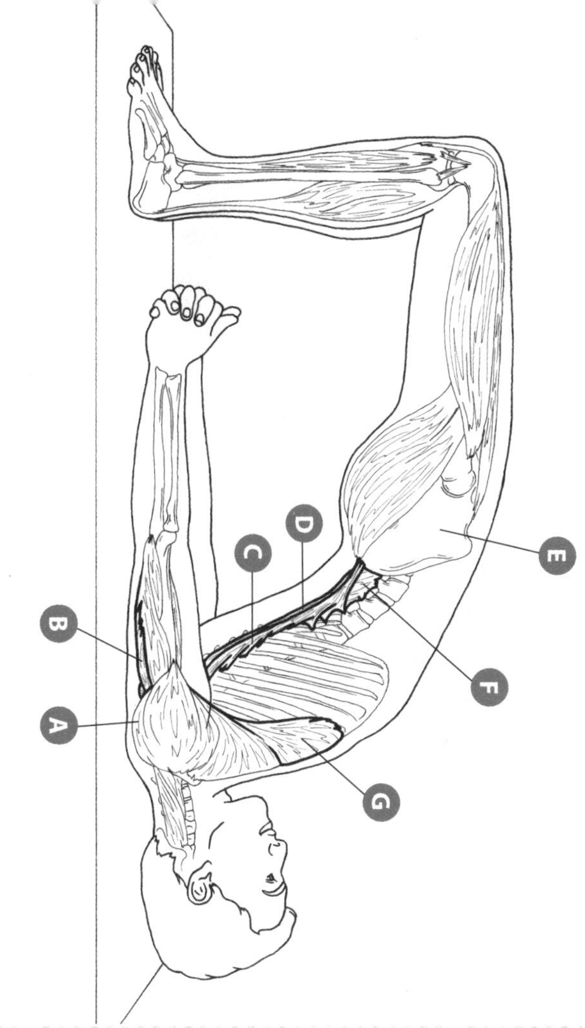
A
B
C
D
E
F
G

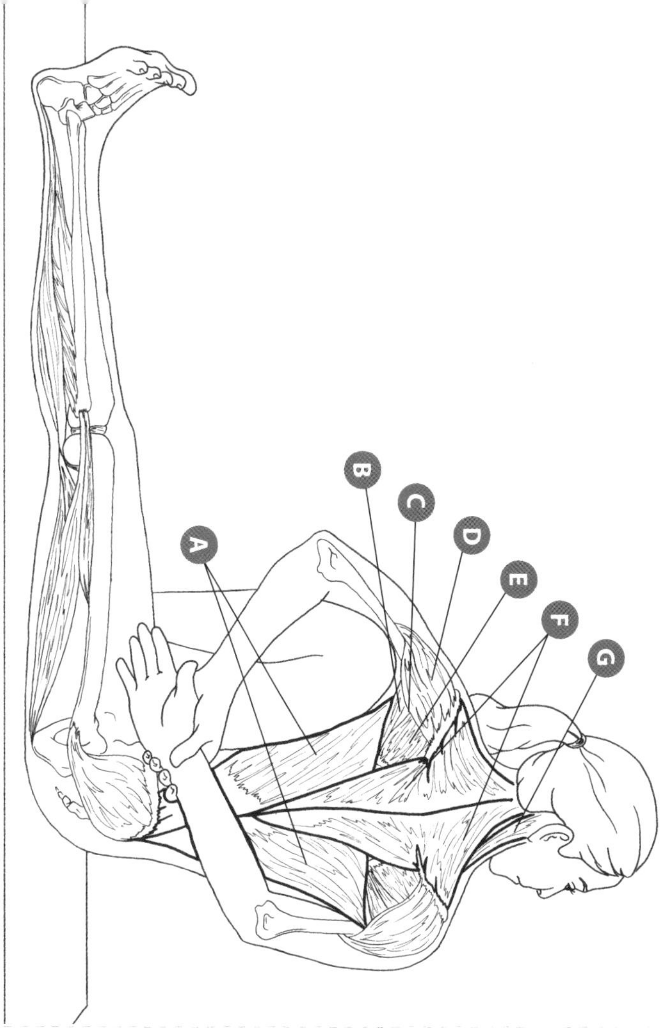
A
B
C
D
E
F
G

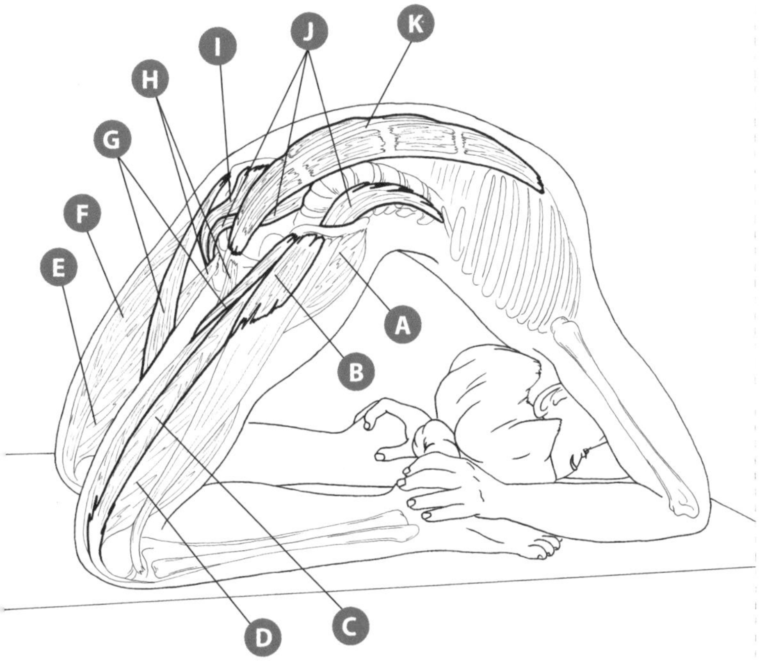
A
B
C
D
E
F
G
H
I
J
K

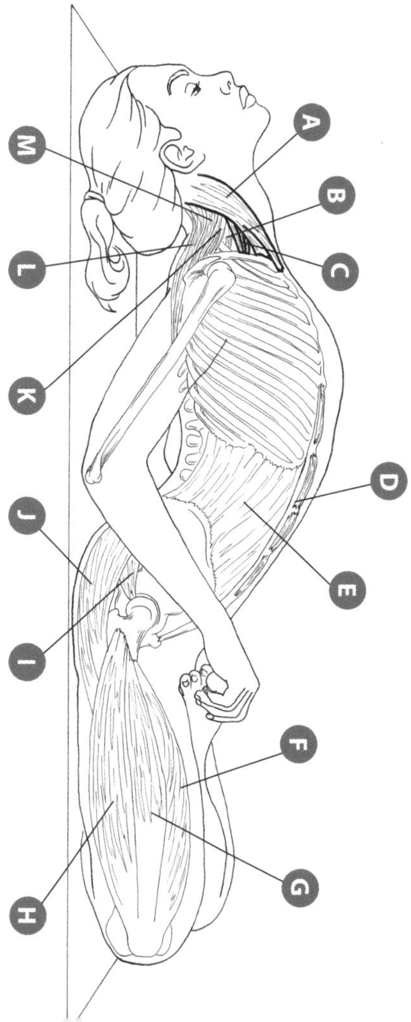
A
B
C
D
E
F
G
H
I
J
K
L
M

Marichyasana C
Marichi's Pose C

A .... Latissimus dorsi

B .... Teres major

C .... Teres minor

D .... Posterior deltoid

E .... Infraspinatus

F .... Trapezius

G .... Sternocleidomastoid (SCM)

Setu Bandha Sarvangasana
Bridge

A .... Posterior deltoid

B .... Triceps brachii

C .... Iliocostalis

D .... Longissimus

E .... Pelvis

F .... Quadratus lumborum

G .... Pectoralis major (lower fibers)

Matsyasana
Fish

A .... Sternocleidomastoid (SCM)

B .... Levator scapula

C .... Scalenes

D .... Rectus abdominis

E .... Internal oblique

F .... Vastus medialis

G .... Vastus intermedius

H .... Vastus lateralis

I .... Piriformis

J .... Gluteus maximus

K .... Splenius cervicis

L .... Trapezius (upper fibers)

M .... Splenius capitis

Kapotasana
Pigeon

A .... Gluteus medius

B .... Tensor fasciae latae (TFL)

C .... Rectus femoris

D .... Vastus lateralis

E .... Vastus medialis

F .... Vastus intermedius

G .... Sartorius

H .... Adductor longus

I .... Iliacus

J .... Psoas

K .... Rectus abdominis